Imaging of White Matter Lesions

Editor

SANGAM KANEKAR

RADIOLOGIC CLINICS
OF NORTH AMERICA

www.radiologic.theclinics.com

Consulting Editor
FRANK H. MILLER

March 2014 • Volume 52 • Number 2

ELSEVIER

1600 John F. Kennedy Boulevard • Suite 1800 • Philadelphia, Pennsylvania, 19103-2899

http://www.theclinics.com

RADIOLOGIC CLINICS OF NORTH AMERICA Volume 52, Number 2
March 2014 ISSN 0033-8389, ISBN 13: 978-0-323-28720-3

Editor: John Vassallo (j.vassallo@elsevier.com)
Developmental Editor: Donald Mumford

Radiologic Clinics of North America (ISSN 0033-8389) is published bimonthly by Elsevier Inc., 360 Park Avenue South, New York, NY 10010-1710. Months of issue are January, March, May, July, September, and November. Periodicals postage paid at New York, NY and additional mailing offices. Subscription prices are USD 460 per year for US individuals, USD 709 per year for US institutions, USD 220 per year for US students and residents, USD 535 per year for Canadian individuals, USD 905 per year for Canadian institutions, USD 660 per year for international individuals, USD 905 per year for international institutions, and USD 315 per year for Canadian and foreign students/residents. To receive student and resident rate, orders must be accompanied by name of affiliated institution, date of term and the signature of program/residency coordinatior on institution letterhead. Orders will be billed at individual rate until proof of status is received. Foreign air speed delivery is included in all *Clinics* subscription prices. All prices are subject to change without notice. **POSTMASTER:** Send address changes to *Radiologic Clinics of North America*, Elsevier Health Sciences Division, Subscription Customer Service, 3251 Riverport Lane, Maryland Heights, MO63043. **Customer Service: Telephone: 1-800-654-2452** (U.S. and Canada); **1-314-447-8871** (outside U.S. and Canada). **Fax: 1-314-447-8029. E-mail: journalscustomerservice-usa@elsevier.com** (for print support); **journalsonlinesupport-usa@elsevier.com** (for online support).

Reprints. For copies of 100 or more of articles in this publication, please contact the Commercial Reprints Department, Elsevier Inc., 360 Park Avenue South, New York, New York 10010-1710. Tel.: +1-212-633-3874; Fax: +1-212-633-3820; E-mail: reprints@elsevier.com.

Radiologic Clinics of North America also published in Greek Paschalidis Medical Publications, Athens, Greece.

Radiologic Clinics of North America is covered in *MEDLINE/PubMed (Index Medicus), EMBASE/Excerpta Medica, Current Contents/Life Sciences, Current Contents/Clinical Medicine, RSNA Index to Imaging Literature, BIOSIS, Science Citation Index,* and *ISI/BIOMED.*

Printed and bound by CPI Group (UK) Ltd, Croydon, CR0 4YY

Contributors

CONSULTING EDITOR

FRANK H. MILLER, MD
Professor of Radiology; Chief, Body Imaging,
Section and Fellowship Program and GI,
Radiology; Medical Director MRI, Department
of Radiology, Feinberg School of Medicine,
Northwestern University, Chicago, Illinois

EDITOR

SANGAM KANEKAR, MD
Section of Neuroradiology; Associate
Professor, Departments of Radiology,
Neurology and Otolaryngology, Penn State
Milton S. Hershey Medical Center and College
of Medicine, The Pennsylvania State
University, Hershey, Pennsylvania

AUTHORS

ARI M. BLITZ, MD
Assistant Professor, Division of
Neuroradiology, Department of Radiology and
Radiological Science, Johns Hopkins
University, Baltimore, Maryland

MACEY D. BRAY, DO
Assistant Professor, Department of Radiology,
University of New Mexico, Albuquerque,
New Mexico

ARISTIDES CAPIZZANO, MD
Assistant Professor, Department of Radiology,
University of Iowa Hospitals and Clinics,
Iowa City, Iowa

ERIC M. CHIN, BS
Department of Radiology, University of
Tennessee Health Science Center, Memphis,
Tennessee

ASIM F. CHOUDHRI, MD
Assistant Chair of Research Affairs; Assistant
Professor, Departments of Radiology,
Neurosurgery, and Ophthalmology, University
of Tennessee Health Science Center; Director
of Neuroradiology, Le Bonheur Neuroscience
Institute, Le Bonheur Children's Hospital,
Memphis, Tennessee

NILESH K. DESAI, MD
Assistant Professor; Director of Pediatric
Neuroradiology Services, Children's
Healthcare of Atlanta at Egleston and Town
Center; Division of Neuroradiology,
Department of Radiology and Imaging
Sciences, Emory University School of
Medicine, Atlanta, Georgia

PUNEET DEVGUN, DO
Department of Radiology, Penn State Milton S.
Hershey Medical Center and College of
Medicine, The Pennsylvania State University,
Hershey, Pennsylvania

DHEERAJ GANDHI, MD
Professor, Division of Neuroradiology,
Department of Radiology; Departments of
Neurology and Neurosurgery, University of
Maryland Medical Center, Baltimore, Maryland

ALLISON M. GRAYEV, MD
Assistant Professor of Radiology, Section of
Neuroradiology, University of Wisconsin
School of Medicine and Public Health,
Madison, Wisconsin

SAURABH GULERIA, MD
Pediatric Radiologist, Children's of Alabama;
Clinical Assistant Professor of Radiology,
University of Alabama at Birmingham,
Birmingham, Alabama

MOHANNAD IBRAHIM, MD
Department of Radiology, University of
Michigan Health System, Ann Arbor,
Michigan

GAURAV JINDAL, MD
Neuroradiology Division, Department of
Radiology, University of Maryland Medical
Center, Baltimore, Maryland

SANGAM KANEKAR, MD
Section of Neuroradiology; Associate
Professor, Departments of Radiology,
Neurology and Otolaryngology, Penn State
Milton S. Hershey Medical Center and College
of Medicine, The Pennsylvania State
University, Hershey, Pennsylvania

TERESA GROSS KELLY, MD
Pediatric Neuroradiologist, Imaging, Children's
Hospital of Wisconsin; Assistant Professor of
Radiology, Medical College of Wisconsin,
Milwaukee, Wisconsin

PATRICIA KIRBY, MD
Clinical Professor, Department of Pathology,
University of Iowa Hospitals & Clinics,
Iowa City, Iowa

JENNIFER KISSANE, MD
Radiology Resident, Department of Radiology,
Penn State Milton S. Hershey Medical Center
and College of Medicine, The Pennsylvania
State University, Hershey, Pennsylvania

TIMOTHY R. MILLER, MD
Neuroradiology Division, Department of
Radiology, University of Maryland Medical
Center, Baltimore, Maryland

SUYASH MOHAN, MD
Neuroradiology Division, Department of
Radiology, University of Pennsylvania,
Philadelphia, Pennsylvania

TOSHIO MORITANI, MD, PhD
Clinical Professor, Department of Radiology,
University of Iowa Hospitals & Clinics,
Iowa City, Iowa

MARK E. MULLINS, MD, PhD
Associate Professor; Vice Chair for Education;
Director of Medical Student Radiology
Education; Program Director of Radiology
Residency Program, Division of
Neuroradiology, Department of Radiology and
Imaging Sciences, Emory University School of
Medicine, Atlanta, Georgia

HEMANT A. PARMAR, MD
Department of Radiology, University of
Michigan Health System, Ann Arbor, Michigan

BRUNO POLICENI, MD
Clinical Associate Professor, Department of
Radiology, University of Iowa Hospitals &
Clinics, Iowa City, Iowa

JEFFREY D. POOT, DO
Department of Radiology, Penn State Milton S.
Hershey Medical Center and College of
Medicine, The Pennsylvania State University,
Hershey, Pennsylvania

**SANJAY P. PRABHU, MBBS, MRCPCH,
FRCR**
Staff Neuroradiologist, Department of
Radiology, Boston Children's Hospital;
Assistant Professor of Radiology, Harvard
Medical School, Boston, Massachusetts

MICHAEL RYAN, MD
Department of Radiology, University of
Michigan Health System, Ann Arbor, Michigan

EDWARD YANG, MD, PhD
Staff Neuroradiologist, Department of
Radiology, Boston Children's Hospital;
Instructor of Radiology, Harvard Medical
School, Boston, Massachusetts

Contents

matter involvement patterns. Special emphasis is placed on pattern recognition and unusual combinations of findings that may suggest a specific diagnosis.

Multiple sclerosis (MS) and its variants are inflammatory as well as neurodegenerative diseases that diffusely affect the central nervous system (CNS). There is a poor correlation between traditional imaging findings and symptoms in patients with MS. Current research in conventional magnetic resonance (MR) imaging of MS and related diseases includes optimization of hardware and pulse sequences and the development of automated and semiautomated techniques to measure and quantify disease burden. Advanced nonconventional MR techniques such as diffusion tensor and functional MR imaging probe the changes found in the CNS, and correlate these findings with clinical measures of disease.

Demyelinating disorders of the central nervous system are characterized by the breakdown of myelin, with or without preservation of the associated axons. Primary demyelinating diseases typically involve loss of myelin with relative sparing of axons. Secondary demyelinating disorders represent a spectrum of white matter disease characterized by damage to neurons or axons with the resultant breakdown of myelin. The pathologic changes seen in secondary demyelinating disorders are varied, ranging from pure demyelination to necrosis with subsequent demyelination. Secondary demyelinating diseases are associated with a wide variety of conditions, including infections/vaccinations, nutritional/vitamin deficiencies, chemical agents, genetic abnormalities, and vascular insult.

This article discusses imaging findings in virus-related infectious and noninfectious encephalitis/encephalopathy with white matter involvement, as well as the differential diagnosis based on the characteristic distribution. Acute viral encephalitis/encephalopathy is a medical emergency. Prompt introduction of treatment has a significant influence on survival and the extent of permanent brain injury. Differentiation between infectious and noninfectious central nervous system involvement is paramount. Neuroimaging provides many clues for the specific diagnosis. Understanding the underlying disorder and pathophysiology is important for the interpretation of the images and therefore the treatment.

When atrophy is seen on imaging in adult patients, it does not necessarily represent Alzheimer disease. Many cases of dementia or cognitive decline could be caused by reversible or preventable diseases, such as vascular dementia. This article familiarizes the physician with various types of vascular lesions leading to dementia and cognitive decline and their imaging appearances. Neuroimaging plays an important role in identifying vascular lesions of the brain early, even before the clinical manifestation of the cognitive decline symptoms and, thus, can help to prevent or delay the symptoms related to the various vascular pathologic conditions.

Magnetic resonance spectroscopy (MRS) can be useful as an adjuvant diagnostic tool to traditional MR imaging of the brain. MRS can provide both quantitative and qualitative information about white matter pathologic abnormality. It is important to interpret MRS in conjunction with other clinical factors including but not limited to additional diagnostic neuroimaging, history and physical examination findings, and genetics.

Diffusion tensor imaging is a magnetic resonance imaging technique that provides insight into the anatomy and integrity of white matter pathways in the brain. Further processing of these data can help map individual tracts, which can aid in surgical planning. Understanding the basics of this technique can improve characterization of white matter development and disorders.

In clinically suspected cases of myelopathy, magnetic resonance imaging without and with gadolinium remains the modality of choice. The first and best imaging approach in the evaluation of myelopathy is to identify whether the cause of myelopathy is compressive or noncompressive. The commonest imaging finding in myelopathy is either focal or diffuse cord hyperintensity on the T2-weighted magnetic resonance images. Detailed clinical history, acuity of symptoms (acute vs insidious onset), distribution of the signal abnormalities, including length of cord involvement, specific tract involvement, and the region of the spinal cord that is affected, are very useful in making the diagnosis.

PROGRAM OBJECTIVE
The objective of the Radiologic Clinics of North America is to keep practicing radiologists and radiology residents up to date with current clinical practice in radiology by providing timely articles reviewing the state of the art in patient care.

TARGET AUDIENCE
Practicing radiologists, radiology residents, and other health care professionals who provide patient care utilizing radiologic findings.

LEARNING OBJECTIVES
Upon completion of this activity, participants will be able to:
1. Review imaging manifestations of the leukodystrophies.
2. Discuss conventional and newer imaging techniques in multiple sclerosis.
3. Recognize viral infections and white matter lesions.

ACCREDITATION
The Elsevier Office of Continuing Medical Education (EOCME) is accredited by the Accreditation Council for Continuing Medical Education (ACCME) to provide continuing medical education for physicians.

The EOCME designates this enduring material for a maximum of 15 *AMA PRA Category 1 Credit*(s)™. Physicians should claim only the credit commensurate with the extent of their participation in the activity.

All other health care professionals requesting continuing education credit for this enduring material will be issued a certificate of participation.

DISCLOSURE OF CONFLICTS OF INTEREST
The EOCME assesses conflict of interest with its instructors, faculty, planners, and other individuals who are in a position to control the content of CME activities. All relevant conflicts of interest that are identified are thoroughly vetted by EOCME for fair balance, scientific objectivity, and patient care recommendations. EOCME is committed to providing its learners with CME activities that promote improvements or quality in healthcare and not a specific proprietary business or a commercial interest.

The planning committee, staff, authors and editors listed below have identified no financial relationships or relationships to products or devices they or their spouse/life partner have with commercial interest related to the content of this CME activity:

Ari M. Blitz, MD; Macey D. Bray, DO; Adrianne Brigido; Aristides Capizzano, MD; Eric M. Chin, BS; Asim F. Choudhri, MD; Nilesh K. Desai, MD; Puneet Devgun, DO; Dheeraj Gandhi, MD; Saurabh Guleria, MD; Kristen Helm; Brynne Hunter; Mohannad Ibrahim, MD; Sangam Kanekar, MD; Teresa Gross Kelly, MD; Patricia Kirby, MD; Jennifer Kissane, MD; Sandy Lavery; Jill McNair; Frank H. Miller, MD; Timothy R. Miller, MD; Suyash Mohan, MD; Toshio Moritani, MD, PhD; Mark E. Mullins, MD, PhD; Hemant A. Parmar, MD; Bruno Policeni, MD; Jeffrey D. Poot, DO; Sanjay P. Prabhu, MBBS, MRCPCH, FRCR; Karthikeyan Subramaniam; Michael Ryan, MD; Edward Yang, MD, PhD.

The planning committee, staff, authors and editors listed below have identified financial relationships or relationships to products or devices they or their spouse/life partner have with commercial interest related to the content of this CME activity:

Allison M. Grayev, MD has a research grant from Bayer AG and royalties/patents with McGraw Hill Publishers.
Gaurav Jindal, MD has a research grant from Stryker and a research grant from Microvention Inc.

UNAPPROVED/OFF-LABEL USE DISCLOSURE
The EOCME requires CME faculty to disclose to the participants:
1. When products or procedures being discussed are off-label, unlabelled, experimental, and/or investigational (not US Food and Drug Administration (FDA) approved); and
2. Any limitations on the information presented, such as data that are preliminary or that represent ongoing research, interim analyses, and/or unsupported opinions. Faculty may discuss information about pharmaceutical agents that is outside of FDA-approved labelling. This information is intended solely for CME and is not intended to promote off-label use of these medications. If you have any questions, contact the medical affairs department of the manufacturer for the most recent prescribing information.

TO ENROLL
To enroll in the *Radiologic Clinics of North America* Continuing Medical Education program, call customer service at 1-800-654-2452 or sign up online at http://www.theclinics.com/home/cme. The CME program is available to subscribers for an additional annual fee of USD $315.

METHOD OF PARTICIPATION
In order to claim credit, participants must complete the following:
1. Complete enrolment as indicated above.
2. Read the activity.
3. Complete the CME Test and Evaluation. Participants must achieve a score of 70% on the test. All CME Tests and Evaluations must be completed online.

CME INQUIRIES/SPECIAL NEEDS
For all CME inquiries or special needs, please contact elsevierCME@elsevier.com.

RADIOLOGIC CLINICS OF NORTH AMERICA

Preface
Imaging of White Matter Lesions

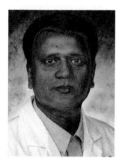

Sangam Kanekar, MD
Editor

Virtually all categories of pathologic conditions may cause white matter abnormalities. For the last four decades magnetic resonance (MR) imaging has established its role in the evaluation of white matter. The sensitivity of MR in identifying white matter is excellent. However, negotiating the exact cause of either the focal or the diffuse white matter remains challenging for the radiologist even on MR and is more so because many of the diseases appear similar, or one disease may have multiple white matter patterns on MR. For the last decade and a half, the evaluation of white matter has been further refined by advanced MR imaging techniques such as MR spectroscopy, diffusion tensor imaging (DTI), thin high-resolution sections, and MR perfusion imaging. These imaging modalities have significantly improved our ability to understand the basic etiopathogenesis of white matter disorders.

Clinical evaluation and diagnosis of central nervous system disorders have always been challenging for clinicians. Imaging modalities play a vital role in diagnosing and directing the clinicians for appropriate clinical testing. The focus of this issue of *Radiology Clinics of North America* is to present a comprehensive review on "Imaging of White Matter."

This issue has a total of 11 articles and is balanced with conventional and high-end modalities in diagnosis and characterization of white matter diseases. The first article describes the for-

mation of the white matter, myelination, and corresponding changes on MR imaging. The next two articles give a very practical imaging approach on how to negotiate the focal and diffuse white matter lesions. The article on leukodystrophy is a very comprehensive approach to pediatric white matter diseases. White matter lesions, due to either multiple sclerosis or secondary demyelination disorders, are commonly encountered in the day-to-day practice. The fifth and sixth articles describe in detail the conventional and newer imaging techniques in regards to various demyelination disorders. Both articles also discuss and describe the various variants and differential diagnosis with diagnostic pearls to the specific diagnosis. Because viral infections often involve the white matter, clinical and imaging features of various viral infections are discussed in detail in the article on viral infection and white matter lesions.

Dementia, due to various reversible and irreversible conditions, is thought to be the next big epidemic of the 21st century. Understanding the various reversible and preventable causes is important so that the appropriate intervention can be performed. Vascular dementia alone, or in combination with other neurodegenerative disorders like Alzheimer disease, is thought to be one of the leading causes of preventable dementia. The article on vascular dementia describes in detail the causes, pathogenesis, and various imaging findings. The next two articles are

Radiol Clin N Am 52 (2014) xi–xii
http://dx.doi.org/10.1016/j.rcl.2013.12.005
0033-8389/14/$ – see front matter © 2014 Elsevier Inc. All rights reserved.

radiologic.theclinics.com

dedicated to the application of the advanced imaging techniques: MR spectroscopy and DTI in various white matter lesions. These articles also describe the basics of these techniques and relevant physics.

Like negotiating white matter of the brain, negotiating the hyperintensity in the spinal cord is also challenging. The last article describes the algorithmic approach to the spinal cord hyperintensity in both acute and chronic onset of myelopathy.

I thank all the authors for their excellent contributions that make this issue an outstanding and comprehensive review on "Imaging of White Matter." I would like to thank Dr Frank Miller for giving me an opportunity to be the guest editor on this issue and bringing this topic to a wider audience. Finally, I thank my wife, Revati, and my children, Samika and Rachita, for their support and love.

I hope you will enjoy reading this issue.

Sangam Kanekar, MD
Section of Neuroradiology
Departments of Radiology, Neurology and
Otolaryngology
The Pennsylvania State University
Milton S. Hershey Medical Center and
College of Medicine
500 University Drive
Hershey, PA 17033, USA

E-mail address:
skanekar@hmc.psu.edu

Myelin, Myelination, and Corresponding Magnetic Resonance Imaging Changes

Saurabh Guleria, MD[a],*, Teresa Gross Kelly, MD[b]

KEYWORDS

- White matter • Myelination • Magnetic resonance imaging

KEY POINTS

- Myelination of the white matter occurs in an orderly and predictable fashion.
- Magnetic resonance (MR) imaging is the most useful modality for in vivo imaging of white matter maturation.
- The anatomic standard MR imaging sequences detect myelination during the early years of life, whereas advanced imaging techniques that include diffusion-weighted imaging, diffusion tensor imaging, and spectroscopy, are most useful later.
- Familiarity with these normal imaging patterns of myelination is essential for providing an accurate assessment of normal myelination and thus identification of disease processes.

INTRODUCTION

An important component of brain maturation involves myelination of white matter, which is essential for normal brain function and enables rapid conduction of nerve signals across the neural systems responsible for higher order motor, sensory, and cognitive functioning. Myelination begins during the fifth month of fetal life and continues throughout life in an orderly pattern thought to be consistent with evolving neural functionality.[1] Detailed postmortem histologic studies provide the most accurate analysis of normal or abnormal myelination but are not suited to investigating the longitudinal relationship between myelination and behavioral maturation. Magnetic resonance (MR) imaging is superior in assessing myelination of the brain noninvasively and it surpasses both computed tomography[2] and ultrasound in contrast resolution. In the past decade there have been rapid advancements in technology

resulting in more sophisticated and higher strength magnets, introduction of new imaging sequences, and refinements of existing sequence protocols that have furthered interest and understanding of myelination. This article discusses the composition of myelin, the process of myelination, and the usefulness of MR imaging for assessment of white matter maturation.

MYELIN STRUCTURE

The structure of myelin is rich in lipid and protein, and it is seen in both the central nervous system (CNS) and peripheral nervous system.[3,4] In the CNS, myelin is primarily found in white matter, although it is also present in gray matter, but in smaller quantities. The long sheets of CNS myelin are composed of several segments of myelin that are modified extensions of oligodendroglial cell processes that wrap around the axon in a concentric lamellar fashion (**Fig. 1**). The axon is not

Disclosures: The authors have no disclosures.
[a] Pediatric Radiology, Children's of Alabama, University of Alabama at Birmingham, 1600 7th Avenue South, Lowder Building Ste. 306, Birmingham, AL 35233, USA; [b] Imaging, Children's Hospital of Wisconsin, Medical College of Wisconsin, 9000 W Wisconsin Avenue, Milwaukee, WI 53226, USA
* Corresponding author.
E-mail address: saurabh.guleria@childrensal.org

radiologic.theclinics.com

continuously wrapped by myelin; gaps are interposed in which the bare axon is exposed to the interstitial space, termed nodes of Ranvier. The nodes of Ranvier are also the sites of multiple sodium channels.[5] The myelinated portion of the axon located between the nodes of Ranvier is called the internodal region, which can further be divided into 2 distinct domains, namely the paranodal loops and compact myelin. Paranodal loops facilitate ion exchange at the node of Ranvier, whereas compact myelin inhibits ion exchange during nerve conduction.

The myelin bilayer is made up of approximately 80% lipid and 20% protein (Fig. 2). The intracellular and extracellular space between the bilayers is filled with water, which makes up approximately 40% of the weight of myelin.

The protein components of myelin's ultrastructure include[5]:
1. Myelin basic protein, which comprises approximately 30% of the myelin proteins and is localized at the cytoplasmic surface of compact myelin.
2. Proteolipid protein (PLP), which has 4 membrane-spanning domains that make up about 50% of the myelin proteins. The PLP maintains the extracellular spacing of compact myelin by virtue of its electrostatic interactions with myelin lipids.
3. Cyclic nucleotide phosphodiesterase, which is the least abundant protein and makes up about 4% of the myelin proteins. It is concentrated on the cytoplasmic side of the myelin lamellae.
4. Myelin-associated glycoprotein, which constitutes less than 1% of the myelin proteins, but probably helps oligodendrocyte processes distinguish between myelinated and unmyelinated axons in the CNS.
5. Myelin oligodendrocyte glycoprotein (MOG), which is mainly confined to oligodendrocyte bodies and is seen in the outermost surface of the myelin sheath. The precise function of MOG is unknown, but it may have a role in defining the structural integrity of the myelin sheath.

The lipid components of myelin's ultrastructure include[6]:
1. Cholesterol, which plays a critical role in the assembly and integrity of myelin and is mostly found in the outer layer of the cell membrane.
2. Phospholipids, which comprise approximately one-third of the total lipids, which are hydrophobic and are located on the cytoplasmic side of the cell membrane.
3. Glycosphingolipids, which account for approximately one-third of the total lipids and include cerebrosides, sulfatides, globosides, and gangliosides. The concentration of cerebroside in the brain has been shown to correlate proportionally with the amount of myelin present.[7]

The composition of myelin is largely preserved among mammalian species. There are also regional variations within a single species such as spinal cord myelin, which has a higher lipid/protein ratio than myelin from brain tissue.[6]

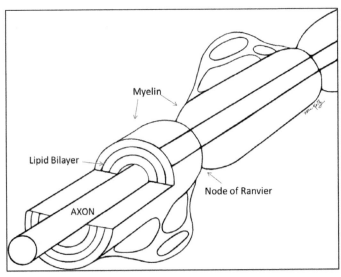

Fig. 1. Cross section of a myelinated axon showing formation of myelin sheath from extension of a cell process from an oligodendrocyte.

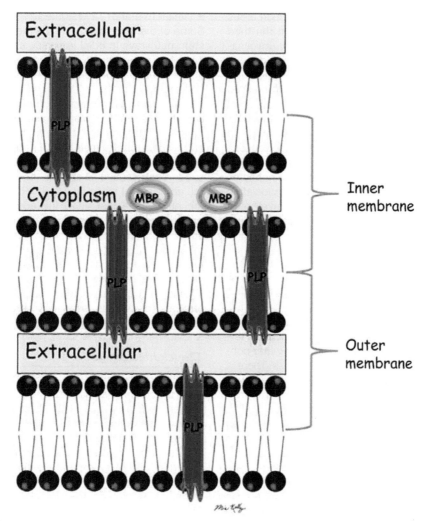

Fig. 2. The layers of myelin. Myelin is composed of multiple layers having alternating protein-lipid layered structure. The lipid bilayer includes a variety of proteins including proteolipid protein (PLP) and myelin basic protein (MBP).

MYELIN FUNCTION

Myelin acts as an electrical insulator for neurons and increases the speed of action potential transmission 100-fold compared with transmission along an unmyelinated axon. Myelin is of critical importance because speed of conduction is fundamental in allowing complex motor, sensory, and behavior of neuronal functions to occur.

The action potential is generated by voltage-gated sodium channels at the nodes of Ranvier, but the presence of myelin prevents ions from entering or leaving the axon along myelinated segments. Instead, the ionic current from an action potential at one node of Ranvier provokes another action potential at the next node, which results in jumping of action potential from one node of Ranvier to another, with the internodal myelin acting as an insulator of high electrical resistance. This process results in a highly efficient saltatory conduction of the action potential, much faster than the continuous conduction by sodium channels evenly distributed along the unmyelinated axon. Myelin also contains many enzymes and has been implicated in maintaining axonal integrity, as well as regulating axonal transport.[8] Hence, myelin has an intimate relationship with the underlying axon and any injury to myelin is associated with axonal dysfunction.[9]

THE PROCESS OF MYELINATION

Myelination of the brain begins during the fifth fetal month, progresses rapidly for the first 2 years of life, and then slows markedly after 2 years. In contrast, fibers to and from the association areas of the brain continue to myelinate into the third and fourth decades of life.[10] In general, myelination progresses from the caudal to cephalad, posterior to anterior, and central to peripheral directions. As an example, myelination progresses from the brainstem to the cerebellum and basal ganglia, and then to the cerebral hemispheres. In a particular location, the dorsal region tends to myelinate before the ventral regions. The process of myelination also relates to functional outcomes such that the somatosensory system in neonates myelinates earlier than motor and association pathways.[11,12] A rapid growth of the myelinated white matter volume is observed between birth and 9 months of age.

IMAGING OF MYELINATION
T1-weighted Images

Anatomic MR imaging sequences (T1 and T2 weighted) play an important role in the evaluation of the white matter, because they can depict alterations that are secondary to change in water content as a result of the myelination process. There is reduction in T1 and T2 relaxation times with continued white matter maturation that corresponds with reduction in tissue water as well as the interaction of water with myelin lipids.[13] As previously mentioned, these imaging sequences are more helpful early in life and have limited application for patients older than 2 years of age.

On T1-weighted images, most of the white matter in the newborn brain is hypointense compared with gray matter, and the appearance is similar to that of T2-weighted images in adults. Some of the exceptions include the dorsal brainstem pathways (medial lemnisci, medial longitudinal fasciculi) (**Fig. 3**B), and the posterior limb of the internal capsules (see **Fig. 3**D), which are myelinated at birth.

During the following months, the T1 signal intensity of white matter increases as myelination progresses. This increase in signal intensity begins in the sensorimotor (see **Fig. 3**F) and visual pathways (see **Fig. 3**L, N), then continues to the subcortical association areas in the frontal, temporal, and parietal lobes (see **Fig. 3**P, R, and T). By the end of the first year, the adult myelination pattern is reached almost everywhere, except for some subcortical regions of the anteromedial frontal lobes, which may remain isointense to gray matter until the middle of the second postnatal year.[10] This increase in T1 signal, as a result of T1 shortening, is attributed to increasing cholesterol and glycolipids (especially cerebrosides) on the myelin surface.[1]

T2-weighted Images

The changes seen on T2-weighted images have been proposed to be caused by decrease in water content, primarily as a result of increased hydrophobic interaction within the lipid bilayer. On T2-weighted images of term neonates, the unmyelinated white matter is hyperintense compared with gray matter, with the exception of the areas mentioned earlier (the posterior limbs of the internal capsules and the dorsal brainstem (see **Fig. 3**A, C, and E)).

Table 1
MR imaging appearance of myelination on T1-weighted and T2-weighted sequences

Anatomic Structure	T1-weighted Images	T2-weighted Images
Dorsal brainstem (superior cerebellar peduncle, MLF, medial and lateral lemnisci)	26–29 wk of gestation	27–30 wk of gestation
Middle cerebellar peduncle	0–1 mo	0–2 mo
Posterior limb of internal capsule	0–1 mo	0–3 mo
Anterior limb of internal capsule	2–3 mo	7–11 mo
Genu of corpus callosum	4–6 mo	5–8 mo
Splenium of corpus callosum	3–4 mo	4–6 mo
Centrum semiovale	2–4 mo	7–11 mo
Occipital white matter, deep	3–5 mo	7–14 mo
Occipital white matter, subcortical	4–7 mo	7–12 mo
Frontal white matter, deep	3–7 mo	11–16 mo
Frontal white matter, subcortical	7–11 mo	12–24 mo

Abbreviation: MLF, medial longitudinal fasciculus.
Data from Barkovich AJ. Normal development of the neonatal and infant brain, skull, and spine. In: Barkovich AJ, editor. Pediatric neuroimaging. 5th edition. Philadelphia: Lippincott Williams & Wilkins; 2011.

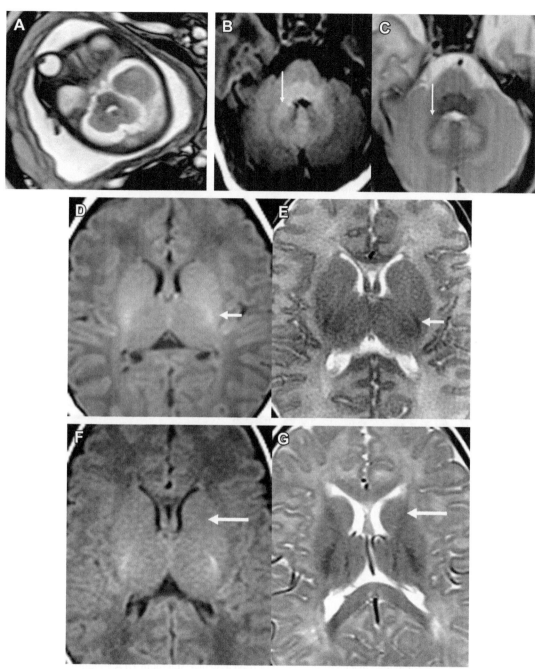

Fig. 3. (*A*) T2 fast imaging with steady state precession axial fetal MR image of 27 week estimated gestation age fetus showing hypointense dorsal brainstem. (*B*) A 9-day-old neonate shows the T1 hyperintense myelinated appearance of the middle cerebellar peduncle (*arrow*). (*C*) There is low signal on T2-weighted images in the middle cerebellar peduncle of the same neonate (*arrow*). (*D*) T1-weighted image in 11-day-old term neonate showing hyperintensity (*arrow*) within the posterior limb of the left internal capsule with greater signal noted in the dorsal fibers. (*E*) Axial T2-weighted fast spin echo (FSE) image in 12-week-old girl showing low-signal myelin (*arrow*) within the posterior limb of the left internal capsule. (*F*) T1-weighted image in 2-month-old girl demonstrates intermediate T1 signal in the anterior limb of the left internal capsule, compatible with the early stages of myelination (*white arrow*). The bilateral posterior limbs of the internal capsules are T1 hyperintense, representing near complete myelination. (*G*) FSE T2-weighted image of 8-month-old showing near complete T2 hypointense myelination of the left anterior limb (*arrow*).

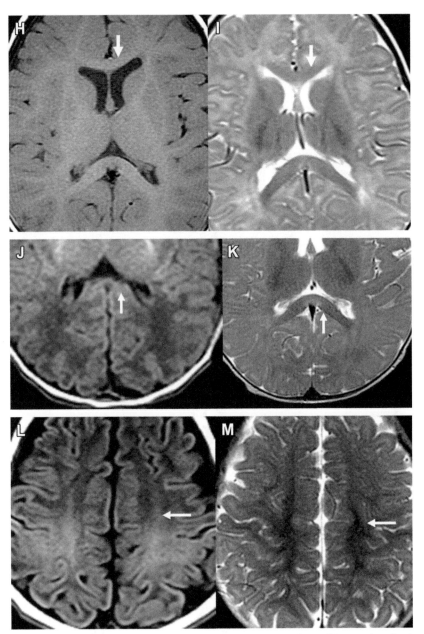

Fig. 3. (*continued.*). (*H*) The myelination of genu begins at about 4 months and is complete by 6 months. Note near complete myelination of genu in this T1-weighted image of a 6-month-old (*arrow*). (*I*) T2-weighted image in this 8-month-old shows completed myelination in genu (*arrow*) as well as splenium. (*J*) A 3-month-old with developing T1 hyperintensities in splenium from myelination (*arrow*). (*K*) There is uniform T2 hypointensity within splenium in this 6-month-old (*arrow*). There is minimal if any delay in myelination changes of corpus callosum in fluid-attenuated inversion recovery (FLAIR) sequence compared with FSE T2-weighted images. (*L*) A 3-month-old boy showing hyperintensity (*arrow*) within central semiovale, consistent with myelination. (*M*) T2-weighted imaging in this 11-month-old showing marked T2 hypointensity (*arrow*). Note the posterior subcortical myelination predominance.

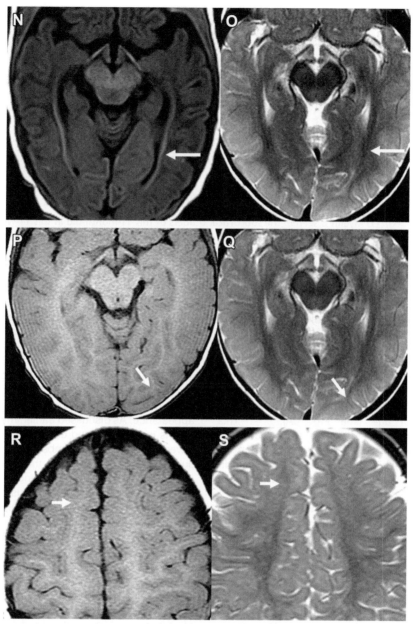

Fig. 3. *(continued)*. (*N*) T1-weighted image showing myelination developing in occipital deep white matter (*arrow*) in a 3-month-old infant. (*O*) The myelination is usually complete by 12 months of age, as in this FSE T2-weighted image (*arrow*), and may lag behind a few months when using conventional spin echo technique. (*P*) A 6-month-old with myelinated subcortical fibers of the occipital lobe appearing as hyperintensity on T1-weighted image (*arrow*). The myelination extends from the perirolandic region to the subcortical U fibers of the occipital lobe by 6 to 7 months. (*Q*) An 11-month-old with myelinated subcortical U fibers on FSE T2-weighted image (*arrow*). Hemispheric white matter begins myelination centrally with slow peripheral U fiber extension. The occipital lobe is the first to complete myelination by the end of the first year. (*R*) A 6-month-old with beginning T1 hyperintensity (*arrow*) in the central white matter of the frontal lobes. (*S*) The myelination changes are delayed in T2-weighted images and progress more slowly in the frontal and temporal lobes, as seen in this 14-month-old (*arrow*).

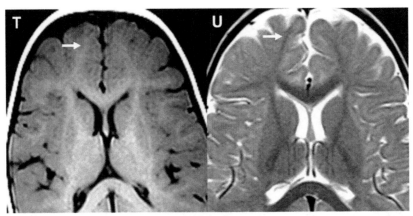

Fig. 3. (*continued*). (*T*) Myelin is seen in the subcortical U fibers of this 11-month-old in this T1-weighted image (*arrow*). In general, the adult pattern of myelination is achieved by 1 year of age. (*U*) A 14-month-old with beginning myelination in the anterior U fibers (*arrow*). The process of myelination is complete by 2 years of age with the exception of terminal zones of myelination, which can be seen until early adulthood. However, occasional scattered unmyelinated lobar white matter fibers may be seen until the age of 40 months.

With the widespread application of the fast spin echo (FSE) technique (which uses longer echo train lengths, echo times, and recovery times), the corpus callosum (genu and splenium) is routinely visible as a hypointense structure on T2-weighted images at birth,[14] in contrast with prior reports, in which it was not visible until 4 to 8 months of age (see **Fig. 6A**).[1,15,16] This difference could be attributed to the conventional spin echo techniques used to acquire T2-weighted images in the earlier studies. In addition, the anterior limb of the internal capsule and the deep occipital and frontal white matter are also visible as hypointense structures on T2-weighted images several months earlier than expected. It is now established that myelination is visible sooner on FSE-acquired T2-weighted images than on conventional spin echo T2-weighted images.[14] In general, white matter is almost completely hypointense compared with gray matter on T2-weighted images by the age of 24 months (**Table 1**).[1,17] However, the subcortical white matter in the anteromedial frontal and temporal lobes and in the parietal lobes may remain slightly hyperintense compared with gray matter until the middle of the third year of life, and this is considered to be a normal finding so long as follow-up studies show progression of myelination. However, caution is needed in children with epilepsy or developmental abnormalities, because subcortical hyperintensities may be the only abnormality seen in some inborn errors of metabolism[17,18] or focal cortical dysplasia (malformation of cortical development).[19] Such cases need close follow-up for further evaluation and are discussed in detail elsewhere in this issue.

T1-weighted images can best assess the process of myelination during the first 6 months of life, and T2-weighted images should be used between the ages of 6 and 18 months. The qualitative evaluation of T1-weighted or T2-weighted images has consistently detected a temporal order in which different brain structures attain a myelinated appearance. As discussed earlier, myelination first begins in the pons and cerebellar peduncles followed by the posterior limbs of the internal capsules, optic radiations, and the splenium of the corpus callosum. Next, the anterior limbs of the internal capsules, genu of the corpus callosum, and then the white matter of the frontal, parietal, and occipital lobes become myelinated. Although this temporal sequence is consistent across studies, the times vary widely depending on the grading scheme and MR sequence used. In addition, the functionally and structurally related axons that originate in the same brain region, such as the anterior limb of the internal capsule and the genu of corpus callosum, myelinate at about the same time.

Barkovich[20] charted the ages at which the changes of myelination appear on T1-weighted and T2-weighted images and established milestones to determine whether myelination is normal or delayed at various times up to 2 years of age. These milestones apply to children who were born at term (40 gestational weeks). If a child is born prematurely, then the adjusted age should be used. The adjusted age is calculated by subtracting the number of months that the child was born prematurely from the current age. For example, a child born at 32 weeks' gestational age (2 months before the due date) and imaged at age 8 months should meet the myelination milestones for a 6-month-old child (current age [8 months] minus months born prematurely [2 months]). However, it is not clear whether the brain develops differently in the ex utero environment under the influence of endogenous steroids, which might exaggerate maturation in the early months of life.

Various other approaches to assessing milestones of white matter maturation have been advocated in the literature. Some investigators have analyzed the images in terms of patterns and have attempted to assess maturation from these patterns.[21,22] Other investigators have used age at which gray and white matter are isointense as a critical factor in evaluating the patient for developmental delay.[23–26] Irrespective of the system used, consistent use of a system is more important than the system itself.

Fluid-attenuated Inversion Recovery Sequence

The fluid-attenuated inversion recovery (FLAIR) sequence is now widely used and has become an important part of pediatric MR examinations. The FLAIR pulse sequence produces heavily T2-weighted images with cerebrospinal fluid signal suppression, thus enhancing the conspicuity of white matter lesions. A few studies have evaluated the white matter signal changes of myelination as seen on FLAIR images. On the FLAIR sequence, myelination generally lags behind conventional T2-weighted images. This apparent lag in myelination is attributed to T1 sensitivity of the FLAIR sequence. In addition, a triphasic pattern in FLAIR signal intensity has been observed in the deep white matter (in contrast with white matter elsewhere), appearing hypointense at birth, becoming hyperintense in the first few months, and later reconverting to being hypointense relative to adjacent gray matter during the second year of life (Fig. 4).[14] A higher content of free water in the deep white matter early in life has been postulated.[14]

Diffusion-weighted Imaging

Diffusion-weighted imaging (DWI) is sensitive to the microscopic diffusion of water within tissues, thus providing information on molecular displacements over distances comparable with cell dimensions.[27] The diffusion of water molecules in the white matter fiber is restricted by physical barriers such as cell membranes, chemical interactions of water and macromolecules, and action potential. The process of myelination results in an initial decrease in apparent diffusion coefficient (ADC) signal and an increase in anisotropy. These changes predate the T1-weighted and T2-weighted signal intensity alterations and are thought to represent the changes of premyelination.[28,29] Because diffusion-weighted images are also T2-weighted, the influence of T2 signal have to be separated from pure diffusion effects, by calculating a map of ADC values. Low ADC corresponds with high DWI signal intensity (restricted diffusion), and high ADC correlates with low DWI signal intensity. During sequential white matter myelination, there is an increase in ADC and these changes in brain water diffusion have been attributed to decreasing total water content.[29] In diffusion-weighted images, the posterior limbs of the internal capsules, which myelinate at birth, are ADC hypointense compared with unmyelinated hemispheric white matter (Fig. 5A, C). As myelination continues, contrast between gray and white matter slowly diminishes until they become isointense by 9 months of age (see Fig. 5B, D). Similar to changes occurring on T2-weighted images, the early maturing sensorimotor pathways become hypointense compared with

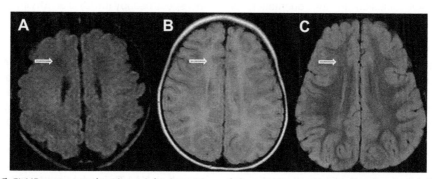

Fig. 4. (A–C) FLAIR sequence showing triphasic pattern of deep white matter myelination (*arrows*). The signal changes from hypointense at 2 weeks old to hyperintense at 7 months old, and attaining an adult hypointense pattern at 2.5 years old.

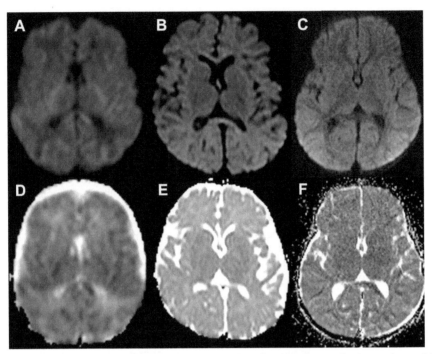

Fig. 5. Diffusion-weighted images (*A–C*) and ADC maps (*D–F*) at the age of 2 weeks, 9 months, and 2.5 years. In DWI, the white matter is hypointense in neonates, converting to isointense at about 9 months of age, with mature white matter being hypointense to gray matter. The ADC maps show increased signal in unmyelinated white matter, but appears isointense to gray matter after myelination.

cortex by about 9 months. Beyond the first year of age, the cerebral cortex and cerebral white matter are largely isointense except for peritrigonal and frontal subcortical white matter hyperintensity, which persists until the end of the second year (see **Fig. 5**C, E). Beyond the second year of life, there has been increasing interest in diffusion MR imaging, when changes seen on conventional T1-weighted and T2-weighted MR images are largely complete.[1]

Diffusion Tensor Imaging

Within normal tissue, there is a directional component of water diffusion in the orientation of preferred motion, termed anisotropy, which can be quantitatively measured via diffusion tensor imaging (DTI) to provide information about the tissue microstructure.[30] Many structural and biochemical changes of the myelinating oligodendrocytes contribute to the formation of an environment that restricts the directionality of the water diffusion.[31] At birth, there are greater magnitudes of anisotropy in central gray matter compared with white matter structures. The amount of white matter anisotropy increases over the first decade of life, such that the compact white matter pathways such as corticospinal tracts develop anisotropy at an earlier age (**Fig. 6**) than the noncompact white

matter tracts of the centrum semiovale.[32] In contrast, there is continued increase in anisotropy of the slowest-maturing subcortical white matter and the frontal white matter, even beyond the first decade of life. Myelination is thought to enhance the speed and fidelity of the transmission of action potentials along neurons, explaining age-related improvements in cognition. DTI studies of older children suggest that there is continued improvement in the diffusion anisotropy from childhood through adolescence.[33–35]

Proton MR Spectroscopy

MR spectroscopy (MRS) is an MR imaging modality that determines relative concentrations of target brain metabolites. The signal is not only derived from protons in water but also from protons in molecules such as creatine, *N*-acetylaspartate (NAA), choline (Cho), and glutamate (Glu). The data suggest that there are age-related increases in levels of NAA that begin at low levels around the immediate postnatal period and then increase rapidly during the first 24 months, becoming less pronounced thereafter.[36,37] There is similarly a linear increase in the NAA/Cho ratio as well as NAA/Cr in white matter with advancing age.[36] Technical differences result in differing appearances of the MR spectra. The techniques

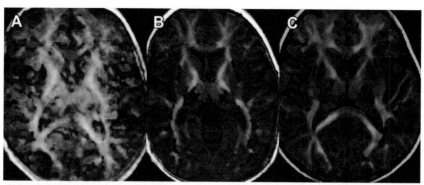

Fig. 6. DTI with directionally color coded fractional anisotropy (FA) maps from 51 days (A), 7 months (B), and 13 months of age (C). Superior to inferior direction is coded blue, anterior to posterior tracts are coded green, and mediolaterally directed tracts are coded in red. Note the increasing thickness and color of fiber tracts with age. Maturation of these fibers results in increased FA, which can be seen as increasing color in these regions.

with short echo times have a different appearances compared with techniques with long echo times, because T2 relaxation and J coupling cause broadening and decreased amplitude of peaks.[36] The increase in number of sharp peaks obtained with the short echo time technique is helpful in patients with suspected inborn errors of metabolism. In contrast, a stable baseline is more easily obtained and peaks are more easily quantified using long echo times, which are critical in the evaluation of maturity and are best performed with long-echo spectra. Also, different regions of the brain provide differing compositions of spectra. These spatial as well as temporal changes in spectra closely correlate with myelination, beginning in the thalami, followed by basal ganglia, then sensorimotor and visual pathways, with association regions in the anterior frontal, anterior temporal, and posterior parietal lobes maturing last.[38,39]

TERMINAL ZONES OF MYELINATION

The periatrial bundles of white matter are the last areas to be mature and are consistently seen along the dorsal and superior aspects of atria of lateral ventricles.[40] This normal variant should not be confused with periventricular leukomalacia (PVL). A helpful feature is the presence of normally myelinated white matter that separates these regions from the ventricles, a feature that is not seen with PVL.[41] In the coronal plane, the terminal zones have a triangular configuration with the tip oriented superiorly. Location is sometimes helpful for differentiation, given that PVL is seen inferolaterally along the optic radiations, compared with the terminal zones, which are seen more superiorly.[41] In addition to periatrial terminal zones, persistent unmyelinated areas in anterior frontal

and temporal lobes have been described as a normal finding in some children, and may not mature until 40 months of age.[40]

SUMMARY

Noninvasive imaging techniques permit investigation of the anatomic and functional maturation of the white matter. Understanding healthy developmental trajectories of white matter structure and function is of crucial importance for identification of various disorders. Although the pathophysiologic processes are complex, the process of development is orderly and follows a regular pattern over time. Familiarity with these normal patterns of myelination is essential for providing an accurate assessment of normal myelination. It is also important to be aware of the pulse sequences that are most useful during various stages of development. Ongoing investigations point to newer MR imaging techniques such as diffusion (ADC) imaging, DTI, and spectroscopy as useful imaging tools for accurate determination of normal myelination in the developing brain.

ACKNOWLEDGMENTS

The authors would like to thank Mia S. Kelly, BA, for the medical illustrations.

REFERENCES

1. Barkovich AJ, Kjos BO, Jackson DE Jr, et al. Normal maturation of the neonatal and infant brain: MR imaging at 1.5T. Radiology 1988;166:173–80.
2. Brant-Zawadzki M, Enzmann DR. Using computed tomography of the brain to correlate low white matter attenuation with early gestational age in neonates. Radiology 1981;139:105–8.

3. Morell P, Quarles RH, Norton W. Formation, structure, and biochemistry of myelin. In: Siegel J, editor. Basic neurochemistry: molecular, cellular, and medical aspects. 4th edition. New York: Raven Press; 1989. p. 109–36.

4. Van De Graff KM. Nervous tissue and the central nervous system. In: Van De Graff KM, editor. Human anatomy. 6th edition. New York: McGraw-Hill; 2002. p. 351.

5. Trapp B, Kidd G. Structure of the myelinated axon. In: Lazzarini R, editor. Myelin biology and disorders, vol. 1. London: Elsevier Academic Press; 2004. p. 3–27.

6. Taylor C, Marta C, Bansal R, et al. The transport, assembly, and function of myelin lipids. In: Lazzarini R, editor. Myelin biology and disorders, vol. 1. London: Elsevier Academic Press; 2004. p. 57–88.

7. Morell P, Quarles RH. Myelin formation, structure and biochemistry. In: Siegel GJ, Agrano¡ BW, Albers RW, et al, editors. Basic neurochemistry: molecular, cellular and medical aspects. 6th edition. New York: Lippincott Williams & Wilkins; 1999. p. 69–93.

8. Edgar JM, McLaughlin M, Yool D, et al. Oligodendroglial modulation of fast axonal transport in a mouse model of hereditary spastic paraplegia. J Cell Biol 2004;166:121–31.

9. Tsunoda I, Fujinami RS. Inside-out versus outside-in models for virus induced demyelination: axonal damage triggering demyelination. Springer Semin Immunopathol 2002;24:105–25.

10. Barkovich AJ. Magnetic resonance techniques in the assessment of myelin and myelination. J Inherit Metab Dis 2005;28:311–43.

11. Yakovlev P, Lecours A. The myelogenic cycles of regional maturation of the brain. In: Minkowski A, editor. Regional development of the brain in early life. Oxford (United Kingdom): Blackwell; 1967. p. 3–70.

12. Brody BA, Kinney HC, Kloman AS, et al. Sequence of central nervous system myelination in human infancy. I. An autopsy study of myelination. J Neuropathol Exp Neurol 1987;46:283–301.

13. Fatouros PP, Marmarou A. Use of magnetic resonance imaging for in vivo measurements of water content in human brain: method and normal values. J Neurosurg 1999;90:109–15.

14. Murakami JW, Weinberger E, Shaw DW. Normal myelination of the pediatric brain imaged with fluid-attenuated inversion-recovery (FLAIR) MR imaging. AJNR Am J Neuroradiol 1999;20:1406–11.

15. Grodd W. Normal and abnormal patterns of myelin development of the fetal and infantile human brain using magnetic resonance imaging. Curr Opin Neurol Neurosurg 1993;6:393–7.

16. Shaw DW, Weinberger E, Astley SJ, et al. Quantitative comparison of conventional spin echo and fast spin echo during brain myelination. J Comput Assist Tomogr 1997;21:867–71.

17. Barkovich AJ. Concepts of myelin and myelination in neuroradiology. AJNR Am J Neuroradiol 2000;21:1099–109.

18. Van der Knaap MS, Valk J. Magnetic resonance of myelin, myelination, and myelin disorders. 2nd edition. Berlin: Springer; 1995.

19. Bronen RA, Vives KP, Kim JH, et al. Focal cortical dysplasia of Taylor, balloon cell subtype: MR differentiation from low-grade tumors. AJNR Am J Neuroradiol 1997;18:1141–51.

20. Barkovich AJ, Raybaud C. Normal development of the neonatal and infant brain, skull, and spine. In: Barkovich AJ, Raybaud C, editors. Pediatric neuroimaging. 5th edition. Philadelphia: Lippincott Williams & Wilkins; 2012. p. 20–80.

21. Martin E, Boesch C, Zuerrer M, et al. MR imaging of brain maturation in normal and developmentally handicapped children. J Comput Assist Tomogr 1990;14:685–92.

22. Van der Knaap MS. Myelination and myelin disorders: a magnetic resonance study in infants, children and young adults [PhD thesis]. Amsterdam, Netherlands: Free University of Amsterdam and University of Utrecht; 1991.

23. Bird C, Hedberg M, Drayer BP, et al. MR assessment of myelination in infants and children: usefulness of marker sites. Am J Neuroradiol 1989;10:731–40.

24. Dietrich RB, Bradley WG, Zagaroza EJ, et al. MR evaluation of early myelination patterns in normal and developmentally delayed infants. AJNR Am J Neuroradiol 1988;9:69–76.

25. Staudt M, Schropp C, Staudt F, et al. Myelination of the brain in MRI: a staging system. Pediatr Radiol 1993;23:169–76.

26. Staudt M, Schropp C, Staudt F, et al. MRI assessment of myelination: an age standardization. Pediatr Radiol 1994;24:122–7.

27. Le Bihan D. Molecular diffusion, tissue microdynamics and microstructure. NMR Biomed 1995;8:375–86.

28. Nomura Y, Sakuma H, Tagami T, et al. Diffusional anisotropy of the human brain assessed with diffusion-weighted MR: relation with normal brain development and aging. AJNR Am J Neuroradiol 1994;15:231–8.

29. Neil JJ, Shiran SI, McKinstry RC, et al. Normal brain in human newborns: apparent diffusion coefficient and diffusion anisotropy measured by using diffusion tensor MR imaging. Radiology 1998;209:57–66.

30. Pierpaoli C, Jezzard P, Basser PJ, et al. Diffusion tensor MR imaging of the human brain. Radiology 1996;201:637–48.

31. Baumann N, Pham-Dinh D. Biology of oligodendrocyte and myelin in the mammalian central nervous system. Physiol Rev 2001;81:871–927.

32. McGraw P, Liang L, Provenzale J. Evaluation of normal age-related changes in anisotropy during

infancy and childhood as shown by diffusion tensor imaging. AJR Am J Roentgenol 2002;179:1515–22.

33. Barnea-Goraly N, Menon V, Eckert M, et al. White matter development during childhood and adolescence: a cross-sectional diffusion tensor imaging study. Cereb Cortex 2005;15:1848–54.

34. Ben Bashat D, Ben Sira L, Graif M, et al. Normal white matter development from infancy to adulthood: comparing diffusion tensor and high b value diffusion weighted MR images. J Magn Reson Imaging 2005;21:503–11.

35. Schmithorst VJ, Wilke M, Dardzinski BJ, et al. Correlation of white matter diffusivity and anisotropy with age during childhood and adolescence: a cross-sectional diffusion-tensor MR imaging study. Radiology 2002;222:212–8.

36. Kreis R, Ernst T, Ross BD. Development of the human brain: in vivo quantification of metabolite and water content with proton magnetic resonance spectroscopy. Magn Reson Med 1993;30:424–37.

37. Toft PB, Leth H, Lou HC, et al. Metabolite concentrations in the developing brain estimated with proton MR spectroscopy. J Magn Reson Imaging 1994;4: 674–80.

38. Kreis R, Hofmann L, Kuhlmann B, et al. Brain metabolite composition during early human brain development as measured by quantitative in vivo 1H magnetic resonance spectroscopy. Magn Reson Med 2002;48:949–58.

39. Vigneron DB, Barkovich AJ, Noworolski SM, et al. Three-dimensional proton MR spectroscopic imaging of premature and term neonates. AJNR Am J Neuroradiol 2001;22:1424–33.

40. Parazzini C, Baldoli C, Scotti G, et al. Terminal zones of myelination: MR evaluation of children aged 20–40 months. AJNR Am J Neuroradiol 2002;23:1669–73.

41. Baker LL, Stevenson DK, Enzmann DR. End-stage periventricular leukomalacia: MR evaluation. Radiology 1988;168(3):809–15.

A Pattern Approach to Focal White Matter Hyperintensities on Magnetic Resonance Imaging

Sangam Kanekar, MD[a,b,*], Puneet Devgun, DO[a]

KEYWORDS

- Focal white matter hyperintensity • Multiple sclerosis • Acute disseminated encephalomyelitis
- CNS vasculitis • Lyme • Sarcoid

KEY POINTS

- Evaluation of focal white matter hyperintensities on magnetic resonance (MR) imaging in any age group is always challenging.
- It is important to have a specific imaging approach, including age, pattern of distribution, signal characteristics on various sequences, enhancement pattern, and other ancillary findings, to infer to a correct cause for white matter hyperintensities.
- Normal MR imaging almost always excludes intracranial vasculitis. However, there are no pathognomonic MR imaging findings in vasculitis.
- Asymptomatic (silent) lacunar infarcts are at least 5 times more common than symptomatic infarcts.
- The risk of dementia and severity of cognitive impairment is preferentially associated with periventricular white matter lesions, whereas mood disorders are more likely seen with deep white matter lesions.

INTRODUCTION

Evaluation of focal white matter hyperintensities (WMH) on magnetic resonance (MR) imaging in any age group is always challenging because the cause of these hyperintensities may vary from infectious, inflammatory, neoplastic, or demyelinating findings to nonspecific findings related to aging and other systemic conditions (Box 1, Table 1). Most clinicians look to the imager for a specific diagnosis or to limit the differential diagnosis so that an appropriate test may be advised to confirm the cause or underlying disease process. Without an appropriate clinical history and findings, these nonspecific WMH can be challenging to differentiate. An understanding of the clinical presentation, pathophysiology, and associated imaging findings can allow the radiologist to limit the differential. It is important to have a specific imaging approach, including age, pattern of distribution, signal characteristics on various sequences, enhancement pattern, and other ancillary findings, to infer a correct cause for these hyperintensities. Many times in clinical practice it may not be able to characterize these hyperintensities, and in such cases discussion with the clinicians with appropriate follow-up may be the best

[a] Department of Radiology, Penn State Milton S. Hershey Medical Center and College of Medicine, The Pennsylvania State University, 500 University Drive, Hershey, PA 17033, USA; [b] Department of Neurology, Penn State Milton S. Hershey Medical Center and College of Medicine, The Pennsylvania State University, 500 University Drive, Hershey, PA 17033, USA
* Corresponding author. Department of Radiology, College of Medicine, Penn State Milton S. Hershey Medical Center and College of Medicine, The Pennsylvania State University, 500 University Drive, Hershey, PA 17033.
E-mail address: skanekar@hmc.psu.edu

Radiol Clin N Am 52 (2014) 241–261
http://dx.doi.org/10.1016/j.rcl.2013.11.010

Box 1
Differential diagnosis of focal white matter hyperintensities on T2-weighted imaging

1. Virchow-Robin spaces
2. Migrainous ischemia
3. Multiple sclerosis
4. Acute disseminated encephalomyelitis
5. Central nervous system (CNS) vasculitis
   Primary vasculitis
   a. Giant-cell arteritis
   b. Primary angiitis of the CNS
   c. Takayasu disease
   d. Polyarteritis nodosa
   e. Kawasaki disease
   f. Churg-Strauss syndrome
   g. Wegener granulomatosis
   Secondary vasculitis
   h. Collagen vascular diseases
   i. Systemic lupus erythematosus
   j. Scleroderma
   k. Rheumatoid arthritis
   l. Sjögren syndrome
   m. Mixed connective tissue disease
   n. Behçet disease
   o. Infection
   p. Illicit drugs
   q. Malignancy
   r. Other systemic conditions
6. Cerebrovascular disease
   a. Lacunar infarcts
   b. Watershed infarctions
7. CADASIL (cerebral autosomal dominant arteriopathy with subcortical infarcts and leukoencephalopathy)
8. Sarcoidosis
9. Lyme disease
10. Progressive multifocal leukoencephalopathy
11. Age-related changes
12. Effects of radiation therapy or drugs
13. Metastatic disease
14. Inherited white matter diseases
15. CNS lymphoma

solution. The purpose of this article is to provide a pattern approach to differentiate various common and a few uncommon diseases presenting as focal WMH.

PERIVASCULAR SPACES OR VIRCHOW-ROBIN SPACES

Perivascular spaces (PVS) or Virchow-Robin spaces (VRS) are pial-lined, fluid-filled structures surrounding penetrating arteries and arterioles. These spaces are seen most commonly along the path of lenticulostriate arteries entering the basal ganglia, or along the perforating medullary arteries entering the cortical gray matter. Other areas where prominent PVS can be seen include the subinsular region, dentate nuclei, and cerebellum. The exact etiology of these PVS has yet to be delineated. Multiple hypotheses have been suggested, including spiral elongation of the penetrating blood vessels, increased cerebrospinal fluid (CSF) pulsations, sequelae of ex vacuo phenomenon, abnormality of arterial wall permeability, and accumulation of brain interstitial fluid between the vessel and pia or interpial space.[1]

PVS become prominent and dilated with the age of the patient. Prominence of PVS in older patients is thought to be due to 2 main reasons. First, VRS are a direct extension of the subarachnoid space, and aging is associated with enlargement of ventricles and sulci, resulting in prominence of the subarachnoid space. Second, atherosclerotic changes, particularly in hypertensive patients, result in unfolding and tortuosity of the vessels, leading to prominence of PVS.

On MR imaging PVS appear as round to oval, smoothly demarcated fluid-filled cysts, typically less than 5 mm in diameter, and often occur in clusters.[1] PVS are isointense to CSF on all pulse sequences including fluid-attenuated inversion recovery (FLAIR), and demonstrate no enhancement after contrast administration (Fig. 1). PVS do not cause focal mass effect or restriction on diffusion-weighted (DW) images. On axial images they are typically seen around the lateral portion of the anterior commissure. Although most show normal signal intensity in the adjacent brain; 25% may have a small rim of slightly increased signal intensity. VRS in the midbrain surrounding the branches of the collicular and accessory collicular arteries are slightly hyperintense to CSF on FLAIR images.

One of the common clinical challenges is to differentiate PVS from lacunar infarction. Location, morphology, and signal intensity tend to differentiate these 2 conditions. Dilated PVS usually are isointense to CSF on all pulse sequences,

Table 1
Salient distinguishing features of commonly seen focal white matter lesions on T2-weighted imaging

	Clinical Features	Imaging Features	Ancillary Findings
VRS	Asymptomatic	Smoothly demarcated lesions isointense to CSF on all pulse sequences, no enhancement, bilateral symmetric involvement of the basal ganglia, subinsular region, dentate nuclei, and cerebellum	No mass effect or DWI restriction, relative stability over time
Migraine	Female, 10–45 y, headache with aura	T2/FLAIR hyperintensities in juxtacortical, periventricular region, sparing the callosal and subcallosal region	Family history of migraine, increasing headache frequency
MS	Young woman, 30–40 y	Ovoid lesions involving the corpus callosum, periventricular, juxtacortical, infratentorial, subcortical U fibers, optic nerves, and spinal cord	CSF oligoglonal bands ++, optic neuritis
ADEM	Pediatric age group	Multiple asymmetric, poorly defined subcortical WM lesions involving the subcortical and deep WM, basal ganglia and thalamus, posterior fossa (brainstem, middle cerebellar peduncles, and cerebellar WM)	Postviral or vaccination, decrease in size and number on follow-up, bilateral optic neuritis
CNS vasculitis	Middle-aged female>>male	Small hyperintensities in the deep and subcortical WM with areas of microhemorrhages or infarcts. Multiple segmental narrowing and dilations along the vessel, avascular areas, hazy vessel margins, collateral formation, intracerebral aneurysms	DSA gold standard for evaluation of vessels. Definitive diagnosis by tissue biopsy
Lacunes	Focal motor or sensory symptoms, sensorimotor, ataxic hemiparesis, and dysarthria	Deep, sharply marginated, focal lesions, 3–20 mm in diameter. Acute: focal areas of DWI restriction. Chronic: multiple WMH in deep WM	Atherosclerosis, ipsilateral high-grade carotid stenosis, aortic arch atheroma
Watershed infarcts	Elderly with atherosclerosis in setting of hypotension	Confluent lesions parallel to lateral ventricle, unilateral (beads of pearls)	Shock, cardiac arrest, or cardiac bypass
CADASIL	Middle age	Diffuse symmetric periventricular WM, basal ganglia, temporal lobes, thalamus, internal capsule, and pons	Autosomal dominant, absence of optic nerve or spinal cord involvement
Sarcoidosis	Aseptic meningitis, isolated cranial neuropathies	Diffuse meningeal and parenchymal WM lesions, periventricular and deep WMH, cranial nerve enhancement	Enhancing sella masses, thickening of the infundibulum, communicating or obstructive hydrocephalus

(continued on next page)

Table 1
(continued)

	Clinical Features	Imaging Features	Ancillary Findings
Lyme	Tick exposure, flu symptoms, arthritis, erythema migrans, CVS and CNS signs and symptoms	Normal to multiple bilateral periventricular and/or subcortical T2 hyperintensities, cranial nerve involvement (CN III, V, VII)	Positive Lyme titers, clinical history
PML	Immunocompromised patients, on natalizumab for MS	Bilateral, multiple hyperintensities with involvement of subcortical U fibers, no mass effect or hemorrhage Lesions lack enhancement or restricted diffusion on DWI	JCV DNA PCR in CSF
Age-related WMH	Elderly patient	Focal or diffuse periventricular or deep WMH	Enlargement of ventricles and cerebral sulci
Radiation induced	RT ± CT	Focal, patchy, or diffuse T2 hyperintensities in the periventricular WM, centrum semiovale with sparing the subcortical arcuate fibers, cerebral cortex, and deep gray	May show cognitive decline

Abbreviations: ADEM, acute disseminated encephalomyelitis; CADASIL, cerebral autosomal dominant arteriopathy with subcortical infarcts and leukoencephalopathy; CN, cranial nerve; CSF, cerebrospinal fluid; CT, chemotherapy; CVS, cardiovascular system; DSA, digital subtraction angiography; DWI, diffusion-weighted imaging; FLAIR, fluid-attenuated inversion recovery; JCV, John Cunningham virus; MS, multiple sclerosis; PCR, polymerase chain reaction; PML, progressive multifocal leukoencephalopathy; RT, radiotherapy; VRS, Virchow-Robin spaces; WM, white matter; WMH, white matter hyperintensities.

symmetric bilaterally, less than 5 mm in diameter, and located in the inferior one-third of the putamen. Lacunes, on the other hand, are often larger than 5 mm, asymmetric, located in the upper two-thirds of the putamen, and are not isointense to CSF on all imaging sequences unless they have undergone complete cystic change. Occasionally PVS may become very large and appear bizarre,

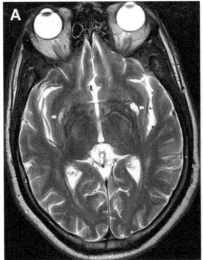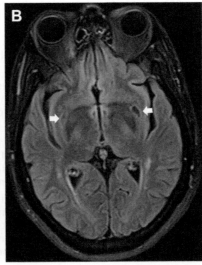

Fig. 1. Virchow-Robin spaces (VRS) in a 47-year-old male patient with history of headache. (*A*) Axial T2-weighted and (*B*) fluid-attenuated inversion recovery (FLAIR) images reveal oval shape, smoothly demarcated, cystic spaces, isointense to cerebrospinal fluid (CSF), around the lateral portion of the anterior commissure (*arrows*).

causing focal mass effect and occasionally hydro-cephalus, known as giant or tumefactive PVS.[2] Giant PVS need to be differentiated from cystic neoplasm such as like dysembryoplastic neuroe-pithelial tumor and infection, which may otherwise lead to unnecessary biopsy and the associated risks. The key features distinguishing these lesions from neoplasm are their isointensity to CSF on all sequences, their characteristic location, their lack of associated neurologic dysfunction, and their relative stability over time (Fig. 2). Dilatation of VRS within the white matter of the cerebral con-vexities is less common, and has been shown to correlate with hypertension and dementia in the aging brain. In children, dilated VRS within the ce-rebral white matter has been described in patients with mucopolysaccharidosis, whereby foam cells distend the perivascular spaces (Fig. 3). In an endemic area, dilated PVS needs to be differenti-ated from infection such as neurocysticercosis. Neurocysticercosis cysts may be multiple, scat-tered throughout the brain, have a scolex (parasite head), and often have an enhancing cystic wall.

MIGRAINE-RELATED HYPERINTENSITIES

Migraines are a complex and disabling brain disor-der characterized by recurrent episodes of cere-bral disturbance that are often influenced by lifestyle and genetic factors. The prevalence in the United States is reported as 17.1% in females and 5.6% in males.[3] It is more common between

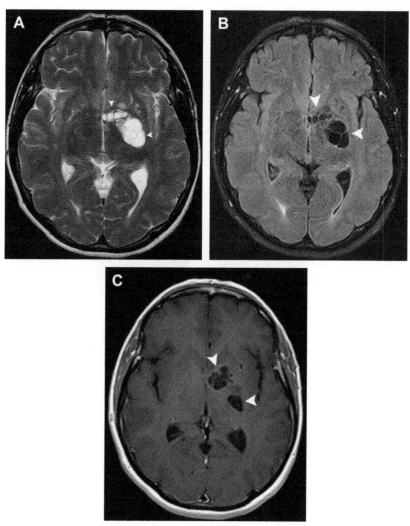

Fig. 2. Giant VRS mimicking a mass. A 32-year-old male patient presented with chronic headache. (A) Axial T2-weighted and (B) FLAIR images show large cystic lesions (arrowheads), isointense to CSF in the left deep gray mat-ter nuclei and internal capsule. There is no perilesional edema. (C) Contrast-enhanced axial T1-weighted image shows no enhancement (arrowheads).

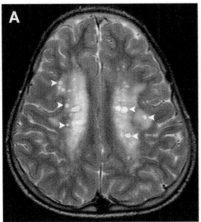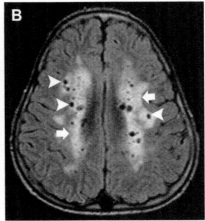

Fig. 3. Mucopolysaccharidosis with dilated VRS in a 5-year-old child. (*A*) Axial T2-weighted and (*B*) FLAIR images show multiple dilated, round, well-defined, cystic spaces isointense to CSF (*arrowheads*). Diffuse hyperintensity (*arrows*) is also noted in the cerebral white matter bilaterally.

the ages of 10 and 45 years and may run in the family. The pathophysiology of migraine is still debatable. For many years it has been centered on whether it is primarily a neural or vascular (cerebral vasoconstriction causing aura through cerebral ischemia and subsequent vasodilatation producing headache) disorder. Clinically various types of migraines have been described. One of the important clinical features that determine effective treatment and outcome is the presence or absence of aura (visual hallucinations). Migraine with an aura is considered to have a higher incidence of WMH and an increased risk for ischemic stroke in females.[4]

The pathophysiology of these WMH in migraine is elusive. Prolonged and repeated oligemia during migraine attacks is thought to affect the vulnerable small deep penetrating arteries and local critical hypoperfusion, leading to ischemic brain injuries that are seen as WMH on MR. The CAMERA study showed that females with migraines had a significantly increased risk of WMH in the brain, including pons and subclinical infarcts in the posterior circulation. It is important to recognize and characterize these hyperintensities in a patient with headache.[5] WMH in migraine are seen predominantly in the deep white matter (47%) and periventricular region (19%) on T2-weighted and FLAIR images (**Fig. 4**). Involvement of the callosal and subcallosal region is extremely rare, but juxtacortical hyperintensities are not uncommon.[6] Most deep WMH are located within the frontal lobes, followed by parietal, temporal, and occipital lobes. These lesions are multiple (≥9) hyperintensities in 63% of the patients. Increasing age, family history of migraine, and increasing headache frequency were found to be the factors associated with WMH.

MULTIPLE SCLEROSIS

More than 100 years has passed since Charcot, Carswell, Cruveilhier, and others described the clinical and pathologic characteristics of multiple sclerosis (MS).[7] MS is a chronic demyelinating disease of unknown etiology. Women are affected twice as often as men, and disease onset is usually in the third or fourth decade.[8,9] MS remains a

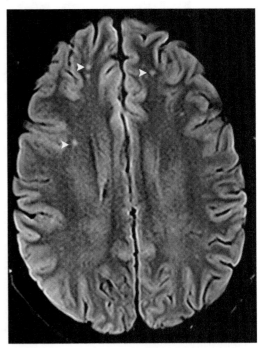

Fig. 4. A 43-year-old woman with migraine headache. Axial FLAIR image shows tiny nonspecific hyperintensities (*arrowheads*) in the subcortical region in the frontal white matter bilaterally.

clinical diagnosis and is supplemented by imaging and CSF findings. MS is characterized by neurologic symptoms disseminated in space and time. Many criteria have been proposed, but the most widely accepted and used are the McDonald criteria. Under the current revised 2010 McDonald guidelines, demonstration of dissemination in space is defined as more than 1 T2 lesion in at least 2 of the 4 areas periventricular, juxtacortical, infratentorial, or spinal cord; dissemination in time is defined as a new T2 and/or gadolinium-enhancing lesion(s) on follow-up MR imaging, with reference to a baseline scan, irrespective of the timing of the baseline or simultaneous presence of asymptomatic gadolinium-enhancing and nonenhancing lesions at any time.[10]

Axial and sagittal FLAIR images remain the main preferred sequence for evaluation of periventricular and juxtacortical MS lesions, whereas posterior fossa lesions are best seen on T2-weighted images. Contrast can be helpful in establishing an early diagnosis by detecting new lesion activity and ruling out alternative diagnoses. The characteristic findings of MS lesions have a predilection for the periventricular white matter. These lesions tend to be ovoid in configuration with the major axes perpendicular to the ventricular surface, also known as Dawson fingers (**Fig. 5**). Other characteristic locations where lesions are frequently found are the corpus callosum, initially involving the callososeptal margins, subcortical region, brainstem, subcortical U fibers, optic nerves, and visual pathway (**Fig. 6**).[11] Lesions in the corpus callosum occur frequently in all stages of MS with its involvement ranging between 25% and

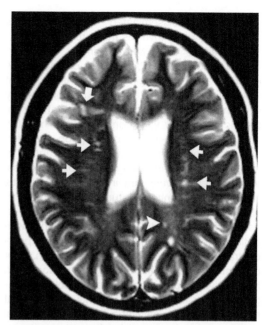

Fig. 6. A 29-year-old female patient with MS. Axial T2-weighted image shows juxtacortical plaque in the right frontal lobe (*thick arrow*) and bilateral periventricular demyelinating plaques (*arrows*). Increased signal intensity similar to that of gray matter is seen in the peritrigonal white matter (*arrowhead*) (dirty-appearing white matter [DAWM]).

93% of MS patients, compared with only 2% of patients with white matter disease from other causes such as stroke, cerebral autosomal dominant arteriopathy with subcortical infarcts and leukoencephalopathy (CADASIL), lymphoma, and progressive multifocal leukoencephalopathy

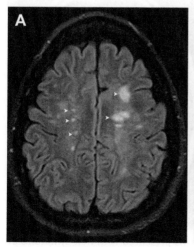
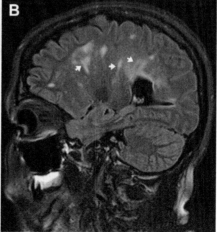

Fig. 5. Classic multiple sclerosis (MS) plaques in a 36-year-old female patient with a history of optic neuritis and weakness. (*A*) Axial and (*B*) sagittal FLAIR images reveal multiple flame-shaped periventricular lesions, most of which are perpendicular to the lateral margin of the lateral ventricle, characteristic of MS (*arrowheads*). Appearance of the lesions on sagittal view is called Dowson fingers (*arrows*).

(PML). Acute disseminated encephalomyelitis (ADEM) very rarely involves the corpus callosum.

In a verified case, MR imaging is often performed to look for progression or diagnose new lesions. New or enlarging T2 lesions represent new inflammation and provide complementary information on disease activity. Pattern of enhancement may vary from diffuse to nodular, ring or horseshoe-like, depending on evolution and resolution of inflammation and disruption of the blood-brain barrier (Fig. 7). Leptomeningeal enhancement is very rare in MS. Optic neuritis may be a presenting feature in MS and may show a hyperintense, edematous optic nerve on coronal fat-saturated T2-weighted imaging, with optic nerve and sheath enhancement on post-contrast fat-saturated T1-weighted images. Four percent of healthy individuals of all ages can have periventricular changes that cannot be distinguished from MS. In these patients, findings that may favor MS are periventricular and juxtacortical lesions, and lesions involving the anterior tips of the temporal lobes, posterior fossa, or spinal cord.

Besides classic small lesions, additional MR imaging features that are commonly seen in MS include T1-weighted black holes and diffusely abnormal white matter. MS may show large diffuse lesions with poorly defined boundaries on T2-weighted images. These areas of diffusely abnormal or dirty-appearing white matter (DAWM) have intensity similar to that of gray matter on T2-weighted scans and are most commonly found around the ventricles, adjacent to the trigone and occipital horn, the body of the lateral ventricles, and the centrum semiovale (see Fig. 6).

ACUTE DISSEMINATED ENCEPHALOMYELITIS

ADEM is defined as the first episode of inflammatory demyelination associated with multifocal neurologic deficits, with involvement of multiple sites in the central nervous system (CNS) and accompanied by encephalopathy. ADEM may be seen following a wide range of conditions such as nonspecific respiratory infections, specific viral illness (such as measles, rubella, mumps, and chickenpox), and vaccinations (including diphtheria, smallpox, tetanus, and typhoid), and may even arise spontaneously.[7]

The exact pathogenesis of ADEM is unclear. The 2 most common mechanisms hypothesized are the inflammatory cascade theory and the molecular mimicry theory.[12,13] In the inflammatory cascade theory, viral infection results in nervous tissue damage, which causes segregated antigens to leak into the systemic circulation through a damaged blood-brain barrier; these antigens are processed in the lymphatic organs and elicit a T-cell response, which in turn damages the CNS and perpetuates inflammation. Whereas in the molecular mimicry theory there is a structural similarity between the pathogen and the myelin proteins of the host, B and T cells that are activated during the immune response to infection enter the CNS and react against the presumed foreign antigen represented by the homologue myelin protein. ADEM is

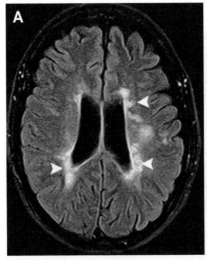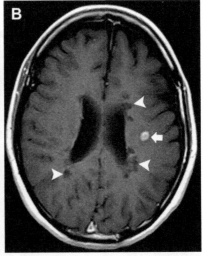

Fig. 7. A 33-year-old female patient with a known case of MS presented with new symptoms of weakness. (*A*) Axial FLAIR images show multiple areas of demyelinating plaques in the periventricular white matter bilaterally (*arrowheads*). (*B*) Postcontrast T1-weighted image shows multiple hypointense lesions corresponding to the chronic demyelinating plaques (*arrowheads*). Nodular enhancing lesion seen in the left deep white matter is most suggestive of active plaque (*thick arrow*).

characterized histologically by perivenous edema, demyelination, and infiltration with macrophages and lymphocytes, with relative axonal sparing. In the later stages, disease is characterized by perivascular gliosis. The CSF may be normal or show a pleocytosis of 1000 or more cells per mm³.

Imaging findings of ADEM are very nonspecific and at times could be challenging to differentiate from other demyelination conditions such as MS, especially in the pediatric age group. In a typical case, MR shows multiple, asymmetrically distributed, poorly defined, hyperintense lesions on T2-weighted/FLAIR images involving the subcortical and deep white matter (Fig. 8). There is frequent involvement of the deep gray matter nuclei (ie, thalamus and basal ganglia) in acute stages. Involvement of the cerebral cortex and posterior fossa is seen in up to 30% and 50% cases, respectively. In the posterior fossa, ADEM lesions mostly involve the brainstem, middle cerebellar peduncles, and cerebellar white matter. DW imaging may show restricted diffusion in the first 7 days of clinical onset, owing to swelling of the myelin sheaths, reduced vascular

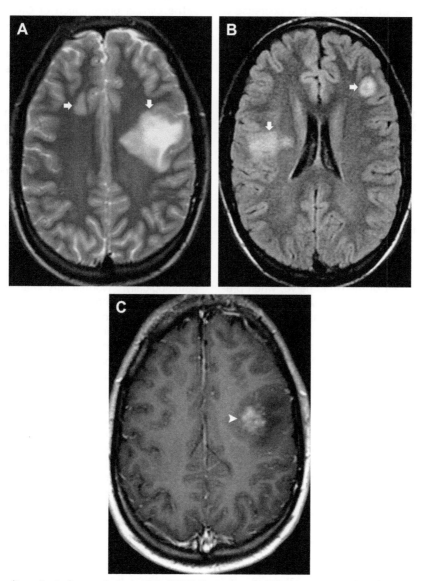

Fig. 8. Acute disseminated encephalomyelitis (ADEM). A 14-year-old boy presented with a history of acute changes in mental status. (A) Axial T2-weighted and (B) FLAIR images show multiple, asymmetric hyperintense areas (arrows) involving the subcortical and deep white matter in the frontal lobes bilaterally. (C) Contrast-enhanced axial T1-weighted image shows focal irregular central enhancement within the demyelinating area (arrowhead).

supply, and dense inflammatory cell infiltration in the acute phase of ADEM. Unlike stroke, this restricted diffusion does not seem to imply irreversible damage in ADEM. In the subacute (>7 days) stage, increased diffusivity with higher apparent diffusion coefficient (ADC) values are seen because of axonal loss, demyelination, and edema, causing an expansion of the extracellular space.[14] On the postcontrast scan, most of the lesions do not enhance. Larger lesions may show peripheral or focal irregular central enhancement (see Fig. 8C). Changes on MR spectroscopy largely depend on the stage of the disease. In the acute stages of ADEM there is a decrease in N-acetylaspartate (NAA), with normal levels of choline. Lesions in the subacute stage show reduction of NAA in regions corresponding to the areas of high T2 signal intensity, with an increase in choline resulting from transient neuroaxonal dysfunction and partial breakdown of myelin.[15] Various imaging features are used to differentiate ADEM from MS, which is important from the point of view of treatment and prognosis. MS lesions are usually small, somewhat symmetric, and commonly involve the corpus callosum and pericallosal region. ADEM lesions are subcortical or are in the deep white matter with less predilection for the corpus callosum. Involvement of the gray matter, cortical as well as deep, is early and frequent in ADEM. At times this involvement of the basal ganglia and thalami may be symmetric, mimicking metabolic disorders such as Leigh disease. Involvement of the optic nerve, when present, is usually unilateral in MS whereas it is mostly bilateral in ADEM. At present, there are no absolute clinical features, or radiologic, serum, or CSF biomarkers that can distinguish ADEM from pediatric MS. Thus, sequential MR imaging plays an important role in diagnosing ADEM, establishing its monophasic nature, and distinguishing it from MS. Unfortunately there are no clear guidelines on interval and duration of studies. On follow-up imaging, after treatment with steroids, there is typically a decrease in the size and number of lesions or complete resolution of ADEM lesions, whereas MS lesions may show new, often asymptomatic lesions. Appearance of new lesions strongly suggests MS.

CNS VASCULITIS

CNS vasculitis represents a heterogeneous group of inflammatory diseases that primarily affect the small leptomeningeal and parenchymal blood vessels of the brain. CNS vasculitis can be classified as primary vasculitis (giant-cell arteritis, primary angiitis of the CNS, Takayasu disease, polyarteritis nodosa, Kawasaki disease, Churg-Strauss syndrome, Wegener granulomatosis) and secondary vasculitis (collagen vascular diseases, infection, illicit drugs, malignancy, and other systemic conditions). The exact pathogenesis of these vasculitides is still not completely understood. Recent advances have pointed toward the immune and cytokine-mediated damage to the vessel wall leading to endothelial damage, production of chemotactic factors, infiltration of neutrophils and monocytes, stimulation of clotting and kinin pathways, and release of cytokines, oxygen radicals, and proteolytic enzymes.

The clinical presentation of CNS vasculitis is variable. It is most commonly seen in middle-aged female patients. Clinically the patient may present with headache, cranial nerve palsies, encephalopathy, seizures, psychosis, myelitis, stroke, intracranial hemorrhage, and aseptic meningoencephalitis.

Almost all forms of vasculitis can involve the vessels feeding the brain parenchyma and can cause either focal or diffuse white matter changes or stroke-like episodes. Imaging plays an important role in identifying both parenchymal and vessel abnormalities. Although MR imaging is most sensitive in detecting the parenchymal changes attributable to vasculitis, MR angiography and computed tomography (CT) angiography remain insufficient to disclose the vessel changes. Digital subtraction angiography still remains the gold standard to define the vessel pathologically.[7] Normal MR imaging almost always excludes intracranial vasculitis. However, there are no pathognomonic MR imaging findings in vasculitis. Multiple nonspecific small hyperintensities involving the deep and the subcortical white matter and deep gray matter on T2-weighted/FLAIR imaging are one of the most frequent presentations of vasculitis on MR imaging (Fig. 9A).[7,16] Multiple infarcts in various vascular territories and of different ages in young patients must raise the suspicion for cerebral vasculitis. In addition, multiple, tiny, scattered foci of hemorrhages on blood-sensitive sequences such as gradient echo (GRE)/susceptibility-weighted (SW) imaging are common. GRE/SW imaging sequences may also show focal areas of subarachnoid hemorrhages.[17] Careful evaluation of the vessel on the conventional sequences may show increased thickness of vessel wall on T1-weighted images, vessel wall edema on T2-weighted images, and mural enhancement on postcontrast T1-weighted images. In advanced cases, MR or CT angiography may show nonatherosclerotic arterial stenosis and occlusions (see Fig. 9B, C).

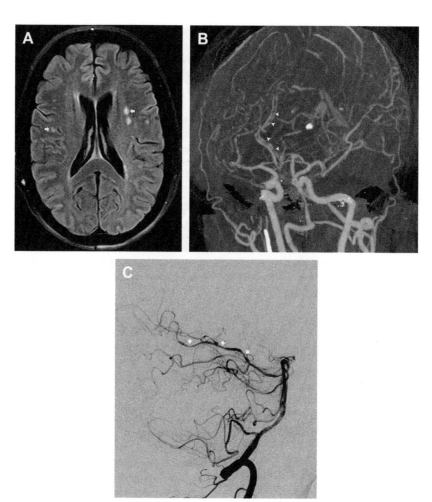

Fig. 9. A 41-year-old female patient with primary central nervous system vasculitis. (A) Axial FLAIR image shows multiple tiny scattered hyperintensities in the subcortical and deep white matter bilaterally (arrows). (B) Oblique view of the computed tomography angiogram and (C) lateral view of digital subtraction angiogram show multiple short-segment areas of narrowing in the anterior cerebral arteries (arrowheads) and posterior cerebral arteries (arrows) bilaterally.

LACUNAR INFARCTS

Lacunar infarcts are defined pathologically as deep, sharply margined, focal lesions ranging from 3 to 4 mm to 15 to 20 mm in size.[18] For a long time, lacunar infarcts were thought to be caused by intrinsic disease of the small vessels, called lipohyalinosis, resulting from hypertension and diabetes. However, this hypothesis, called the lacunar hypothesis, does not explain why 50% of lacunar infarcts are seen in normotensive patients.[19] Lacunes are now thought to result from focal ischemic infarcts caused by thrombi or emboli composed of platelets or fibrin (often with incorporated red blood cells) against a background of diffuse atherosclerotic narrowing of small vessels. Ipsilateral high-grade carotid stenosis and aortic-arch atheroma have been shown to be risk factors for lacunar stroke.

Asymptomatic (silent) lacunar infarcts are at least 5 times more common than symptomatic infarcts.[20] When symptomatic, lacunar infarcts may present with classic lacunar syndromes: pure motor stroke, pure sensory stroke, sensorimotor stroke, ataxic hemiparesis, and dysarthria.[18,20] MR imaging is more sensitive than CT for the diagnosis of acute and chronic lacunar infarctions. Acute lacunes (Fig. 10) show focal areas of restricted diffusion, most commonly in the deep white matter, whereas chronic lacunes typically present as multiple WMH on T2-weighted and FLAIR images.[18,20] A common differential diagnosis includes VRS, which follows CSF signal on all MR imaging sequences. Sometimes an old lacune may show CSF density in the center with surrounding hyperintensity on FLAIR images (Fig. 11).[18,20]

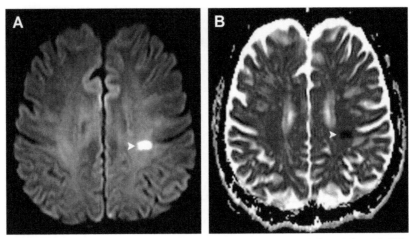

Fig. 10. Acute lacunar stroke in 61-year-old man with sudden onset of motor deficit. (*A*) Axial diffusion-weighted (DW) image and (*B*) apparent diffusion coefficient (ADC) image show focal area of restricted diffusion in the left frontal deep white matter with corresponding low ADC (*arrowhead*).

WATERSHED INFARCTIONS

Watershed infarctions are seen at the junction of the distal fields of the 2 nonanatomizing major cerebral arteries. Watershed infarctions are classified into cortical watershed infarcts and internal watershed infarcts.[21] Cortical watershed infarcts are classically between the anterior cerebral artery (ACA) and middle cerebral artery (MCA) territories, and between the ACA, MCA, and posterior cerebral artery junctional zones. Based on imaging, internal watershed infarcts can be further classified into confluent internal watershed or partial internal watershed infarctions.[22] Confluent internal watershed infarctions are confluent lesions running parallel to the lateral ventricle. These lesions are usually unilateral owing to extensive involvement of white matter, and typically present with stepwise onset of contralateral hemiplegia that recovers poorly. Partial internal watershed infarction appears as a single or multiple discrete, rounded lesions in the same distribution as confluent internal watershed infarction, and usually presents as episodes of brachiofacial sensory and motor deficit, with good recovery.[21,22]

The mechanisms of cortical watershed infarct and internal watershed infarct are presumed to be due to the result of microembolization from either carotid artery atherosclerosis or vulnerable plaque, or from artery-to-artery emboli precipitated by an

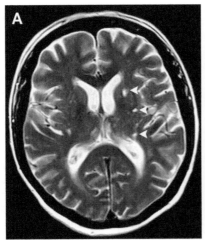
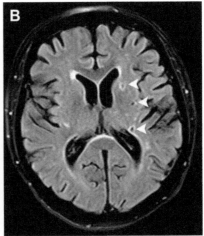

Fig. 11. Chronic lacunar infarctions in a 59-year-old male patient. (*A*) Axial T2-weighted image reveals multiple hyperintensities in the left deep gray matter nuclei and left thalamus. (*B*) Axial FLAIR image of these lesions shows peripheral hyperintensity with central area of hypointensity (*arrowheads*).

episode of systemic arterial hypotension (ie, shock, cardiac arrest, or cardiopulmonary bypass surgery).[21–23] Internal watershed infarcts are caused by a combination of hypoperfusion of the internal border zone, severe carotid disease, and a hemodynamic event.

In acute events, DW imaging is very sensitive for the diagnosis of internal watershed infarct. Internal watershed infarcts are seen as hyperintensities running parallel to the lateral ventricles, either confluent or focal, and may be unilateral or bilateral (Fig. 12A).[18] In the chronic stages they are seen as linear hyperintensities parallel to the lateral ventricles (beads of pearl) on T2-weighted and FLAIR images (see Fig. 12B).

CADASIL

CADASIL is a hereditary, monogenic form of small-vessel disease, caused by mutations in the NOTCH3 gene.[24] It is the most common hereditary form of stroke leading to progressive dementia. The pathologic changes are specifically located in cerebral arterioles, which show thickening of the media and degeneration of smooth muscle, and deposition of granular osmiophilic material, leading to narrowing of the vessel lumen.[25] Genetic testing is the gold standard for diagnosing CADASIL.

MR imaging is the most relevant tool for monitoring the cerebral changes in CADASIL. MR abnormalities may be seen in childhood, but are definitely positive by 35 years of age. MR imaging reveals white matter and a microangiopathic pattern of signal abnormalities suggestive of ischemic infarcts, lacunes, and diffuse leukoencephalopathy. T2-weighted/FLAIR imaging reveals increased signal intensity located within the periventricular white matter, basal ganglia, thalamus, internal capsule, and pons (Fig. 13). The severity of the signal abnormalities is highly variable and increases with age. In patients younger than 40 years, T2 hyperintensities are usually punctate or nodular with a symmetric distribution, and predominate in the periventricular areas and within the centrum semiovale.[26,27] The abnormalities become more diffuse with time, symmetric, and occur in the external capsule and the anterior part of the temporal lobes (see Fig. 13B). Other MR imaging findings include prominent VRS and microbleeds (in 25%–69% of patients) on GRE/SW images (see Fig. 13C). Perfusion imaging with CT, MR, or single-photon emission computed tomography (SPECT) shows marked reduction in cerebral blood flow (CBF) in the affected portion of the brain. This CBF deficit is in turn inversely correlated with disability and cognitive impairment. Proton MR spectroscopy within the hyperintense lesions shows reduced NAA, choline-containing compounds, total creatine, and total metabolite content in CADASIL patients in comparison with control subjects.[28]

CADASIL may be difficult to distinguish from relapsing-remitting MS. The autosomal dominant pattern of inheritance, absence of optic nerve or spinal cord involvement, and the symmetric pattern of white matter abnormalities on brain

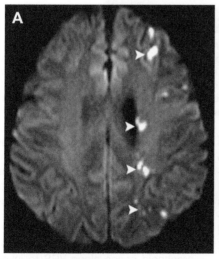
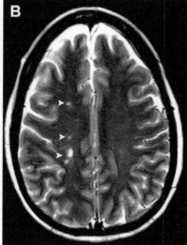

Fig. 12. Cortical watershed infarctions in a 58-year-old male patient who presented with right-side weakness following cardiac surgery. (A) Axial DW image shows multiple areas of restricted diffusion (arrowheads) in the left deep white matter parallel to the lateral ventricles. (B) Axial T2-weighted image of another patient shows chronic, multiple linear hyperintensities parallel to the lateral ventricles, with beads of pearl appearance (arrowheads).

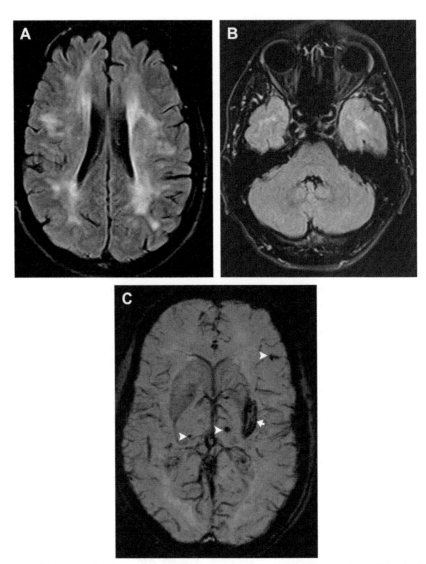

Fig. 13. A 36-year-old male patient presented with transient neurologic deficits, mild cognitive decline, and pseudobulbar palsy (cerebral autosomal dominant arteriopathy with subcortical infarcts and leukoencephalopathy [CADASIL]). (*A*) Axial FLAIR image shows abnormally high signal in the white matter bilaterally. (*B*) Axial FLAIR image shows confluent regions of high signal in the anterior part of the temporal lobe. (*C*) Axial susceptibility-weighted image shows multiple scattered small hemorrhagic lesions (*arrowheads*) in the cerebral parenchyma with large chronic bleed in the left putamen (*arrow*).

MR imaging are key factors in differentiating the 2 conditions. The other differential diagnosis in young patient with stroke is a mitochondrial encephalopathy such as mitochondrial encephalopathy, lactic acidosis, and stroke-like episodes (MELAS). However, infarcts in MELAS, a maternally transmitted condition, are usually cortical and are located in the posterior parts of the brain.

SARCOIDOSIS

Sarcoidosis is a systemic disorder with the propensity to involve multiple organs. Neurosarcoidosis,

generally seen as a part of the systemic disease, is an uncommon but serious manifestation of sarcoidosis. Meningeal infiltration (found in 64%–100% of patients) by inflammatory cells is the primary target of involvement that may lead to cranial neuropathies, hydrocephalus, encephalopathy, and hypothalamic dysfunction.[29,30] These inflammatory exudates may further extend from the subarachnoid space along VRS to involve the brain parenchyma. Patients with neurosarcoidosis may show an acute presentation with isolated cranial neuropathies (found in 75% of patients) or aseptic meningitis.[29,30]

The pathophysiologic mechanism behind sarcoidosis remains elusive. It is suggested to be due to heightened immunity, which is mediated primarily by CD4+ helper cells and macrophages.[31] The histologic hallmark of sarcoidosis is discrete, compact, noncaseating epithelioid cell granuloma. Epithelioid cell granulomas consist of highly differentiated mononuclear phagocytes (epithelioid cells and giant cells) surrounded by CD4 and CD8 lymphocytes.

MR imaging remains the modality of choice for the diagnosis of neurosarcoidosis, but remains less specific. The common MR imaging findings include diffuse meningeal enhancement and focal nonenhancing and enhancing white matter lesions. Diffuse or nodular leptomeningeal enhancement is perhaps the most common manifestation of neurosarcoidosis, seen in about 40% of cases.[32] Periventricular and deep white matter lesions are frequently seen on T2-weighted/FLAIR images in neurosarcoidosis (**Fig. 14**). On the contrast-enhanced study, these lesions can be divided into enhancing and nonenhancing lesions. Enhancing parenchymal lesions or granulomas are a fairly common manifestation of neurosarcoidosis, with 35% of cases presenting as multiple supratentorial and/or infratentorial masses. These lesions are thought to be due to centripetal spread of the disease from leptomeningeal involvement. Nonenhancing brain parenchymal lesions are less common and occur most frequently in the periventricular white matter, but may also be seen in the brainstem and basal ganglia. These lesions are thought to be due to small areas of infarction caused by granulomatous angiopathy.

Besides white matter lesions, other findings frequently seen with neurosarcoidosis include enhancing masses within the sella, with or without thickening and enhancement of the infundibulum; communicating or obstructive hydrocephalus secondary to leptomeningeal/dural involvement or secondary to ventricular system adhesions or loculations, respectively; and cranial nerve involvement (up to 50% of patients), especially the optic nerve, which shows enhancement and thickening with or without associated leptomeningeal involvement.[32] MR imaging is not only useful for narrowing the differential diagnosis but also can be helpful for monitoring the response to immuno-modulatory therapy. At times these lesions are difficult to differentiate from MS on MR imaging and on CSF study, as elevated oligoclonal bands typically seen with MS are often seen with neurosarcoidosis as well.

LYME

Lyme disease is a tick-transmitted multisystem inflammatory disease caused by the spirochete *Borrelia burgdorferi* in the United States and *Borrelia garinii* and *Borrelia afzelii* in Europe.[33,34] Approximately 20,000 new cases are reported each year. Lyme disease is the most common vector-borne disease in the United States. *Borrelia* species are transmitted by the bite of infected *Ixodes* ticks. Transmission of *B burgdorferi* requires at least 24 to 48 hours of tick attachment. In the United States, the highest incidence is seen in the coastal Northeast states (from Massachusetts to Maryland), the Midwest (Minnesota

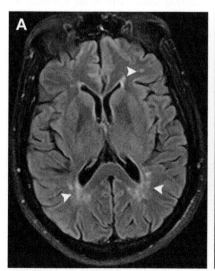
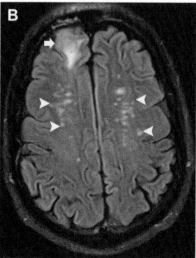

Fig. 14. A 41-year-old female patient with systemic sarcoidosis presented with hypothalamic dysfunction. (*A, B*) Axial FLAIR images show multiple hyperintensities (*arrowheads*) in the periventricular and deep white matter bilaterally. A focal hyperintense mass (*arrow*) is seen in the right frontal cortex with perilesional edema.

and Wisconsin), and the West (California, Oregon, Utah, and Nevada). Most of Lyme disease exposures are in May through July when the nymphal stage of the ticks is most active, which primarily transmits B burgdorferi to human beings.

The disease process has 3 stages. Stage 1 occurs 2 to 30 days after the tick bite. Clinically, patients may have flu-like symptoms and an expanding skin lesion (erythema chronicum migrans). Stage 2 presents 1 to 4 months after infection, and consists of cardiac and neurologic symptoms. Stage 3 occurs up to a few years later, and manifests as arthritic and chronic neurologic symptoms. Neurologic symptoms may consist of peripheral neuropathies, radiculoneuropathies, myelopathies, encephalitis, lymphocytic meningitis, pain syndromes, cerebellar signs, cognitive disorders, movement disorders, and cranial nerve palsies. Facial palsy is very common in neuro-Lyme disease and may be responsible for 25% of new-onset Bell palsy in endemic areas.[33]

CNS involvement in Lyme disease is thought to be due to direct cytotoxicity, neurotoxic mediators secreted by leukocytes and glial cells (indirect cytotoxicity), or triggered autoimmune reactions via molecular mimicry.[35] Neuroimaging may be completely normal even in patients with known Lyme disease who have neurologic manifestation. The most common abnormality seen on MR is multiple bilateral periventricular and/or subcortical foci of T2 prolongation (Fig. 15A).[36] These findings usually mimic MS; however, multiple enhancing cranial nerves (third, fifth, and seventh cranial nerve), nerve root, or meningeal enhancement may favor Lyme over MS (see Fig. 15B).[37,38] Facial nerve enhancement may be most prominent at the fundus of the internal auditory canal and along the labyrinthine and tympanic segments.[37] The diagnosis of Lyme neuroborreliosis is difficult and is essentially clinical, based on a history of tick exposure, epidemiology, and clinical signs and symptoms as well as serologic confirmation with a sensitive enzyme immunoassay.

PROGRESSIVE MULTIFOCAL LEUKOENCEPHALOPATHY

PML is considered to be due to reactivation of the John Cunningham virus (JCV) systemically in an immunosuppressed patient, causing dissemination to the brain.[39] In the CNS oligodendrocytes repair the worn-out myelin, and its destruction leads to a demyelination process. PML is a destructive infection of oligodendrocytes by the JCV, leading to demyelination.[39,40] This demyelination is predominantly seen to involve the cerebral hemispheres, cerebellum, or brainstem. PML is encountered in patients with human immunodeficiency virus (HIV) infection, those with hematologic diseases undergoing chemotherapy, those with autoimmune disorders, and patients with liver or renal impairment caused by reduction in CD4 T-lymphocyte count. PML may also be seen following rituximab therapy directed at treating B-cell neoplasms or connective tissue disorders, and treatment with the immunomodulating monoclonal antibody natalizumab for MS.[41]

On histologic specimens, infected oligodendrocytes show nuclear enlargement filled with JC virions, which leads to lytic death of the oligodendrocytes and release of the virus to infect neighboring cells. The virus spreads in a centrifugal

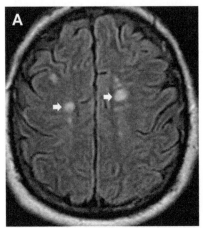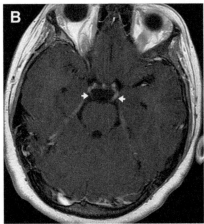

Fig. 15. A 46-year-old female patient with Lyme disease presented with a history of diplopia and facial nerve palsy. (A) Axial FLAIR image reveals multiple white matter hyperintensities (arrows) involving the cerebral white matter bilaterally. (B) Contrast-enhanced T1-weighted image demonstrates enhancement of third cranial nerve bilaterally (arrows).

direction, leading to a circumferential expansion of demyelination.[39,40] The clinical presentation of PML is extremely varied, with neurologic and psychiatric symptoms. It typically results in a progressive neurologic decline during which patients develop cognitive impairment, altered mental status, and personality changes. Without treatment, patients have a progressive downhill course, with death occurring within 1 year of diagnosis of PML in 90% of cases.

The diagnosis of PML is confirmed by detection of JCV DNA by polymerase chain reaction in CSF. However, imaging, especially MR imaging, certainly gives a lead to the diagnosis of PML from the pattern and distribution of the abnormality. The diagnostic hallmark of PML is the presence of multiple foci of demyelination found initially sparsely distributed in the subcortical white matter, but also in the cortex and deep gray structures (Fig. 16).[40,42] These lesions are frequently bilateral and multiple, with involvement of the subcortical U fiber. Mass effect and hemorrhage are unusual. Demyelination is predominately seen to involve the parietal, occipital, and frontal lobes. Lesions lack enhancement and restricted diffusion. Rarely demyelination may be symmetric, involving either the frontal or parietal lobes, or both, as well as the periventricular white matter, mimicking the appearance of toxic leukoencephalopathy. Another common site for PML is the posterior fossa and deep gray matter nuclei. PML may also be seen in patients with MS undergoing treatment with immunomodulating drugs (Fig. 17). Proton MR spectroscopy shows low levels of NAA owing to axonal and neuronal damage, high levels of choline resulting from frank demyelination and cell membrane breakdown, and lactate and lipid peaks attributable to tissue necrosis. A myoinositol peak may be elevated because of an increase in glial activity.[43,44]

Occasionally on imaging, PML may be difficult to distinguish from HIV encephalopathy. PML is more often discrete, multifocal, and asymmetric, with scalloping, and has a greater predilection for the subcortical white matter, whereas HIV encephalitis is more often ill defined, diffuse, symmetric, and periventricular in location. Clinically HIV encephalitis most often presents with global cognitive disturbances and dementia, whereas PML presents with a focal motor or sensory deficit.

AGE-RELATED WHITE MATTER LESIONS

With aging, the brain, like the rest of the body's organs, shows a variety of changes that may or may not be associated with neurologic or neuropsychological deficits. These changes include enlargement of the ventricles and the cerebral sulci reflecting gray and white matter loss, a decrease in neurons and synapses, and an increase in lipofuscin and mineral deposits in brain structures.[45] White matter changes, either focal or diffuse, are commonly seen on pathology and on MR imaging. Incidental WMH on T2-weighted MR images are frequently seen in elderly patients. In the general population the prevalence of WMH ranges from 11% to 21% in adults aged around 64 years to 94% at age 82 years.[45,46]

White matter changes are variable and include periventricular caps or rims, and periventricular and deep white matter multiple punctate, patchy, or confluent lesions. Age-related white matter lesions can be categorized into periventricular white matter lesions (PVWMLs), which are attached to the ventricular system; and deep white matter lesions (DWMLs), which are located apart from the cerebral ventricle in subcortical white matter.[46] On T2-weighted/FLAIR images, PVWMLs may be further differentiated into smooth, well-defined hyperintensities versus irregular PVWMLs.

The etiology, histopathology, and clinical presentations of these hyperintensities differ. Smooth PVWMLs including caps and halos are more likely

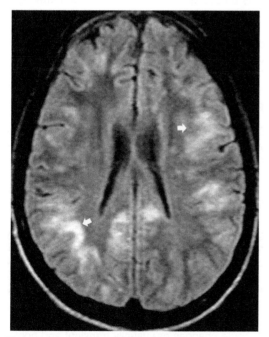

Fig. 16. Progressive multifocal leukoencephalopathy (PML). A 36-year-old male patient positive for human immunodeficiency virus presented with acute cognitive decline. Axial FLAIR image shows abnormal signal intensity in the subcortical white matter (*arrows*) in the right parietal and left frontal lobes.

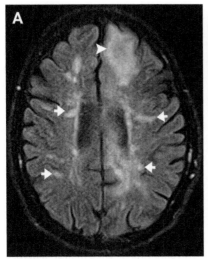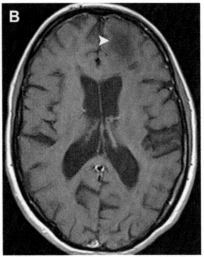

Fig. 17. MS with PML. A 41-year-old female patient with a known case of MS on natalizumab therapy presented with acute encephalopathy. (*A*) Axial FLAIR and (*B*) contrast-enhanced axial T1-weighted images demonstrate multiple demyelinating plaques in the periventricular white matter bilaterally (*arrows*). Large abnormal signal-intensity lesion is seen in the left frontal lobe involving subcortical and subjacent white matter. No mass effect or contrast enhancement is apparent (*arrowhead*).

to be nonischemic, whereas DWMLs and irregular PVWMLs are more likely to be due to microcystic ischemic lesions. Smooth PVWMLs are due to either ependymal loss or differing degrees of mye-lination in adjacent fiber tracts.[45,46] Irregular PVWMLs are more frequently seen with athero-sclerosis and are thought to be more hemodynam-ically determined, whereas DWMLs might be more attributable to small-vessel disease, which is seen more commonly with hypertension. Studies have shown that the risk of dementia and severity of cognitive impairment is preferentially associated with PVWMLs, whereas mood disorders are more likely seen with DWMLs.

Imaging, especially MR imaging, plays a vital role in the diagnosis of white matter lesions in symp-tomatic patients. T2-weighted and FLAIR images are very sensitive in diagnosing and characterizing these changes. Not all the hyperintensities seen in elderly patients are clinically significant or symp-tomatic. For example, periventricular caps, which are seen in almost all normal patients, are totally asymptomatic. These caps are uniform triangular-shaped hyperintense foci, with the base resting on the tops of the frontal horns and with the apex pointing anteriorly into the adjacent white matter. The medial aspect of the triangle is defined by the genu of the corpus callosum, whereas the lateral border extends along the white matter. Periventric-ular caps are thought to be due to loss of myelin content, breakdown of the ependymal lining with adjacent astrocytic gliosis (ependymitis granula-ris), and increased periependymal and extracellular

fluid. Irregular PVWMLs are seen within 1 cm of the lateral margin of the lateral ventricle and are more commonly seen with hypertension.[45,46] Punctate, early confluent, and confluent hyperintense lesions may be seen involving the deep white matter and are mostly associated with small-vessel disease (Fig. 18). Because of the age of the patient, most of these lesions are self-explanatory; however, careful evaluation of the DW imaging ADC is impor-tant to exclude acute ischemic lesions.

RADIATION-INDUCED EFFECTS

Despite continuous improvements in cancer ther-apy, treatment-related CNS toxicity/complica-tions remain an important issue. White matter is one of the primary targets of radiation, chemo-therapy, or a combination of these treatments. This effect is thought to be multifactorial, with damage to the vascular endothelial cells and oli-godendrocytes being regarded as direct primary targets of radiation. Depending on the time of occurrence and clinical presentation, these neuro-logic effects are divided into acute (during radia-tion), subacute or early delayed (up to 12 weeks after radiation ends), and late (months to years after radiation).[47]

Acute changes are usually transient and nonle-thal and, therefore, the amount of information avail-able on the histopathologic features is limited. In the early delayed phase, there is a breakdown in the blood-brain barrier and production of tumor ne-crosis factor α by microglial cells and astrocytes.

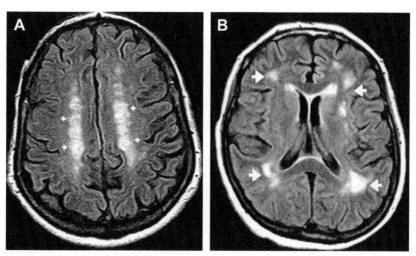

Fig. 18. Age-related white matter changes in a 71-year-old man with mild cognitive decline. (*A, B*) Axial FLAIR images show multiple hyperintensities (*arrows*) scattered through the deep and periventricular white matter.

Histology shows multifocal areas of demyelinated plaques resulting from damage to oligodendroglia, with an intense marginal microglial and astrocytic reaction and perivascular cell reaction. In the late delayed phase, besides breakdown in the blood-brain barrier there is also damage to the endothelium, leading to its proliferation and changes in the vessel wall, with subsequent obliteration of the lumen leading to ischemia. Radiotherapy produces hyalinization and fibrinoid necrosis of small arteries and arterioles with endothelial proliferation and calcium deposition. A CT scan may show abnormal, periventricular hypodensities with or without ventricular enlargement. MR imaging is very sensitive in identifying the early and late delayed changes in white matter. MR imaging shows focal, patchy, or diffuse T2 hyperintensities in the periventricular white matter and the centrum semiovale, with sparing of the subcortical arcuate fibers, the cerebral cortex, and deep gray matter structures (**Fig. 19**).[48,49] Later stages may show deposition of iron salts and calcium in the vessel walls as well as in the deep gray matter nuclei and subcortical tissue. There may be concomitant dilatation of the ventricles. The degree of the MR hyperintensities grossly correlates with neuropsychological examinations. White matter changes may become compounded by chemotherapy.

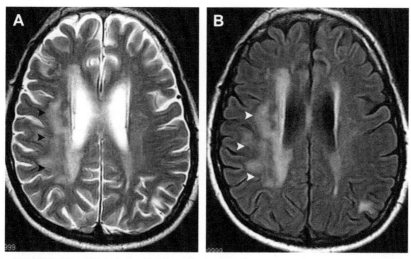

Fig. 19. A 52-year-old male patient treated with radiotherapy for metastasis presented with left-side weakness and mild cognitive decline. (*A*) Axial T2-weighted and (*B*) FLAIR images reveal increased signal intensity (*arrowheads*) in the right frontoparietal white matter.

REFERENCES

1. Heier LA, Bauer CJ, Schwartz L, et al. Large Virchow-Robin spaces: MR-clinical correlation. AJNR Am J Neuroradiol 1989;10(5):929–36.
2. Stephens T, Parmar H, Cornblath W. Giant tumefactive perivascular spaces. J Neurol Sci 2008; 266(1–2):171–3.
3. Diamond S, Bigel ME, Silberstein S, et al. Patterns of diagnosis and acute and preventive treatment for migraine in the United States: results from the American Migraine Prevalence and Prevention study. Headache 2007;47:355–63.
4. Seneviratne U, Chong W, Billimoria PH. Brain white matter hyperintensities in migraine: clinical and radiological correlates. Clin Neurol Neurosurg 2013;115(7):1040–3.
5. Kruit MC, van Buchem MA, Launer LJ, et al. Migraine is associated with an increased risk of deep white matter lesions, subclinical posterior circulation infarcts and brain iron accumulation: the population-based MRI CAMERA study. Cephalalgia 2010;30:129–36.
6. Rossato G, Adami A, Thijs VN, et al. Cerebral distribution of white matter lesions in migraine with aura patients. Cephalalgia 2010;30:855–9.
7. Smith KJ, McDonald WI. The pathophysiology of multiple sclerosis: the mechanisms underlying the production of symptoms and the natural history of the disease. Philos Trans R Soc Lond B Biol Sci 1999;354(1390):1649–73.
8. Nusbaum A, Rapalino O, Fung K, et al. White matter disease and inherited metabolic disorders. In: Atlas SW, editor. Magnetic resonance imaging of the brain and spine, vol. 1, 4th edition. Philadelphia: Williams & Wilkins; 2009. p. 343–444.
9. Debouverie M, Pittion-Vouyovitch S, Louis S, et al. Natural history of multiple sclerosis in a population-based cohort. Eur J Neurol 2008;15(9):916–21.
10. Polman CH, Reingold SC, Banwell B, et al. Diagnostic criteria for multiple sclerosis: 2010 revisions to the McDonald criteria. Ann Neurol 2011;69(2):292–302.
11. Traboulsee A, Li DK. Conventional MR imaging. Neuroimaging Clin N Am 2008;18(4):651–73.
12. Menge T, Hemmer B, Nessler S, et al. Acute disseminated encephalomyelitis: an update. Arch Neurol 2005;62:1673–80.
13. Rossi A. Imaging of acute disseminated encephalomyelitis. Neuroimaging Clin N Am 2008;18(1):149–61.
14. Balasubramanya KS, Kovoor JM, Jayakumar PN, et al. Diffusion-weighted imaging and proton MR spectroscopy in the characterization of acute disseminated encephalomyelitis. Neuroradiology 2007;49:177–83.
15. Bizzi A, Ulug AM, Crawford TO, et al. Quantitative proton MR spectroscopic imaging in acute disseminated encephalomyelitis. AJNR Am J Neuroradiol 2001;22:1125–30.
16. Salvarani C, Brown RD Jr, Calamia KT, et al. Primary central nervous system vasculitis: analysis of 101 patients. Ann Neurol 2007;62:442–51.
17. Albayram S, Saip S, Hasiloglu ZI, et al. Evaluation of parenchymal neuro-Behçet disease by using susceptibility-weighted imaging. AJNR Am J Neuroradiol 2011;32(6):1050–5.
18. Marks MP. Cerebral ischemia and infarction. In: Atlas SW, editor. Magnetic resonance imaging of the brain and spine, vol. 1, 4th edition. Philadelphia: Williams & Wilkins; 2009. p. 772–825.
19. Horowitz DR, Tuhrim S, Weinberger JM, et al. Mechanisms in lacunar infarction. Stroke 1992;23:325–7.
20. Ay H, Oliveira-Filho J, Buonanno F, et al. Diffusion-weighted imaging identifies a subset of lacunar infarction associated with embolic source. Stroke 1999;30:2644–50.
21. Momjian-Mayor I, Baron JC. The pathophysiology of watershed infarction in internal carotid artery: review of cerebral perfusion studies. Stroke 2005;36:567–77.
22. Bladin CF, Chambers BR. Clinical features, pathogenesis, and computed tomographic characteristics of internal watershed infarction. Stroke 1993;24:1925–32.
23. Bladin CF, Chambers BR. Frequency and pathogenesis of hemodynamic stroke. Stroke 1994;25:2179–82.
24. Tournier-Lasserve E, Joutel A, Melki J, et al. Cerebral autosomal dominant arteriopathy with subcortical infarcts and leukoencephalopathy maps to chromosome 19q12. Nat Genet 1993;3:256–9.
25. Ruchoux MM, Maurage CA. CADASIL: cerebral autosomal dominant arteriopathy with subcortical infarcts and leukoencephalopathy. J Neuropathol Exp Neurol 1997;56:947–64.
26. Gladstone JP, Dodick DW. Migraine and cerebral white matter lesions: when to suspect cerebral autosomal dominant arteriopathy with subcortical infarcts and leukoencephalopathy (CADASIL). Neurologist 2005;11:19–29.
27. Yousry TA, Seelos K, Mayer M, et al. Characteristic MR lesion pattern and correlation of T1 and T2 lesion volume with neurologic and neuropsychological findings in cerebral autosomal dominant arteriopathy with subcortical infarcts and leukoencephalopathy (CADASIL). AJNR Am J Neuroradiol 1999;20(1):91–100.
28. Auer DP, Schirmer T, Heidenreich JO, et al. Altered white and gray matter metabolism in CADASIL: a proton MR spectroscopy and 1H-MRSI study. Neurology 2001;56(5):635–42.
29. Delaney P. Neurological manifestations in sarcoidosis: review of the literature, with report of 23 cases. Ann Intern Med 1977;87:336–45.

30. Stern BJ, Krumholz A, Johns C, et al. Sarcoidosis and its neurological manifestations. Arch Neurol 1985;42:909–17.

31. Colby TV. Interstitial lung diseases. In: Thurlbeck W, Churg A, editors. Pathology of the lung. 2nd edition. New York: Thieme Medical Publishers; 1995. p. 589–737.

32. Smith JK, Matheus MG, Castillo M. Imaging manifestations of neurosarcoidosis. AJR Am J Roentgenol 2004;182(2):289–95.

33. Agarwal R, Sze G. Neuro-Lyme disease: MR imaging findings. Radiology 2009;253(1):167–73.

34. Hengge UR, Tannapfel A, Tyring SK, et al. Lyme borreliosis. Lancet Infect Dis 2003;3(8):489–500.

35. Rupprecht TA, Koedel U, Fingerle V, et al. The pathogenesis of Lyme neuroborreliosis: from infection to inflammation. Mol Med 2008;14(3–4):205–12.

36. Agosta F, Rocca MA, Benedetti B, et al. MR imaging assessment of brain and cervical cord damage in patients with neuroborreliosis. AJNR Am J Neuroradiol 2006;27(4):892–4.

37. Vanzieleghem B, Lemmerling M, Carton D, et al. Lyme disease in a child presenting with bilateral facial nerve palsy: MRI findings and review of the literature. Neuroradiology 1998;40(11):739–42.

38. Kochling J, Freitag HJ, Bollinger T, et al. Lyme disease with lymphocytic meningitis, trigeminal palsy and silent thalamic lesion. Eur J Paediatr Neurol 2008;12(6):501–4.

39. Berger JR, Concha M. Progressive multifocal leukoencephalopathy: the evolution of a disease once considered rare. J Neurovirol 1995;1:5–18.

40. Thurnher MM, Thurnher SA, Mühlbauer B, et al. Progressive multifocal leukoencephalopathy in AIDS: initial and follow-up CT and MRI. Neuroradiology 1997;39:611–8.

41. Langer-Gould A, Atlas SW, Green AJ, et al. Progressive multifocal leukoencephalopathy in a patient treated with natalizumab. N Engl J Med 2005;353:375–81.

42. Whiteman ML, Post MJ, Berger JR, et al. Progressive multifocal leukoencephalopathy in 47 HIV-seropositive patients: neuroimaging with clinical and pathologic correlation. Radiology 1993;187:233–40.

43. Chang L, Ernst T, Tornatore C, et al. Metabolite abnormalities in progressive multifocal leukoencephalopathy: a proton magnetic resonance spectroscopy study. Neurology 1997;48:836–45.

44. Iranzo A, Moreno A, Pujol J, et al. Proton magnetic resonance spectroscopy pattern of progressive multifocal leukoencephalopathy in AIDS. J Neurol Neurosurg Psychiatry 1999;66:520–3.

45. Vernooij MW, Smits M. Structural neuroimaging in aging and Alzheimer's disease. Neuroimaging Clin N Am 2012;22(1):33–55.

46. Galluzzi S, Lanni C, Pantoni L, et al. White matter lesions in the elderly: pathophysiological hypothesis on the effect on brain plasticity and reserve. J Neurol Sci 2008;273(1–2):3–9.

47. Sheline G. Radiation therapy of brain tumors. Cancer 1977;39:873–81.

48. Postma TJ, Klein M, Verstappen CC, et al. Radiotherapy-induced cerebral abnormalities in patients with low-grade glioma. Neurology 2002;59:121–3.

49. Ball WS Jr, Prenger EC, Ballard ET. Neurotoxicity of radio/chemotherapy in children: pathologic and MR correlation. AJNR Am J Neuroradiol 1992;13(2):761–76.

An Imaging Approach to Diffuse White Matter Changes

Nilesh K. Desai, MD[a,b,*], Mark E. Mullins, MD, PhD[c]

KEYWORDS

• Diffuse • Leukodystrophy • Leukoencephalopathy • MRI • T2 • White matter

KEY POINTS

• Diffuse white matter abnormalities encompass a large number of congenital and acquired disorders.
• Clinical history is paramount to honing the differential in diffuse leukoencephalopathies.
• Approaching white matter disorders categorically and then individually in a standardized fashion will aid greatly in procuring a reasonable differential diagnosis.

INTRODUCTION

White matter disorders represent a large, heterogeneous group of disorders that span the continuum of congenital metabolic disorders (typically presenting early in infancy) to acquired processes, such as chronic ischemic microvascular white matter disease (typically manifesting in the late stages of life). Magnetic resonance (MR) imaging has dramatically revolutionized the diagnostic evaluation of patients with these disease processes, proving to be far more sensitive than any other imaging modality in detecting white matter disease.[1] Furthermore, in those suffering from the same malady, the patterns of MR imaging findings are often objectively similar, greatly aiding diagnosis of such patients even with confounding clinical signs and symptoms that may cloud the diagnosis. Unfortunately, however, imaging patterns of many white matter disorders may overlap, especially in their end stages, posing significant challenges for radiologists. A disciplined, systematic imaging approach to diagnosing white matter disorders is therefore paramount in deriving accurate, complete differentials that will serve to hone the initial clinical workup of these complex patients and possibly, in some cases, even provide a single diagnosis. An initial helpful imaging approach to white matter disease is to first separate focal from diffuse white matter disorders, while remembering that any focal process may progress to eventually become diffuse. For the purposes of this article, a diffuse white matter disorder is defined as any entity that involves the entirety or vast majority of the supratentorial and/or infratentorial white matter as a unit rather than as an isolated, random location within the brain. Also included in this definition, and briefly discussed, are those disorders that characteristically involve typical, symmetric large regions of white matter in persons afflicted with the same disorder. Discussed in this review is the imaging approach to diffuse pediatric and adult white matter disorders.

DEFINITIONS

Terminology in white matter disorders may be quite confusing as different authors commonly use the same terms with slightly different meaning and yet still use various nomenclature

Disclosures: None.
[a] Division of Neuroradiology, Department of Radiology and Imaging Sciences, Emory University School of Medicine, 1364 Clifton Road Northeast, EUH B115, Atlanta, GA 30322, USA; [b] Children's Healthcare of Atlanta at Egleston and Town Center, Atlanta, GA 30329, USA; [c] Division of Neuroradiology, Department of Radiology and Imaging Sciences, Emory University School of Medicine, 1364 Clifton Road Northeast, Room D125A, Atlanta, GA 30322, USA
* Corresponding author.
E-mail address: nilesh.k.desai@emory.edu

interchangeably, further complicating the matter. The terminology used in this discussion coincides with that used in the text by Dr Marjo S. van der Knaap and Dr Jaap Valk in *Magnetic Resonance of Myelination and Myelin Disorders, third edition*, given its authoritative presence in the field and more so, the consistent use of white matter language contained within the text.[2] Briefly, "white matter disorders" and "leukoencephalopathy" are interchangeable umbrella terms that encompass all disorders, no matter the cause, that exclusively or predominately affect the white matter.[2] "Hypomyelination" and "amyelination" are terms that refer to the near complete or complete permanent absence of myelination, respectively, without inclusion of diseases that result in destruction of myelin or the presence of abnormal myelin.[2] "Dysmyelination" is representative of disorders in which dysfunctional myelination results in some degree of abnormal myelin within the white matter with or without the presence of demyelination.[2] "Demyelination" is simply the loss of myelin by whatever insult. Delayed, but progressive myelination is referred to as "retarded myelination" and is typically the result of chronic, reversible, or irreversible diseases that impair timely, but otherwise normal myelination.[2] A more complete discussion of white matter terminology can be found in the article by Guleria and Kelly elsewhere in this issue.

IMAGING TECHNIQUE
Computed Tomography

Computed tomography (CT) of the head is often a first-line modality that patients presenting emergently with diffuse white matter pathology may encounter when the diagnosis of a white matter disorder has not been previously made. It remains a gross survey tool and should primarily act as a screening tool for acute pathologic abnormalities, such as mass lesions, hemorrhage, profound hypoxic ischemic encephalopathy (HIE), and so on, for which immediate attention is typically necessary. Although in some instances CT may serve as a terminal imaging modality, it more commonly acts as a bridge to definitive imaging with MR imaging given CT's poor sensitivity and specificity in evaluating white matter disorders even with the administration of intravenous contrast.[1] CT technique for all indications is commonly performed using axial technique at peak kilovolt of 120 and milliamperes of 250 to 350 with modern multislice scanners, allowing for source slice thicknesses on the order of 0.625 mm, usually reconstructed at 2.5 to 3.0 mm in both brain and algorithm. Pediatric doses are typically lower with common peak kilovolts ranging from 100 to 120 and milliamperes ranging from 100 to 250.

MR Imaging

Conventional sequences including T1-weighted spin-echo-based or inversion recovery, T2-weighted fast spin-echo, and T2-fluid attenuated inversion recovery (FLAIR) at all ages remain the gold standard in and of themselves in evaluating white matter disorders. Diffusion-weighted imaging and postcontrast T1-weighted sequences may also prove helpful in some cases and probably should routinely be performed in patients suspected of having a leukoencephalopathy. When available, it is advisable that multivoxel MR spectroscopy (see the article by Bray and Mullins elsewhere in this issue), at both short and intermediate echo times (TE = 20–30 ms and TE = 135–144 ms, respectively) and diffusion tensor imaging be performed, as the former may aid in the differential diagnosis and both may be helpful in monitoring disease status with or without treatment (see the articles by Bray and Choudhri elsewhere in this issue). Although conventional sequences may offer limited advantages from 1.5 T to 3.0 T, because advanced imaging modalities like MR spectroscopy and diffusion tensor imaging benefit greatly from high-field strength, it is generally advisable that all patients suspected to have a leukoencephalopathy be evaluated at 3.0 T whenever possible.

CLINICAL HISTORY

As challenging as white matter disorders may be, an initial interrogation of the clinical history may be quite helpful in children and adults suspected of having a white matter disorder. In children, family history, birth history, head circumference, psychomotor retardation including issues of speech, motor, or global developmental delay, psychomotor regression, tonicity, seizures, and even results of ophthalmologic examination are all potentially helpful in categorically refining the differential. For both children and adults, age, gender, known toxic exposure including history of radiotherapy, time of onset (ie, infancy vs childhood vs adulthood), acuity or chronicity of sign and symptom onset, and immune status may all be helpful. For example, a child presenting in the infantile period with hypotonia, psychomotor retardation, and macrocephaly may clue the radiologist into the possibility of Canavan or Alexander disease as opposed to an acquired leukoencephalopathy or acute demyelinating inflammatory process, such as acute disseminated encephalomyelitis.

NORMAL MYELINATION

The initial and perhaps most difficult task that a radiologist faces when evaluating for a possible leukoencephalopathy is knowing the normal appearance of CT and MR imaging in the incompletely myelinated brain of a child. Although CT has limited uses for most white matter disorders, radiologists should be aware that the incompletely myelinated infant normally has significantly hypodense white matter that would otherwise represent a leukoencephalopathy in the older child and adult. It is understandable, therefore, that detecting white matter pathology in such young infants may prove quite challenging by CT alone. Myelination begins in utero and is largely complete on MR imaging by 24 months of life.[3] During this dynamic process, the immature white matter progressively increases in signal on T1-weighted sequences and decreases in signal on T2-weighted sequences. Myelination generally occurs from inferior to superior, posterior to anterior, and central to peripheral in a stepwise predictable fashion, such that standard ages of when myelination appears are prescribed to certain anatomic regions and ultimately to clinical stages of development.[3] Generally, T1-weighted images are most useful in evaluating myelination in the first 6 months of life, after which T2-weighted sequences are most useful. It is imperative that the radiologist evaluating for a white matter disorder understand myelination "milestones" on T1- and T2-weighted sequences in significant depth to not only be able to accept normality but to also detect abnormality even in its earliest stages. The general approach to imaging the incompletely myelinated child is to first review the conventional T1- and T2-weighted sequences, and immediately decide the age of the child in months remaining blinded to the age of the child in the medical record. The age of the child in the medical record is then checked to ensure that myelination is indeed age-appropriate. This process avoids the natural tendency to rationalize the myelination based on age (ie, "I think it is probably ok for that age"). Furthermore, this necessitates the radiologist to have in-depth knowledge of MR imaging in the young child. Should myelination appear delayed but otherwise normal, the child's history should be rechecked for prematurity and then re-referenced to MR imaging because this is an often explanation for seemingly "delayed myelination." Such an algorithm is especially important in detecting retarded myelination, amyelination, and hypomyelination syndromes in which significant prolongation of T2 relaxation times may not be present. A more complete discussion of myelination is found in the article, "Myelin, Myelination, and Corresponding MRI Changes" of this text.

Once it has been decided that a normal myelination for the patient's age is not present, the radiologist must decide if the imaging supports that of a lack of myelination as in hypomyelination or retarded myelination or whether there exists a dysmyelinating or even demyelinating process in which dysfunctional myelination or loss of myelin, respectively, is occurring. With a lack of myelination, T2 signal of the white matter is mildly increased but not the usually significant T2 hyperintensity seen with dysmyelination or demyelination. This relative lack of myelination may be more difficult to ascertain on T1-weighted images as T1 white matter signal, whereas commonly low or intermediate compared with cortex in patients with hypomyelination, may sometimes show high signal white matter compared with cortex, depending on the amount of myelination.[4] A generally helpful clue to the presence of a hypomyelinating syndrome is that the appearance of the white matter resembles that of the young infant. To diagnose a hypomyelination disorder, a stable lack of myelination on 2 successive MR imagings, 6 months apart, with at least one having occurred after the age of 1, should be documented.[5] If myelination is progressing, even if at a delayed pace, a diagnosis of retarded myelination should be sought, which may be secondary to a host of entities including, for example, malnutrition and metabolic disorders. A more complete discussion of hypomyelination disorders including the important distinction between leukodystrophies and hypomyelination may be found in the article by Yang and Robson elsewhere in this issue.

Once the radiologist has satisfied this distinction, it is then best to approach white processes in adults and children by deciding if the process is either diffuse in spatiality or symmetric and regional versus multifocal. A discussion of the vast multifocal white matter disorders may be found in the article by Kanekar and Devgun elsewhere in this issue. Furthermore, an extensive discussion of leukodystrophies including inherited metabolic disorders that preferentially affect children may be found in the article by Yang and Robson elsewhere in this issue.

ADULT-ONSET LEUKODYSTROPHIES

Leukodystrophies are an exceptional cause of white matter disorders in the adult population. Such leukodystrophies typically represent adult-onset forms of otherwise infantile or juvenile-onset disorders. It may be extremely difficult to diagnose such patients by clinical means alone and may in fact present with unusual symptoms such as mental illness.[6] To further complicate the matter, neuroradiologic studies may be nonspecific, overlapping with more common primary demyelinating white matter disorders such as multiple sclerosis, or conversely, interpretation of such studies fails to recognize the possibility of such entities given their rarity and incomplete understanding by the reviewing radiologist. A more complete discussion on leukodystrophies may be found in the article by Yang and Robson elsewhere in this issue.

Metachromatic leukodystrophy is an autosomal-recessive lysosomal storage disorder resulting from deficiency of the enzyme arylsufatase A that results in the multiorgan abnormal accumulation of sufatide, including within the central nervous system, that eventually results in progressive demyelination. Although the infantile and juvenile-onset subtypes are most common, adult-onset, defined as onset after the age of 16 years, may occur.[6] Regardless of the subtype, it seems that patients typically manifest in the frontal and parietal periventricular and deep white matter, sparing the subcortical white matter until late in the disease, at which time the subcortical white matter becomes involved and the typical "tigroid" pattern is seen. Corpus callosum involvement is common in metachromatic leukodystrophy but not as significantly as in adrenoleukodystrophy or globoid cell leukodystrophy. In severe cases, the cerebellar white matter and central gray matter may be involved.[7]

Globoid cell leukodystrophy or Krabbe disease (**Fig. 1**) is an autosomal-recessive disorder caused by absence of galactosylceramide beta-galactosidase, an enzyme crucial to myelin breakdown, resulting in inappropriate accumulation of neurologically toxic galactosylsphingosine.[8] Some, if not most, neuroradiologic studies in the literature categorize Krabbe disease as either early onset (<2 years) or late onset (>2 years) and thus imaging findings of both juveniles and adults are contained within this group.[2,9] Although both groups have predominant pyramidal tract involvement along with parieto-occipital periventricular white matter and callosal involvement, cerebellar and deep gray matter involvement are less characteristic with late onset.[9] In a small case series containing only adults, general findings of symmetric or asymmetric T2 prolongation were noted in the corticospinal/pyramidal tracts, thinning at the isthmus of the corpus callosum, and variable degrees of posterior white matter volume loss and T2 hyperintensity.[10] Note should

be made that some adult patients with this disease may have normal neuroradiologic examinations.[2]

Adrenoleukodystrophy (**Fig. 2**) is an x-linked white matter disorder that involves the impaired transport of very long chain fatty acid into peroxisomes. Multiple phenotypes in affected male patients are known including the childhood cerebral form, adult cerebral form, and adrenomyeloneuropathy, the latter primarily involving the spinal cord and peripheral nerves and representing the most common variant in adults.[11] Patients with adrenomyeloneuropathy may have normal neuroradiologic studies or demyelination along multiple tracts, including the corticospinal tract, spinothalamic tract, visual and auditory pathways. Furthermore, male patients with adrenomyeloneuropathy may have severe bilateral lobar involvement mimicking the childhood cerebral form in which large areas of the parieto-occipital white matter including the splenium of the corpus callosum demonstrate demyelination.[12] Periventricular and deep white matter involvement predominate with eventual subcortical involvement. A leading edge of enhancement and reduced diffusivity may or may not be present depending on the activity of the disease at the time of imaging. Frontal and temporal white matter involvement in these patients is certainly possible and, in fact, in a minority of patients there may be a frontal lobar predominant pattern with anterior callosal involvement.[13] Cerebellar white matter involvement with this disease is also possible.[12] Imaging findings in females (heterozygotes), while similar to male counterparts, are usually milder with posterior lobar white matter involvement, or corticospinal tract involvement.[12]

Alexander disease (**Fig. 3**) or fibrinoid leukodystrophy is the result of dysfunction of glial fibrillary acidic protein, resulting in a disease with a broad phenotypic spectrum including infantile, juvenile, and adult subtypes. Although pediatric, especially infantile, patients may present with large areas of T2 prolongation of the supratentorial white matter with frontal lobar predominance, adult-onset patients typically present with medullary, upper cervical signal abnormality and volume loss, and dentate signal abnormality.[14] Most patients however demonstrate some abnormal T2 prolongation in either the frontal or the posterior periventricular white matter.[14]

VASCULAR LEUKOENCEPHALOPATHY

Cerebral autosomal-dominant arteriopathy with subcortical infarcts and leukoencephalopathy (CADASIL; **Fig. 4**) is an inherited condition due to

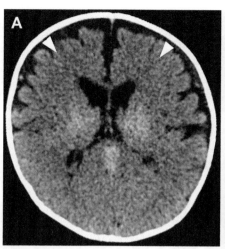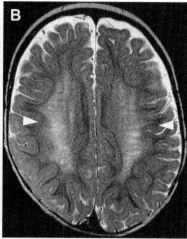

Fig. 1. Example of Krabbe disease. Selected head CT and brain MR images from an approximately 6-month-old patient with Krabbe disease, including axial noncontrast head CT (*A*) and axial T2-weighted images (*B*). *Arrowheads* help to delineate the relatively symmetric abnormal white matter hypodensity on head CT and hyperintensity on the T2-weighted brain MR imaging. No definite abnormal enhancement was appreciated (not shown). Please see the text for additional discussion of this disease entity. (*Courtesy of* Arastoo Vossough, MD, Children's Hospital of Pennsylvania, Philadelphia, PA.)

a Notch3 gene mutation that results in migraine headaches, recurrent subcortical ischemic infarcts, psychiatric symptoms, pseudobulbar palsy, urinary incontinence, and eventual progressive dementia.[15] This nonatherosclerotic, nonamyloid disease process is the result of the deposition of granular osmiophilic material into media of small perforating vessels with concentric wall thickening and eventual stenosis. Although skin biopsy is eventually typically used to confirm the diagnosis, neuroradiologic studies are often the initial examination that can help suggest this entity. Unfortunately, the finding of multiple lacunar infarcts, even with involvement of the basal ganglia, petechial hemorrhage, and diffuse T2 prolongation of the supratentorial white matter as seen in CADASIL, is quite similar to the very common microangiopathic white matter changes predominantly related to atherosclerosis and hypertension encountered in everyday radiologic practice.[16] Key important distinguishing features that can help the radiologist suggest CADASIL include (1) significant, confluent T2 hyperintensity within the anterior temporal lobe, especially when the remainder of the temporal lobe is unaffected; (2) involvement of the external capsule and insula; (3) absence of cortical infarcts; and (4) corpus callosal involvement.[2,16] Clinical history and family history may also be beneficial in such cases as can the relatively young age of patients (usual presentation between ages 40 and 60) that would otherwise be considered premature for microangiopathy.[2]

Cerebral autosomal-recessive arteriopathy with subcortical infarcts and leukoencephalopathy (CARASIL) is a rare arteriopathy similar to CADASIL that predominately involves male patients, with nearly all patient reports thus far of Japanese origin.[17] Clinical presentation is typically earlier than CADASIL, presenting between 20 and 45 years of age. Imaging findings are quite similar; however, white matter changes in CARASIL develop homogenously with sparing of the subcortical U fibers early in the disease, unlike the more heterogenous T2 prolongation seen initially in CADASIL.[17] Callosal involvement and petechial hemorrhage are generally lacking.[17]

Cerebral amyloid angiopathy (CAA; Fig. 5) is a well-known cerebrovascular disorder classically affecting elderly patients in the sporadic form and middle-aged adults in the familial form.[2] CAA is associated with advanced age, dementia including Alzheimer disease, radiation necrosis, and spongiform encephalopathies.[18] CAA is characterized by the inappropriate deposition of congophilic amyloid within arterioles and capillaries of leptomeningeal and cortical vessels, sparing vessels of the white matter.[19] In addition, vessels may demonstrate fibrinoid necrosis, vessel wall fragmentation, and microaneurysms. Such patients may have leukoencephalopathy with severe, diffuse, or patchy white-matter myelin loss, often sparing the subcortical white matter, corpus callosum, and temporal regions.[19] An unusual variant of CAA is the induction of large regions of lobar T2

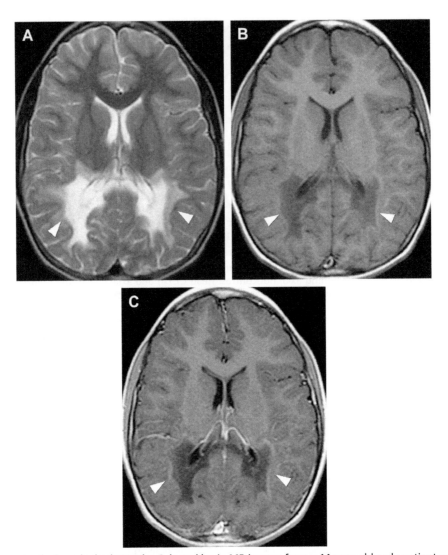

Fig. 2. Example of adrenoleukodystrophy. Selected brain MR images from a 14-year-old male patient with confusion, including axial T2-weighted (*A*) as well as T1-weighted (*B*) and T1 post-contrast-weighted (*C*) images. *Arrowheads* help to delineate the relatively symmetric abnormal white matter hyperintensity. Note the pattern of involvement centered on the splenium of the corpus callosum and the bilateral periatrial white matter as well as the thin, smooth peripheral enhancement. Please see the text for additional discussion of this disease entity. (*Courtesy of* John Hesselink, MD, FACR, University of California San Diego School of Medicine, San Diego, CA.)

hyperintensity with local mass effect without sparing of the subcortical U fibers. This more focal form of CAA leukoencephalopathy has been reported to harbor variable degrees of inflammation and may be reversible with immunosuppressives.[20] CAA is typified by supratentorial cortical petechial hemorrhages, often with small cortical infarcts and lobar hemorrhages. Such extensive pathologic abnormality translates to numerous foci of susceptibility on gradient echo T2* and on susceptibility weighted imaging, especially peripherally rather than centrally, with better sensitivity for the latter.[18]

The reader is referred to the article by Kanekar elsewhere in this issue for an in-depth review of such leukoencephalopathies including the relatively common Binswanger disease.

VIRAL INFECTION

Although a host of infections may affect the brain, including viral, bacterial, fungal, and parasitic, it is primarily viral infections that may produce diffuse white matter disease and is especially true in the immunocompromised individual, as in human immunodeficiency virus and

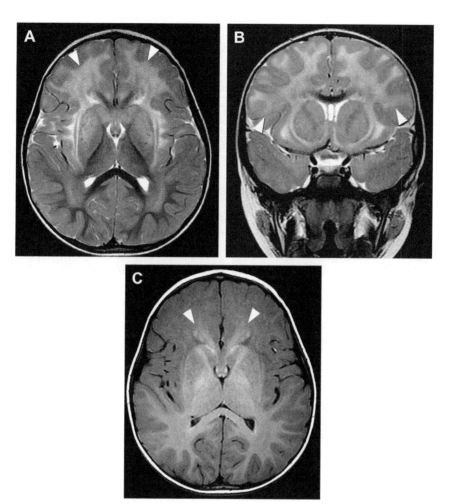

Fig. 3. Example of Alexander disease. Selected brain MR images from a 2-year-old patient with Alexander disease, including axial (*A*) and coronal (*B*) T2-weighted images as well as axial T1 (*C*). *Arrowheads* help to delineate the relatively symmetric abnormal white matter hyperintensity. Note the prominent involvement of the bilateral frontal lobe white matter, including what is sometimes called the "forceps minor." Please see the text for additional discussion of this disease entity. (*Courtesy of* Arastoo Vossough, MD, Children's Hospital of Pennsylvania, Philadelphia, PA.)

cytomegalovirus. A detailed review may be found in the article by Moritani and colleagues elsewhere in this issue.

TOXIC EXPOSURE

A variety of toxic exposures, whether self-induced, accidental, or iatrogenic, may produce reversible or irreversible diffuse leukoencephalopathies, which may result in severe encephalopathy, sometimes with lethal consequences. Clinical history is absolutely paramount in such cases because the findings may be rather nonspecific and while the radiologist may finally be able to suggest a toxic exposure, it is the clinical history that may be able to provide a presumed diagnosis and thereby guide efficient therapy. In the event

of illicit drug use, despite its pervasive presence in modern society, the possibility may go unrecognized.

An underrecognized cause of diffuse leukoencephalopathy is an uncommon complication related to the inhalation of heated heroin vapor, commonly referred to as "chasing the dragon" (**Fig. 6**). In this method, the user heats solid heroin placed on aluminum foil into liquid form to very high temperatures, during which the vapors created by the heating process are inhaled. The exact cause of this spongiform leukoencephalopathy is unclear. Patients may progress through 3 clinical stages with initial cerebellar signs and motor restlessness to pyramidal and pseudobulbar signs and then to spasms, hypotonic paresis, and eventually death.[21] Such patients classically present with

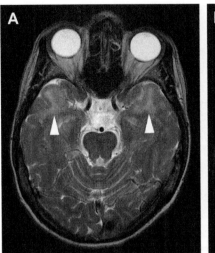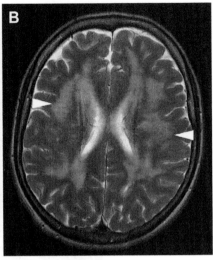

Fig. 4. Example of CADASIL. Selected brain MR images from a 34-year-old patient with a history of multiple strokes, headaches, and cognitive impairment including axial T2 (*A, B*) images. Note the confluent T2 hyperintense signal of the supratentorial white matter with characteristic involvement of the external capsule (not shown) and anterior temporal pole (*arrowheads*). Please see the text for additional discussion of this disease entity. (*Courtesy of* Seena Dehkharghani, MD, Emory University, Atlanta, GA.)

diffuse, symmetric T2 hyperintensity in the cerebellum and posterior limb internal capsule often times with extensive posterior predominant T2 hyperintensity in the supratentorial white matter, sparing the subcortical white matter.[22] The anterior limb of the internal capsule is typically spared. Marked T2 signal is commonly seen within multiple brainstem tracts including the corticospinal, medial lemnisci, and central tegmental. Diffusion-weighted imaging (DWI) may show increased signal but often with high apparent diffusion coefficient (ADC) signal, although true restricted diffusion is possible.[23,24] It is certainly possible that abusers of all illicit drugs may suffer a hypoxic ischemic event that contributes to MR findings.[24] MR spectroscopy may show increased lactate and decreased N-acetyl-aspartate.[23,24] Despite the aforementioned findings on DWI and MR spectroscopy, neither is specifically helpful in establishing the diagnosis, but rather the anatomic regions of T2 prolongation are highly suggestive.[24] As such, the input of the radiologist is paramount in clenching this diagnosis.

Cocaine is well known to cause of a host of adverse neurologic sequelae, including hemorrhagic, ischemic, vasculitic, and vasospastic events, a discussion of which is beyond this review.[25] Of interest, however, is an isolated report of cocaine-induced progressive severe leukoencephalopathy.[25]

Organic compounds and solvents are widely available household items. One of the most common of these agents is toluene, a neurotoxic volatile lipophilic hydrocarbon that may be abused by inhalation, as in the well-publicized form of spray cans.[26] Cerebellar dysfunction, personality changes, emotional instability, neurocognitive impairment, dementia, cranial nerve abnormalities, and pyramidal signs may result. On MR, extensive periventricular white matter T2 signal including involvement of the capsular white matter may be present with variable degrees of atrophy.[27] Although such T2 signal may be impressive, the findings are ultimately nonspecific and may be mimicked by several other leukoencephalopathies. Numerous other organic compounds have been shown to induce a leukoencephalopathy with excessive exposure including paradichlorobenzene, a compound commonly used in household cleaners and pesticides.[28]

TREATMENT-RELATED LEUKOENCEPHALOPATHY

Radiation therapy has increasingly become an independent or adjunctive tool in the treatment of a variety of benign and malignant intracranial neoplasms as well as vascular malformations.[29] Although this treatment has been revolutionary, there are several deleterious effects that can manifest at various time points from weeks to years after the completion of radiotherapy. Examples of such complications include focal white matter injury, as in commonly encountered in radiation necrosis, and diffuse white matter injury, as in radiation leukoencephalopathy and necrotizing

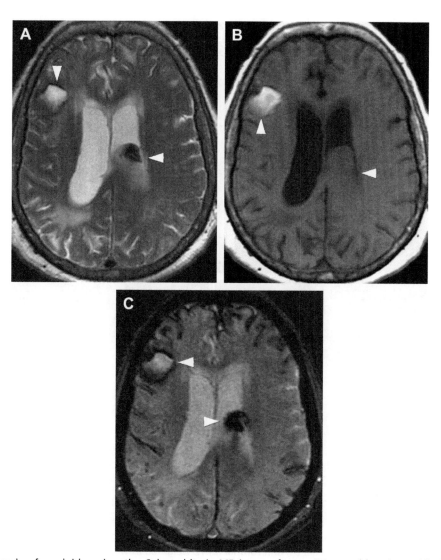

Fig. 5. Example of amyloid angiopathy. Selected brain MR images from a 77-year-old patient with right-sided weakness, including axial T2-weighted (*A*) as well as T1-weighted (*B*) and T2*-weighted (*C*) images. *Arrowheads* help to delineate the multifocal hemorrhages, which include the intraparenchymal and subarachnoid spaces and some of which appear consistent with methemoglobin (intrinsic T1 hyperintensity, also known as T1-shortening). Note the pattern of involvement centered peripherally within the lobes of the supratentorial brain. Please see the text for additional discussion of this disease entity. (*Courtesy of* John Hesselink, MD, FACR, University of California San Diego School of Medicine, San Diego, CA.)

leukoencephalopathy.[30] As is thematic to this article, only diffuse white injury patterns that tend to be late delayed (several months to years) in onset are discussed herein.

Leukoencephalopathy is typically a complication of whole brain rather than focal radiation therapy. The exact incidence of this entity after whole brain radiation therapy varies widely in multiple case series in the literature and is not entirely certain.[31] As previously mentioned, this phenomenon tends to occur in a late delayed fashion; however, there have been reports of some patients

having earlier onset.[31] Risk factors for leukoencephalopathy include older age (>65 years), higher total dose and dose per fraction, larger volumes of brain irradiated, and concurrent chemotherapy.[31] In addition, in a recent small series of patients, the combination of whole brain radiation therapy with stereotactic radiosurgery did result in a significant increase incidence of leukoencephalopathy.[32] The classic pattern of radiation leukoencephalopathy is that of nonenhancing symmetric, confluent diffuse T2 prolongation in the periventricular white matter (**Fig. 7**). The process tends

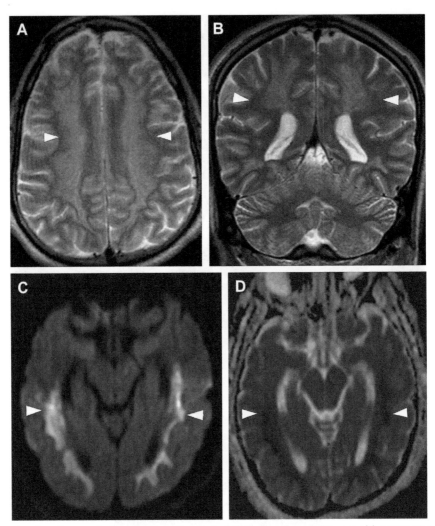

Fig. 6. Example of toxic encephalopathy. Selected brain MR images from a 25-year-old comatose patient with decerebrate posturing, including axial (*A*) and coronal (*B*) T2-weighted as well as axial DWI (*C*) and ADC (*D*) images. *Arrowheads* help to delineate the relatively symmetric abnormal white matter hyperintensity. Note the pattern of restricted diffusion; this restricted diffusion is suggestive of cytotoxic edema and radiographic acuity. In this instance, the imaging findings are consistent with the effects of a combination of prescription and illicit pharmaceuticals. Please see the text for additional discussion of this disease entity. (*Courtesy of* John Hesselink, MD, FACR, University of California San Diego School of Medicine, San Diego, CA.)

to spare the subcortical white matter and corpus callosum. As would be expected, relative cerebral blood volume is decreased in these regions of T2 prolongation.[30] Cerebral atrophy is a common associated finding. Histopathologically, signal changes on MR imaging correspond to a combination of direct white matter injury with demyelination, loss of oligodendrocytes and gliosis, and interrelated vascular injury.[30]

A rarer complication of radiotherapy in combination with chemotherapy is that of disseminated necrotizing leukoencephalopathy (DNL), a more fulminant, typically irreversible process of white matter injury that may be lethal.[33] Clinical deterioration may be rapid with progressive subcortical dementia.[34] DNL may initially appear as multifocal regions of T2 prolongation followed by diffuse white matter T2 hyperintensity. Multifocal regions of enhancement amid the regions of T2 prolongation and possibly with small areas of T2 shortening are characteristic. Histopathologic abnormalities in DNL include demyelination and regions of coagulative necrosis with vascular changes including fibrinoid degeneration.[35]

An increasingly rare entity, mineralizing microangiopathy, is usually seen after chemotherapy and concomitant radiation for childhood malignancies. It is characterized by usually symmetric

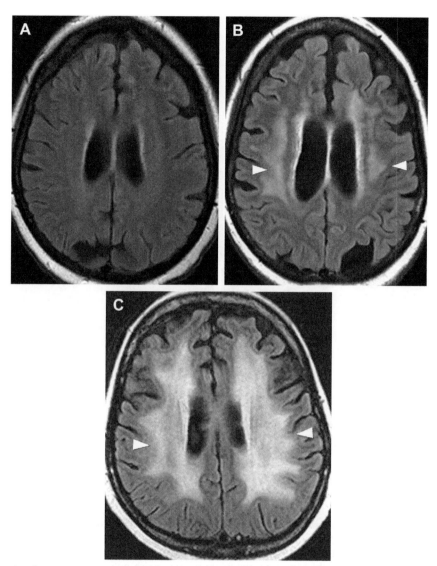

Fig. 7. Example of tumor-treatment-related nonspecific white matter change. Selected brain MR images from a 51-year-old patient with breast cancer and brain metastases, including axial FLAIR images preradiation (*A*) and postradiation therapy at 4 months (*B*) and also at 14 months (*C*). *Arrowheads* help to delineate the nonspecific white matter change. Note the progressive diffuse brain volume loss. Please see the text for additional discussion of this disease entity. (*Courtesy of* John Hesselink, MD, FACR, University of California San Diego School of Medicine, San Diego, CA.)

subcortical white matter, basal ganglia, and deep cerebellar white matter calcification often on a background of diffuse white matter hypodensity or confluent T2 signal.[36]

HIE

HIE (**Fig. 8**) is a catastrophic insult to the brain secondary to decreased or absent cerebral blood flow and poor blood oxygenation.[37] Although in children HIE is typically the result of asphyxia thereby resulting in hypoxemia, in adults, HIE is usually the result of an initial cardiac event or cerebrovascular disease with secondary hypoxia resulting in reduced cerebral blood flow.[37] The pattern of injury on imaging is the result of the severity of the insult, age of the patient, and selective vulnerability of the tissues insulted, with the most metabolically active tissues incurring primary injury. MR imaging remains the gold standard for imaging HIE. Although a detailed review of various injury patterns is beyond the scope of this article, 2 forms of hypoperfusion injury that can result in extensive white matter injury include periventricular leukomalacia (PVL) and severe HIE.[38]

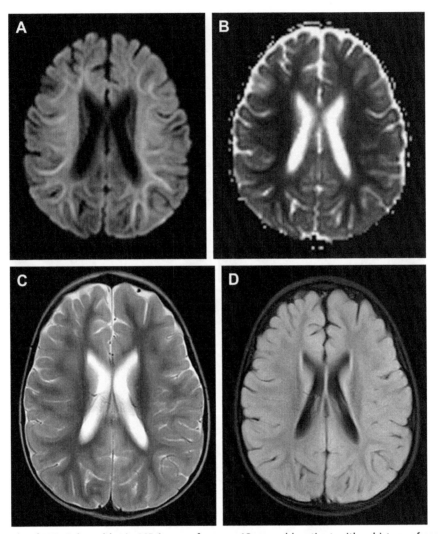

Fig. 8. Example of HIE. Selected brain MR images from an 18-year-old patient with a history of cardiac arrest including axial DWI (*A*), axial ADC map (*B*), axial T2 fast spin-echo (*C*), and axial T2 FLAIR (*D*) images. Note the confluent restricted diffusion of the supratentorial white matter, which only exhibits subtle T2 prolongation. Please see the text for additional discussion of this disease entity.

PVL is a common white matter injury of prematurity.[37] The cause of PVL is quite complex but essentially relates to the inherent vulnerability of periventricular white matter to changes in perfusion. It seems that this is not only due to fewer penetrating arteries in this region[39] but also to inherent vulnerability of regional cells before 32 weeks.[40] The result is regions of T2 prolongation within the periventricular white matter with small foci of T1 shortening with or without T2 shortening.[41] Larger areas of T1 shortening may eventually undergo cavitation with resulting T1 prolongation.[42] Although small regions of abnormal signal intensity eventually transform into small foci of gliosis as do small areas of cavitation, larger areas of gliosis typically result in

diffuse white matter gliosis with secondary callosal volume loss, ex vacuo enlargement of the ventricles, with irregular undulation of the ependymal surface in end-stage PVL.[43] Despite this discussion of MR findings, ultrasound remains the modality of choice for screening premature infants not only for PVL but also for intracranial hemorrhage.[37] With the exception of cystic PVL, however, sensitivity remains low for the typical finding of white matter echogenicity.[41] It is important to remember that not all children with periventricular T2 hyperintensity and white matter volume loss have PVL because a host of other processes may produce similar results, as in the sequelae of ventriculitis and hydrocephalus, among others.[42] Furthermore, the normal presence of

T2 hyperintense zones of terminal myelination, which characteristically spare the ependymal margin and lack the stigmata of regional white matter volume loss, must be differentiated from PVL.[42]

In severe HIE, characteristic patterns of signal abnormality are seen, preferentially affecting regions of high metabolic activity, such as the basal ganglia, cortex to include the perirolandic region, for example, the corticospinal tract. In the acute stage of severe hypoperfusion, regardless of age, should the insult be prolonged or severe enough, T2 prolongation and diffusion restriction should eventually involve the totality of the supratentorial and even infratentorial white matter. Of note however is the entity of delayed white matter injury or postanoxic leukoencephalopathy, which may occur days to weeks after the insulting event, even after the patient is seen to be clinically recovering. In this scenario, there is delayed evolution of extensive white matter T2 signal and diffusion restriction. This entity has been well-documented in carbon monoxide poisoning but may also be seen with any primary event resulting in a severe hypoxic ischemic insult.[37,44]

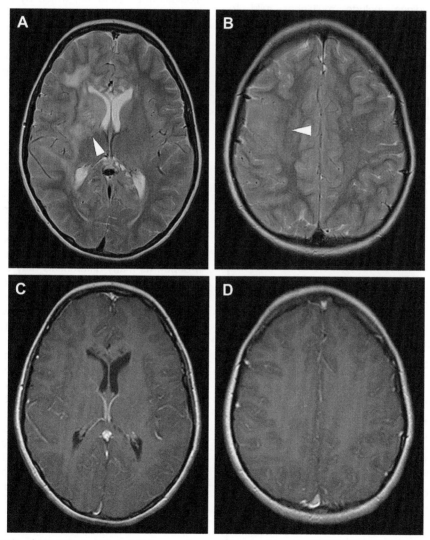

Fig. 9. Example of GC. Selected brain MR images from a 19-year-old patient with a 3-month history of left arm weakness not responding to steroids, including axial T2 fast spin-echo (*A, B*) and axial T1 FLAIR post (*C, D*) images. Note the confluent T2 hyperintense signal of much of the right cerebral white matter with involvement of the basal ganglia. Note the characteristic cortical involvement within the posterior right frontal lobe and enlarged right caudate head (*arrowhead*) without associated enhancement. Please see the text for additional discussion of this disease entity.

NEOPLASIA

Gliomatosis cerebri (GC; **Fig. 9**) is a rare, infiltrative neoplastic process characterized by abnormal glial cell infiltration of the white matter with involvement of at least 2 cerebral lobes.[45] The World Health Organization classifies GC as an astrocytic neoplasm.[46] After biopsy, GC may be classified as World Health Organization grade II-IV depending on histopathologic review. Although clinical presentation of such patients is usually nonspecific and may occur in both adults and children, a sometimes helpful point is that MR imaging findings may be disproportionately extensive to the relatively mild clinical presentation.[45] Key imaging findings include multilobar mild to moderate white matter T2 prolongation, specifically with overlying cortical involvement, which results in blurring of the gray-white matter junction.[45,47] Basal ganglia and brainstem involvement may be present. Enhancement is usually absent.[45] Another key feature is the relatively mild volume positivity of GC despite the extent of abnormal signal that may be present. It is critical to always consider GC in the differential diagnosis of extensive white matter disease because clinical presentation and imaging findings may mimic a variety of nonneoplastic entities including demyelinating diseases, infarction, and even encephalitis (**Box 1**). To clarify, GC is distinct from multicentric glioblastoma multiforme, which by definition involves multiple noncontiguous sites in the brain as opposed to GC, whereby confluent infiltration of parenchyma exists. Admittedly, however, cases of multicentric glioblastoma multiforme and diffuse glioma may be difficult to differentiate from GC.

SUMMARY

The patient with diffuse white matter disease is a commonly encountered entity in everyday neuroradiologic practice. The initial approach in pediatric patients with immature myelination is a confident understanding of the age-appropriate normal appearance of white matter on CT and MR imaging. For both adults and children, clinical history, including known disease states, must be reviewed in depth, as many differentials may be excluded and still others included even before rigorous review of the imaging study. Beyond this initial preparation, the best approach to diffuse white matter disease relies on carefully considering the multitude of possibilities by the umbrella categories listed herein (ie, vascular, neoplastic) and then considering the primary differentials within each category. This approach necessarily relies not only on an educated, broad catchment of possibilities but also on an understanding of key deciphering imaging findings for each diagnosis to then procure the most reasonable differential. Although the ultimate diagnosis may not always be possible by imaging alone, the goal of the radiologist should be at least to guide the clinician toward an efficient pathway of laboratory or other workup so as to ultimately make the diagnosis.

Box 1
Differential diagnosis of diffuse white matter disease

Hypomyelination disorders

Leukodystrophy (geographic)

- Metachromatic leukodystrophy
- Globoid cell leukodystrophy (Krabbe disease)
- Adrenoleukodystrophy/ Adrenomyeloneuropathy
- Alexander disease

Vascular leukoencephalopathy

- CADASIL
- CARASIL
- CAA
- Binswanger disease

Infection

- Viral (HIV, cytomegalovirus, etc)

Toxic exposure

- Heroin
- Cocaine (rare)
- Toluene
- Paradichlorobenzene

Treatment-related (radiochemotherapy) leukoencephalopathy

- Radiation leukoencephalopathy
- Disseminated necrotizing leukoencephalopathy
- Mineralizing microangiopathy

HIE

Neoplasia

- GC

REFERENCES

1. Bradley WG Jr. Magnetic resonance imaging in the central nervous system: comparison with computed tomography. Magn Reson Annu 1986;81–122.

2. Knaap MSvd, Valk J, Barkhof F, et al. 3rd edition. Magnetic resonance of myelination and myelin disorders, vol. xvi. Berlin, New York: Springer; 2005. p. 1084.

3. Barkovich AJ, Kjos BO, Jackson DE Jr, et al. Normal maturation of the neonatal and infant brain: MR imaging at 1.5 T. Radiology 1988;166(1 Pt 1): 173–80.

4. Steenweg ME, Vanderver A, Blaser S, et al. Magnetic resonance imaging pattern recognition in hypomyelinating disorders. Brain 2010;133(10): 2971–82.

5. Schiffmann R, van der Knaap MS. Invited article: an MRI-based approach to the diagnosis of white matter disorders. Neurology 2009;72(8):750–9.

6. Waltz G, Harik SI, Kaufman B. Adult metachromatic leukodystrophy. Value of computed tomographic scanning and magnetic resonance imaging of the brain. Arch Neurol 1987;44(2):225–7.

7. Eichler F, Grodd W, Grant E, et al. Metachromatic leukodystrophy: a scoring system for brain MR imaging observations. AJNR Am J Neuroradiol 2009; 30(10):1893–7.

8. Wenger DA, Rafi MA, Luzi P. Molecular genetics of Krabbe disease (globoid cell leukodystrophy): diagnostic and clinical implications. Hum Mutat 1997; 10(4):268–79.

9. Loes DJ, Peters C, Krivit W. Globoid cell leukodystrophy: distinguishing early-onset from late-onset disease using a brain MR imaging scoring method. AJNR Am J Neuroradiol 1999;20(2):316–23.

10. Farina L, Bizzi A, Finocchiaro G, et al. MR imaging and proton MR spectroscopy in adult Krabbe disease. AJNR Am J Neuroradiol 2000;21(8):1478–82.

11. Griffin JW, Goren E, Schaumburg H, et al. Adrenomyeloneuropathy: a probable variant of adrenoleukodystrophy. I. Clinical and endocrinologic aspects. Neurology 1977;27(12):1107–13.

12. Kumar AJ, Kohler W, Kruse B, et al. MR findings in adult-onset adrenoleukodystrophy. AJNR Am J Neuroradiol 1995;16(6):1227–37.

13. Loes DJ, Hite S, Moser H, et al. Adrenoleukodystrophy: a scoring method for brain MR observations. AJNR Am J Neuroradiol 1994;15(9):1761–6.

14. Farina L, Pareyson D, Minati L, et al. Can MR imaging diagnose adult-onset Alexander disease? AJNR Am J Neuroradiol 2008;29(6):1190–6.

15. Joutel A, Corpechot C, Ducros A, et al. Notch3 mutations in CADASIL, a hereditary adult-onset condition causing stroke and dementia. Nature 1996; 383(6602):707–10.

16. O'Sullivan M, Jarosz JM, Martin RJ, et al. MRI hyperintensities of the temporal lobe and external capsule in patients with CADASIL. Neurology 2001;56(5): 628–34.

17. Fukutake T. Cerebral autosomal recessive arteriopathy with subcortical infarcts and leukoencephalopathy (CARASIL): from discovery to gene identification. J Stroke Cerebrovasc Dis 2011;20(2):85–93.

18. Haacke EM, DelProposto ZS, Chaturvedi S, et al. Imaging cerebral amyloid angiopathy with susceptibility-weighted imaging. AJNR Am J Neuroradiol 2007;28(2):316–7.

19. Gray F, Dubas F, Roullet E, et al. Leukoencephalopathy in diffuse hemorrhagic cerebral amyloid angiopathy. Ann Neurol 1985;18(1):54–9.

20. Oh U, Gupta R, Krakauer JW, et al. Reversible leukoencephalopathy associated with cerebral amyloid angiopathy. Neurology 2004;62(3):494–7.

21. Kriegstein AR, Shungu DC, Millar WS, et al. Leukoencephalopathy and raised brain lactate from heroin vapor inhalation ("chasing the dragon"). Neurology 1999;53(8):1765–73.

22. Keogh CF, Andrews GT, Spacey SD, et al. Neuroimaging features of heroin inhalation toxicity: "chasing the dragon". AJR Am J Roentgenol 2003; 180(3):847–50.

23. Offiah C, Hall E. Heroin-induced leukoencephalopathy: characterization using MRI, diffusion-weighted imaging, and MR spectroscopy. Clin Radiol 2008; 63(2):146–52.

24. Bartlett E, Mikulis DJ. Chasing "chasing the dragon" with MRI: leukoencephalopathy in drug abuse. Br J Radiol 2005;78(935):997–1004.

25. Bianco F, Iacovelli E, Tinelli E, et al. Recurrent leukoencephalopathy in a cocaine abuser. Neurotoxicology 2011;32(4):410–2.

26. Hormes JT, Filley CM, Rosenberg NL. Neurologic sequelae of chronic solvent vapor abuse. Neurology 1986;36(5):698–702.

27. Caldemeyer KS, Pascuzzi RM, Moran CC, et al. Toluene abuse causing reduced MR signal intensity in the brain. AJR Am J Roentgenol 1993;161(6): 1259–61.

28. Hernandez SH, Wiener SW, Smith SW. Case files of the New York City poison control center: paradichlorobenzene-induced leukoencephalopathy. J Med Toxicol 2010;6(2):217–29.

29. Rabin BM, Meyer JR, Berlin JW, et al. Radiation-induced changes in the central nervous system and head and neck. Radiographics 1996;16(5): 1055–72.

30. Pruzincova L, Steno J, Srbecky M, et al. MR imaging of late radiation therapy- and chemotherapy-induced injury: a pictorial essay. Eur Radiol 2009; 19(11):2716–27.

31. Ebi J, Sato H, Nakajima M, et al. Incidence of leukoencephalopathy after whole-brain radiation therapy for brain metastases. Int J Radiat Oncol Biol Phys 2013;85(5):1212–7.

32. Monaco EA 3rd, Faraji AH, Berkowitz O, et al. Leukoencephalopathy after whole-brain radiation therapy plus radiosurgery versus radiosurgery alone for metastatic lung cancer. Cancer 2013;119(1):226–32.

33. Oka M, Terae S, Kobayashi R, et al. MRI in methotrexate-related leukoencephalopathy: disseminated necrotising leukoencephalopathy in comparison with mild leukoencephalopathy. Neuroradiology 2003;45(7):493–7.

34. Lim YJ, Kim HJ, Lee YJ, et al. Clinical features of encephalopathy in children with cancer requiring cranial magnetic resonance imaging. Pediatr Neurol 2011;44(6):433–8.

35. Suzuki K, Takemura T, Okeda R, et al. Vascular changes of methotrexate-related disseminated necrotizing leukoencephalopathy. Acta Neuropathol 1984;65(2):145–9.

36. Shanley DJ. Mineralizing microangiopathy: CT and MRI. Neuroradiology 1995;37(4):331–3.

37. Huang BY, Castillo M. Hypoxic-ischemic brain injury: imaging findings from birth to adulthood. Radiographics 2008;28(2):417–39 [quiz: 617].

38. Rutherford M, Malamateniou C, McGuinness A, et al. Magnetic resonance imaging in hypoxic-ischaemic encephalopathy. Early Hum Dev 2010;86(6):351–60.

39. Ballabh P, Braun A, Nedergaard M. Anatomic analysis of blood vessels in germinal matrix, cerebral cortex, and white matter in developing infants. Pediatr Res 2004;56(1):117–24.

40. Back SA, Luo NL, Borenstein NS, et al. Late oligodendrocyte progenitors coincide with the developmental window of vulnerability for human perinatal white matter injury. J Neurosci 2001;21(4):1302–12.

41. Inder TE, Anderson NJ, Spencer C, et al. White matter injury in the premature infant: a comparison between serial cranial sonographic and MR findings at term. AJNR Am J Neuroradiol 2003;24(5):805–9.

42. Barkovich AJ. 4th edition. Pediatric neuroimaging, vol. xxiv. Philadelphia: Lippincott Williams & Wilkins; 2005. p. 932.

43. Sie LT, Hart AA, van Hof J, et al. Predictive value of neonatal MRI with respect to late MRI findings and clinical outcome. A study in infants with periventricular densities on neonatal ultrasound. Neuropediatrics 2005; 36(2):78–89.

44. Kim JH, Chang KH, Song IC, et al. Delayed encephalopathy of acute carbon monoxide intoxication: diffusivity of cerebral white matter lesions. AJNR Am J Neuroradiol 2003;24(8):1592–7.

45. Freund M, Hahnel S, Sommer C, et al. CT and MRI findings in gliomatosis cerebri: a neuroradiologic and neuropathologic review of diffuse infiltrating brain neoplasms. Eur Radiol 2001;11(2):309–16.

46. Louis DN, Ohgaki H, Wiestler OD, et al. The 2007 WHO classification of tumours of the central nervous system. Acta Neuropathol 2007;114(2):97–109.

47. Bendszus M, Warmuth-Metz M, Klein R, et al. MR spectroscopy in gliomatosis cerebri. AJNR Am J Neuroradiol 2000;21(2):375–80.

Imaging Manifestations of the Leukodystrophies, Inherited Disorders of White Matter

Edward Yang, MD, PhD*,
Sanjay P. Prabhu, MBBS, MRCPCH, FRCR

KEYWORDS

- Leukodystrophy • Inborn error of metabolism • Dysmyelination • Demyelination • Spectroscopy
- White matter

KEY POINTS

- Recognition of leukodystrophies requires a solid understanding of normal myelination.
- When a leukodystrophy is encountered, a pattern-based approach is useful for developing a reasonably sized differential diagnosis. The patterns stressed in this review include globally delayed myelination, subcortical white matter predominant, central white matter predominant, and combined gray/white matter patterns.
- Special emphasis should be placed on recognizing unusual combinations of findings that suggest a specific diagnosis.

INTRODUCTION

In contrast to most other white matter diseases discussed in this issue, leukodystrophies are inherited disorders that result from mutations in a specific gene product or biological pathway. Various working definitions of leukodystrophy have been proposed that further restrict the meaning of this term to inborn errors of metabolism (ie, a specific type of gene product) or demyelination (ie, a specific pathogenic mechanism).[1–3] Matters become more complicated still because some investigators define demyelination as any process leading to myelin loss, whereas some would restrict the meaning of this term to inflammatory disorders such as multiple sclerosis, leaving disorders of myelin synthesis/maintenance under the grouping of 'dysmyelination.'

Because there is considerable overlap in the appearance of inherited white matter diseases regardless of type of gene product or pathogenesis of the signal abnormality seen on imaging, this review uses a pragmatic definition of leukodystrophy, namely any disorder of white matter signal secondary to a defective or absent gene product. Although this definition is fairly broad, it excludes disorders that exclusively affect gray matter structures or at least lack discrete white matter signal abnormality. Therefore, this article excludes some well-known metabolic disorders such as pantothenate kinase deficiency, creatine deficiency syndromes, and many of the organic acidemias (eg, 3-methylgluconic and methylmalonic acidemia). Diffuse white matter disease seen in association with congenital muscular dystrophies has a distinctive clinical presentation,[4–6] and imaging of disorders of peroxisomal biogenesis have been recently reviewed elsewhere[7]; both are also omitted from this review.

As a category, the leukodystrophies usually present a challenge to radiologists because specific disease entities are rarely encountered and there are numerous diseases with overlapping imaging appearance. In this review, a practical approach

Department of Radiology, Boston Children's Hospital, Harvard Medical School, 300 Longwood Avenue, Boston, MA 02115, USA

* Corresponding author. Department of Radiology, Boston Children's Hospital, 300 Longwood Avenue, Boston, MA 02115.

E-mail address: edward.yang@childrens.harvard.edu

Radiol Clin N Am 52 (2014) 279–319
http://dx.doi.org/10.1016/j.rcl.2013.11.008
0033-8389/14/$ – see front matter © 2014 Elsevier Inc. All rights reserved.

to recognizing and categorizing the leukodystrophies is described, focusing on 4 common patterns of signal abnormality in the brain parenchyma (Box 1). Special emphasis is given to unusual imaging features or combinations of features that suggest a specific diagnosis. For the interested reader, additional resources are provided, including reference works dedicated to the topic.[8–10]

IMAGE ACQUISITION

As with other white matter disorders, leukodystrophies are best appreciated on magnetic resonance (MR) imaging.[11] Standard MR imaging protocols should include high-resolution T1-weighted and T2-weighted imaging in at least 2 planes to provide an accurate evaluation of the maturity and integrity of brain myelination. Diffusion-weighted imaging is

---

Box 1
Simplified pattern-based approach to leukodystrophies

Globally Arrested/Absent Myelination

Pelizaeus-Merzbacher disease
18q-deletion syndrome
Free sialic acid storage disorders (Salla)
Trichothiodystrophy
Cockayne syndrome*
Fucosidosis
Hypomyelination with hypodontia and hypogonadotropic hypogonadism (4H syndrome)
Hypomyelination with atrophy of the basal ganglia and cerebellum*
Hypomyelination with congenital cataracts
Nonketotic hyperglycinemia

Subcortical Predominant White Matter Signal Abnormality

Galactosemia
Megalencephalic leukoencephalopathy with subcortical cysts*
Aicardi-Goutières syndrome*

Central White Matter Predominant Signal Abnormality, With or Without Brainstem Involvement

X-linked adrenoleukodystrophy, acyl-coenzyme A oxidase deficiency*
Metachromatic leukodystrophy
Mucopolysaccharidosis
Lowe syndrome*
X-linked Charcot-Marie-Tooth*
Cockayne syndrome+
Vanishing white matter disease (childhood ataxia with central nervous system hypomyelination)
Neuronal ceroid lipofuscinosis+
Leukoencephalopathy with brainstem and spinal cord evolvement and increased lactate*
Phenylketonuria
Sjögren-Larsson syndrome
Nonketotic hyperglycinemia
Hyperhomocysteinemia
Biotinidase (multiple carboxylase) deficiency

Combination of Gray and White Matter Signal Abnormality

Canavan disease*
GM1/GM2 gangliosidoses (Tay-Sachs, Sandhoff syndromes)*
Alexander disease*
Krabbe disease*
Maple syrup urine disease*
Leigh disease and other mitochondrial disorders
Urea cycle disorders*
L-2-hydroxyglutaric aciduria*
Glutaric aciduria type I and II

* indicates a disease with highly characteristic imaging findings.
+ indicates a minority manifestation.
   Data from Barkovich AJ, Patay Z. Metabolic, toxic, and inflammatory brain disorders. In: Barkovich AJ, editor. Pediatric neuroimaging. Philadelphia: Lippincott Williams & Wilkins; 2012. p. 81–239.

also essential because it often shows parenchymal changes to greatest advantage,[12] particularly in the setting of acute clinical deterioration (Box 2). For detection of mineralization (ie, calcium, iron), susceptibility-weighted imaging can increase conspicuity on MR imaging. Gadolinium-based contrast is frequently omitted for workups where a leukodystrophy is a possibility (eg, developmental delay). However, gadolinium-based contrast medium can increase the specificity of the diagnosis because enhancement is a prominent feature in several leukodystrophies (Box 3), and this enhancement can be used to follow disease activity in some disorders (eg, X-linked adrenoleukodystrophy [ALD]).[13] MR spectroscopy is also helpful in building evidence for a metabolic disturbance (ie, lactate)[14,15] and in some cases can suggest a specific diagnosis (Box 4). Two important caveats apply with MR spectroscopy. First, some lactate within the cerebrospinal fluid (CSF) is normal in the first few months of life, and therefore, exclusion of CSF in the interrogated voxel is important for avoiding false-positives. Second, there is evidence that the inverted lactate doublet seen images with intermediate echo time (TE) = 144 millisecond is attenuated at 3 T, and therefore adding a 288-ms acquisition should be considered to avoid this effect.[16]

APPROACH TO IMAGE INTERPRETATION

Recognition that there is an abnormality of white matter is the first obvious step in accurately diagnosing a leukodystrophy. This recognition is more difficult than it might first appear because the patients presenting for leukodystrophy evaluation are usually at an age where immature/incomplete brain myelination is expected. Also, leukodystrophies tend to present in a left-right symmetric fashion similar to immature myelination

---

Box 2
Leukodystrophies featuring restricted diffusion

Leigh disease, mitochondrial disorder

Maple syrup urine disorder

Urea cycle disorders

Canavan

Metachromatic leukodystrophy

Hyperhomocysteinemia

X-linked adrenoleukodystrophy

Nonketotic hyperglycemia

Leukoencephalopathy with brainstem and spinal cord evolvement and increased lactate

Vanishing white matter disease

Data from Barkovich AJ, Patay Z. Metabolic, toxic, and inflammatory brain disorders. In: Barkovich AJ, editor. Pediatric neuroimaging. Philadelphia: Lippincott Williams & Wilkins; 2012. p. 81–239, with permission; and Patay Z. Diffusion-weighted MR imaging in leukodystrophies. Eur Radiol 2005;15(11):2284–303.

Box 3
Leukodystrophies with enhancement

Krabbe disease (cranial nerves, cauda equina)

Metachromatic leukodystrophy (cranial nerves, cauda equina)

X-linked adrenoleukodystrophy, acyl-coenzyme A oxidase deficiency

Alexander disease

Box 4
MR spectroscopy findings in leukodystrophies

Unusual MR Spectroscopy Peaks Associated with Specific Disorders

Phenylketonuria (phenylanaline 7.37 ppm)
Maple syrup urine disease (branched-chain amino acids/ketoacids, 0.9 ppm)
Salla/Canavan disease (increased *N*-acetylaspartate)
Sjögren-Larsson (0.9 and 1.3 ppm peaks that do no suppress with long echo time)
Creatinine deficiency syndromes (decreased creatinine)
Succinate dehydrogenase (Leigh syndrome: 2.4 ppm succinate peak)
Fucosidosis (1.2 ppm doublet, 3.4–3.8 ppm broad peak)
Galactosemia (galactitol 3.67 and 3.74 ppm)
Nonketotic hyperglycinemia (glycine 3.56 ppm)
Urea cycle disorders (glutamine/glutamate 2.05–2.55 and 3.68–3.85 ppm)

Leukodystrophies Where Lactate Is Commonly Encountered

Mitochondrial disorders
Maple syrup urine disease
Krabbe
Alexander
Zellweger disease
Hyperhomocysteinemia
Biotinidase (multiple carboxylase deficiency)
X-linked adrenoleukodystrophy
Vanishing matter disease

Data from Barkovich AJ, Patay Z. Metabolic, toxic, and inflammatory brain disorders. In: Barkovich AJ, editor. Pediatric neuroimaging. Philadelphia: Lippincott Williams & Wilkins; 2012. p. 81–239.

with some rare exceptions.[17,18] As a result, it is easy to incorrectly dismiss hyperintensity in the white mater as immature myelination rather than pathology. To avoid this pitfall, it is essential that an accurate reference for age-specific myelination patterns is readily available to radiologists who interpret pediatric brain imaging studies (see the article by Guleria and Kelly elsewhere in this issue[19]). Knowledge of normal myelination milestones allows accurate detection of delayed myelination and T2 signal abnormality outside expected sites. Specifically, it allows recognition of both delayed myelination as well as cases where the T2 signal has exceeded that expected for immature myelination alone in a particular location.

Most classification systems for leukodystrophies focus on specific biochemical abnormalities (eg, organic acidemias) or the organelle implicated with a specific leukodystrophy (eg, lysosomal disorder).[3,9] However, the imaging appearances of leukodystrophies categorized in this fashion can vary dramatically, and the practicing radiologist usually is most concerned with imaging features. Therefore, in this article, the leukodystrophies are subdivided by imaging pattern and a simplified version of pattern-based approaches is used as described in more detail elsewhere.[10,20]

The 4 patterns to be discussed are summarized in Box 1.

1. Generalized delay or failure in myelination. In these disorders, the myelination has the appearance of a much younger patient and in some cases is entirely absent. The T2 hyperintensity does not typically exceed that seen in brains with immature myelination and lacks focality.
2. Peripheral white matter predominant signal abnormality. Although subcortical white matter is the last to myelinate, disorders in this category feature T2 hyperintensity greater than seen with unmyelinated white matter or focal areas of more pronounced signal increase.
3. Central white matter predominant signal abnormality, with or without brainstem involvement. Here, central white matter is defined as the deep (corona radiata, centrum semiovale) and periventricular white matter. These leukodystrophies tend to spare the subcortical white matter initially and therefore should not be mistaken for globally delayed myelination.
4. Combined gray and white matter signal abnormality. In these disorders, abnormal T2 hyperintensity also affects gray matter structures in either the cortex or deep gray nuclei as well as the white matter.

Within these 4 patterns, particular emphasis should be placed on recognizing disorders with highly characteristic or pathognomonic findings (see asterisks in Box 1). The reason is that most of the leukodystrophies are individually rare, representing at most 10% to 20% of all leukodystrophies (population incidence of leukodystrophies are estimated at 1 in 50 to 100,000 live births with 1 report suggesting 1 in 8000).[21–23] As a result, the relative frequency of a specific disorder is a somewhat unreliable guide to pretest probability: it is generally unknown in any given clinical population and the relative incidence of specific disorders is difficult to ascertain confidently outside the most common disorders (eg, Pelizaeus-Merzbacher, metachromatic leukodystrophy, mitochondrial disorders, and adrenoleukodystrophy). Some additional unique (although not necessarily specific) imaging findings are listed in Box 5. Of particular interest are anterior-posterior and centrifugal/centripetal gradients in the pattern of white matter involvement, something that can be used to differentiate disorders within 1 of the 4 patterns.

Before discussing these 4 patterns in depth, a few general principles should be kept in mind. First, leukodystrophies are generally progressive, leading to diffuse white matter disease and atrophy. Therefore, even highly characteristic imaging patterns become nonspecific at the end stage of disease (Figs. 1 and 2). Second, there is a wide spectrum of severity depending on the degree of functional gene product remaining. As a result, there are usually neonatal, infantile, juvenile, and even adult manifestations of most leukodystrophies. Third, restricted diffusion is a common and helpful finding in patients with leukodystrophy, particularly when imaging is performed during an episode of clinical deterioration. However, these sites of restricted diffusion are not always an indicator of cytotoxic edema and irreversible injury. In many instances, these sites of restricted diffusion actually represent myelin vacuolization[9,12] and may improve with supportive or medical therapy (eg, Fig. 3). Fourth, some humility is required when interpreting studies performed as part of a leukodystrophy evaluation. As noted earlier, these disorders are individually rare. This makes statements on typical imaging manifestations for a specific disorder difficult, and the diversity of causative mutations in any particular disorder make sweeping generalizations even more problematic. Ultimately, communication between the referring physician and the radiologist becomes essential in guiding a sensible workup; for example, dermatologic, auditory, ophthalmologic, and head circumference data may be completely unknown to the interpreting radiologist but in many instances provide critical clues to a specific diagnosis (Box 6).[24] Similarly, newborn screening results vary widely from state

Box 5
Additional imaging findings in the leukodystrophies

Centripetal White Matter Involvement (Subcortical → Periventricular)

L-2-hydroxyglutaric aciduria
Canavan disease
Urea cycle
Kearns-Sayre

Centrifugal White Matter Involvement (Periventricular → Subcortical)

Krabbe disease
Metachromatic leukodystrophy
X-linked adrenoleukodystrophy
Phenylketonuria
Mucopolysaccharidosis
Vanishing white matter disease

Anterior/Posterior Gradient of White Matter disease

Aicardi- Goutières syndrome (anterior)
Alexander disease (anterior)
L-2-hydroxyglutaric aciduria (anterior)
Megencephalic leukoencephalopathy with subcortical cysts (anterior)
Infantile metachromatic leukodystrophy (posterior)
Krabbe disease (posterior)
X-linked adrenoleukodystrophy (posterior)
Mucopolysaccharidoses (posterior)

Parenchymal Calcifications

Aicardi- Goutières (basal ganglia, thalami, dentate, deep/subcortical white matter)
Cockayne syndrome (basal ganglia, dentate, subcortical white matter)
Krabbe disease
X-linked adrenoleukodystrophy (parietooccipital)
TORCH/human immunodeficiency virus

Central Tegmental Tracts Signal Abnormality

Mitochondrial (respiratory chain) diseases
Menkes disease
Vanishing white matter disease
Nonketotic hyperglycinemia
Maple syrup urine disease
Glutaric aciduria I

Data from Barkovich AJ, Patay Z. Metabolic, toxic, and inflammatory brain disorders. In: Barkovich AJ, editor. Pediatric neuroimaging. Philadelphia: Lippincott Williams & Wilkins; 2012. p. 81–239.

to state (see http://www.babysfirsttest.org/new born-screening/states),[25] and as a result the referring clinician may already possess informative biochemical data that pertain to an abnormal brain MR imaging.

PATTERN 1: ARRESTED/ABSENT MYELINATION
Pelizaeus-Merzbacher Disease

Pelizaeus-Merzbacher disease (PMD) is the prototypical disease of arrested or absent myelination, featuring symptoms of nystagmus, ataxia, developmental delay (cognitive as well as psychomotor), and hypotonia that progresses to spasticity.

Patients with the connatal form of the disease present at birth and typically die in early childhood, whereas patients presenting in infancy (usually by 1 year) are said to have the more common classic form of the disease with life expectancy potentially into middle adulthood.[26] PMD is caused by abnormalities in the proteolipid protein 1 (*PLP1*) gene locus located on the X chromosome (Xq22), explaining the predominance of PMD in male patients. *PLP1* is 1 of the 2 major protein constituents of the myelin coat secreted by oligodendrocytes; the other one is myelin basic protein (MBP).[27] Although intuitively deletions or loss of function mutations in *PLP1* might be expected to lead to myelin synthesis failure directly, the

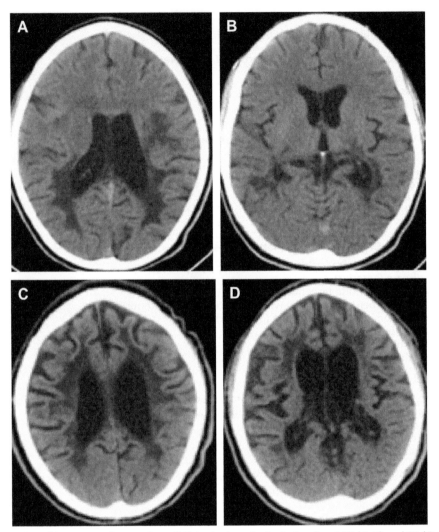

Fig. 1. Progressive white matter changes from X-linked adrenoleukodystrophy at 15 (*A, B*) and 21 (*C, D*) years of age. The classic involvement of the splenium and parietooccipital white matter is obvious on the initial computed tomography study. By the follow-up study, there is nonspecific end-stage white matter disease with volume loss and diffuse hypodensity of the cerebral white matter.

genetics is much more complicated and reflects exquisite sensitivity to gene dosage. Most cases (classic PMD) are caused by duplications of the entire gene locus. Truncating/nonsense mutations or deletions in *PLP1* as well as missense mutations sparing the *PLP1* alternative splicing isoform *DM20* (the embryologically expressed form of *PLP1*) cause mild forms of PMD as well as the related disorder of spastic paraplegia type 2. Missense mutations affecting both *DM20* and *PLP1* lead to the more severe connatal phenotype (hypothesized to reflect an unfolded protein response), as can rare triplications or quintiplication of the *PLP1* locus.[26,28–30] Imaging findings are characterized by absent myelination in the connatal form or arrest of myelination in an early infant pattern for the classic form (**Fig. 4**), the latter associated with some progressive volume loss.[31]

18q Deletion Syndrome

18q deletion syndrome is a somatic chromosome counterpart to PMD, featuring variable dysmorphology (auriculoaural atresia, short stature, midface hypoplasia, extremity deformity) and mental retardation. There is significant phenotypic variability even within pedigrees bearing the same mutation, arguing against simple relationships between specific deletions and phenotype.[32] However, the core phenotypes described earlier seem to best correlate with distal deletions, 18q22.3 through the telomere.[32,33] The fact that

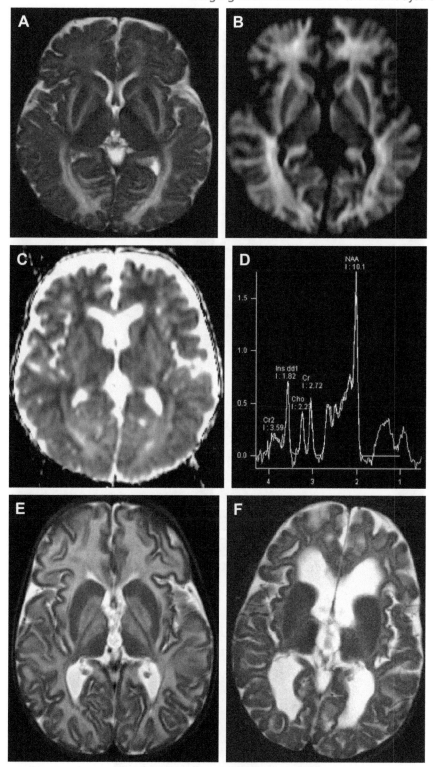

Fig. 2. Eight-month-old with Canavan disease. Axial T2-weighted image (*A*) demonstrates subcortical white matter signal increase greater than expected for immature myelination and signal increase involving the globus pallidus. Apparent diffusion coefficient and diffusion-weighted trace images (*B, C*) demonstrate restricted diffusion in the white matter. MR spectroscopy (*D*) demonstrates marked increase in *N*-acetylaspartate (NAA) relative to choline (Cho), particularly considering patient age. Progressive atrophy of Canavan is demonstrated in another case imaged at 2 years (*E*) and 8 years (*F*) of age. By 8 years of age, there is diffuse white matter atrophy although the globus pallidus signal abnormality has abated.

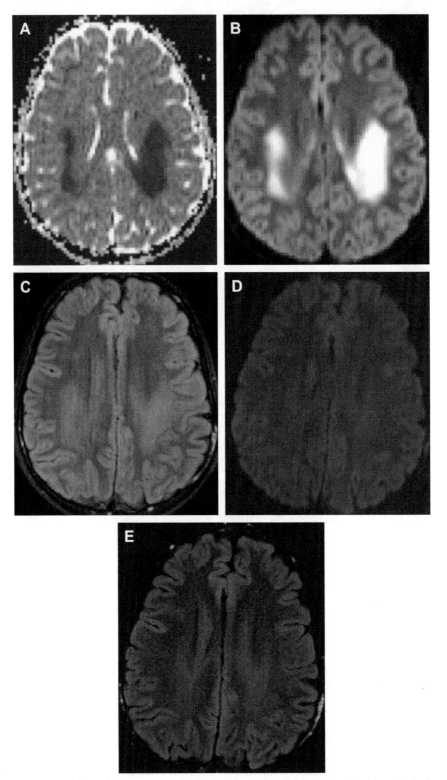

Fig. 3. Fourteen-year-old boy with acute neurologic deficit, eventually diagnosed with X-linked Charcot-Marie-Tooth. Apparent diffusion coefficient and trace diffusion imaging maps (*A, B*) demonstrate profound restricted diffusion in the centrum semiovale with only a faint FLAIR signal abnormality (*C*). Neurologic symptoms spontaneously resolved and the MR imaging 1 year later demonstrates normal diffusion-weighted image trace (*D*) and near normal FLAIR (*E*) appearance.

Box 6
Helpful clinical findings in leukodystrophies

Macrocephaly

Megalencephalic leukoencephalopathy with subcortical cysts
Canavan disease
Alexander disease
Mucopolysaccharidoses (hydrocephalus)
GM2 gangliosidoses (Tay-Sachs, Sandhoff)
L-2-hydroxyglutaric aciduria
Glutaric aciduria type I

Microcephaly

Aicardi-Goutières syndrome
Menkes disease
Cockayne syndrome

Ophthalmologic Abnormalities

Cherry red macule: mucopolysaccharidosis, GM1/GM2 gangliosidoses, Niemann-Pick disease
Retinopathy/vision loss: mucolipidosis, dihydropyramidine dehydrogenase deficiency, trichothiodystrophy, Krabbe, vanishing white matter disease, giant axonal neuropathy, Pelizaeus-Merzbacher, Cockayne syndrome, peroxisomal biogenesis
Strabismus: succinic semialdehyde dehydrogenase
Nystagmus: Pelizaeus-Merzbacher, free sialic acid storage disorders, thiamine deficiency, infantile neuroaxonal dystrophy
Cataracts: Lowe syndrome, Cockayne syndrome, hypomyelination with congenital cataracts, trichothiodystrophy
Glaucoma: Lowe syndrome
Dislocated lens: hyperhomocysteinemia, molybdenum cofactor deficiency, isolated sulfite deficiency
Corneal opacification: mucolipidosis, mucopolysaccharidosis
Extraocular movement abnormalities; 18q deletion, mitochondrial disorder
Coloboma, megalocornea: dihydropyrimidine dehydrogenase deficiency

Dermatologic Abnormalities

Fucosidosis: trunk angiokeratoma
Methylmalonic acidemia: hair loss, desquamative dermatitis
Biotinidase: alopecia, rash
Menkes: sparse coarse hair with split ends, hypopigmented skin
Trichothiodystrophy: brittle hair, teeth/nail dysplasia, ichthyosis
Sjögren-Larsson: ichthyosis
Rhizomelic chondrodysplasia punctata: ichthyosis
Phenylketonuria: dermatitis, eczema
X-linked adrenoleukodystrophy: hyperpigmentation
Cockayne: photosensitivity
Aicardi-Goutières: chilblains (frostbite-like lesions)

Sensorineural hearing loss:

Trichothiodystrophy
Mitochondrial disorders
Peroxisomal biogenesis disorders

Data from Barkovich AJ, Patay Z. Metabolic, toxic, and inflammatory brain disorders. In: Barkovich AJ, editor. Pediatric neuroimaging. Philadelphia: Lippincott Williams & Wilkins; 2012. p. 81–239.

MBP resides in this region suggests a mechanism for the developmental disabilities experienced by these patients. There is an appearance of delayed myelination that is only visible to the naked eye on the T2-weighted images in the deep/subcortical white matter. The myelination pattern resembles an infant aged 1 to 1.5 years and does not progress beyond this point (**Fig. 5**).[34,35] Although the appearance suggests that haploinsufficiency of MBP is the sole explanation for delayed

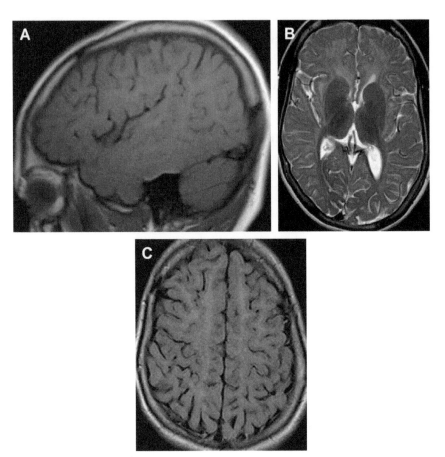

Fig. 4. Fourteen-year-old boy with classic Pelizaeus-Merzbacher disease, diagnosed after nystagmus noticed at 4 months of age. Although there is some myelination visible on sagittal T1-weighted imaging (A), the myelination resembles that of an infant on axial T2-weighted imaging (B). The degree of abnormality is particularly conspicuous on the fluid attenuated inversion recovery image (C), which demonstrates diffuse white matter hyperintensity resembling a T1-weighted image.

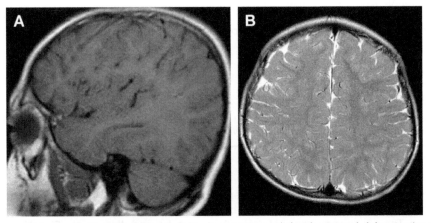

Fig. 5. Six-year-old boy with 18q22 deletion cleft lip, hypotonia, and developmental delay. Notice the normal myelination pattern on the sagittal T1-weighted image (A) but poor deep/subcortical white matter myelination on axial T2-weighted imaging (B).

myelination on T2-weighted images, an autopsy of a patient with 18q deletion syndrome found that the myelin sheaths were grossly intact on electron microscopy and myelin-sensitive stains.[36]

Free Sialic Acid Storage Disorders

Free sialic acid storage disorders are autosomal recessive disorders in which the transporter responsible for egress of sialic acid from lysosomes, sialin encoded by *SLC17A5* (6q13), is defective.[37] As a result, sialic acid builds up in lysosomes and spills into the circulation, where it is eventually excreted into urine. Three forms are recognized, in increasing severity: Salla disease largely as a result of a single point mutation endemic to Finland; an intermediate severity Salla disease; and infantile free sialic storage disease.[38] To avoid confusion with another disorder that lacks severe central nervous system (CNS) involvement and is caused by a separate enzyme, the term sialuria is avoided here.[39] The mild Salla form of the disease presents in early infancy with developmental delays, hypotonia evolving to spasticity, ataxia, and nystagmus; near normal life spans have been reported. The infantile form is more severe with cardiomegaly, hepatomegaly, and even prenatal symptoms of hydrops. MR imaging of the brain in patients with free sialic acid storage resembles PMD in that brain myelination appears arrested with a pattern resembling a child who is a few months old with thinning of the corpus callosum (**Fig. 6**); more severely affected patients appear even more immature and have some cerebellar volume loss.[40,41] The histologic basis of this

MR imaging appearance is unclear. MR spectroscopy has demonstrated increased *N*-acetylaspartate (NAA) levels in patients with Salla disease attributed to overlap from sialic acid metabolites, an MR spectroscopy appearance consistently described for only 1 other disorder (Canavan disease).[42] Although often labeled sialuria, recent reports suggest that mild forms of Salla disease with arrested myelination can have normal urine sialic levels, something that should be considered during the workup of a patient with global myelination delay.[43]

Fucosidosis

Fucosidosis is an autosomal recessive lysosomal disorder caused by mutations in the α-L-fucosidase-1 gene *FUCA1* (1p34). Patients present either in the first year of life or shortly thereafter with intellectual and motor regression, eventually leading to spastic quadraparesis. Coarse facial features similar to mucopolysaccharidoses are also noted.[44] The imaging appearance is predominantly a nonspecific pattern of delayed myelination, but more pronounced periventricular signal increase has also been reported. Another characteristic finding is that of T2 hypointensity in the globus pallidus with variable increase in signal between the medial/lateral lamina of the globus pallidus and the medullary lamina of the thalamus (**Fig. 7**).[44–46] Although the hypointensity of the deep gray matter bears some superficial resemblance to the gangliosidoses and Krabbe disease discussed later, these 2 disorders lack the generalized myelination delay pattern, and

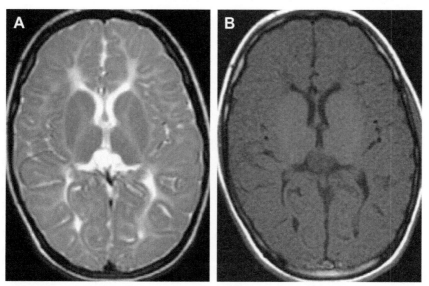

Fig. 6. Seven-year-old girl with developmental delay and Salla disease diagnosed at 3 years of age. Axial T2-weighted (*A*) and T1-weighted (*B*) images demonstrate absence of normal myelination.

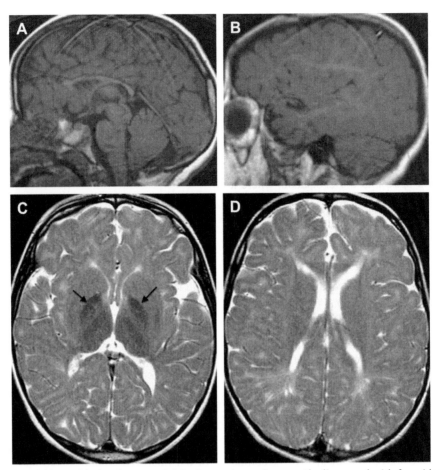

Fig. 7. Five-year-old boy with developmental delay/regression, subsequently diagnosed with fucosidosis. Sagittal T1-weighted images (*A, B*) demonstrate a thin corpus callosum and grossly normal myelination on T1-weighted imaging. Axial T2-weighted images (*C, D*) demonstrate hypointensity of the globus pallidus (*arrows*) for age with global decrease in myelination. Some of the periventricular white matter has increased T2 signal greater than hypomyelination, suggestive of gliosis. Cerebellar volume is intact.

they also have more pronounced basal ganglia hyperintensity. MR spectroscopy is also unique in fucosidase reflecting buildup of fucose with a doublet at 1.2 ppm and 3.4 to 3.8 ppm.[47,48]

Other Disorders with Delayed/Arrested Myelination

Additional monogenic disorders with delayed myelination have been reported. One of these disorders has been dubbed Pelizaeus-Merzbacher like disease (PMLD) and is caused by autosomal recessive mutations in *GJA12/GJC2* (1q42), a gap junction protein.[49,50] Other hypomyelinating disorders that have also been suggested as being Pelizaeus-Merzbacher like include a deletion syndrome involving heat shock protein *HSPD1*,[51] an X-linked deficiency in CNS thyroid transport due to *MCT8*,[52] and a hypomyelinating disorder

caused by mutations in the tRNA synthesis and signaling protein *AIMP1/p43*.[53] The latter 2 disorders could be questioned as PMLDs because they feature some catchup myelination and microcephaly, respectively. Other hypomyelinating disorders are associated with distinctive clinical features: hypodontia and hypogonadism with the so-called 4H syndrome due to RNA polymerase III subunits *POLR3A/B*[54,55]; brittle hair and ichthyosis in the trichothiodystrophies seen with defects in 1 of at least 4 DNA repair enzymes[56]; hypomyelination with congenital cataracts (HCC) caused by mutations in *FAM126A* (7p21)[57]; and deep gray matter and cerebellar atrophy in hypomyelination with atrophy of the basal ganglia and cerebellum (H-ABC) recently mapped to mutations in *TUBB4A* (19p13).[58,59] Another disorder that can present as arrested myelination is nonketotic hyperglycinemia (deficiency of components of the glycine cleavage system at 3p21, 9p24, 16q23).[60] This disorder exhibits restricted diffusion at sites of myelination at the time of imaging (eg, posterior limb of internal capsule and central tegmental tracts at the classic neonatal presentation)[61,62] and exhibits a characteristic glycine peak on MR spectroscopy at 3.56 ppm, suggesting the diagnosis.[10,63,64] An analysis of several hypomyelinating disorders has identified some unique features that may suggest a specific hypomyelinating disorder.[45] For example, 4H syndrome is distinguished from PMD, PMLD, and HCC by myelination of the optic radiations and posterior limb of the internal capsule with cerebellar atrophy and prominent T2 hypointensity of the ventrolateral thalamus (Fig. 8). As explained later under pattern 3 Cockayne syndrome clearly presents as generalized arrest in myelination for many patients, but other patterns can be observed.

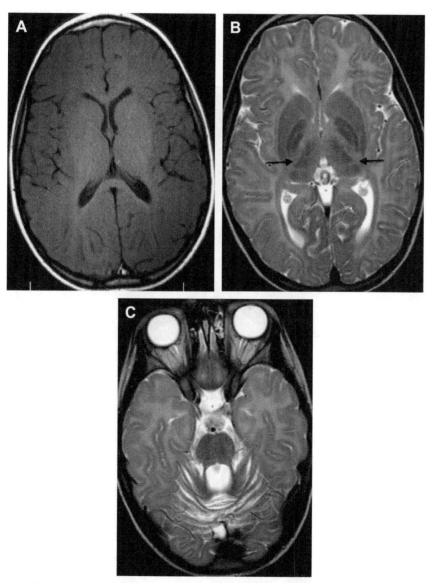

Fig. 8. Five-year-old girl with failure of incisor eruption, motor delay, and (subsequently) delayed puberty. Later diagnosed with 4H syndrome. Although there is global delay of myelination, there is myelination of the posterior limb of the internal capsule on axial T1-weighted images (A) and the optic radiations in both axial T1-weighted and T2-weighted images (A, B). There is characteristic hypointensity of the ventrolateral thalamus on axial T2-weighted images (B, arrows) and volume loss of the cerebellum (C). Hypointensity of the globus pallidus is an inconsistent feature for this disorder.

PATTERN 2: SUBCORTICAL WHITE MATTER PREDOMINANT SIGNAL ABNORMALITY

Although T2 hyperintensity in both the subcortical white matter and gray matter structures is a feature of several disorders (see later discussion), abnormalities concentrated in the subcortical white matter only are relatively uncommon.

Galactosemia

Galactosemia is caused by autosomal recessive mutation in 1 of 3 genes: galactokinase or *GALK* (17q24), galactose galactose-1-phosphate uridyl-transfersase or *GALT* (9p13), or UDP-galactose-4-epimerase known as *GALE* (1p36). The most common form is the classic or type 1 galactosemia caused by *GALT* deficiency, which leads to buildup of galactose-1-phosphate and upstream metabolites such as galactitol.[65] The disease manifests on milk feedings with failure to thrive, poor feeding, lethargy, liver dysfunction, and eventually signs of cerebral edema. Even with institution of a lactose-depleted diet, neurologic sequela are common and include diminished intellectual achievement and decline, delayed speech, and cerebellar signs (ataxia, coordination problems).[66] The MR imaging findings resemble that of delayed terminal myelination with poor myelination in the subcortical white matter on T2-weighted imaging but grossly normal myelination on T1-weighted imaging (**Fig. 9**), corresponding to myelin pallor on pathologic examination.[67]

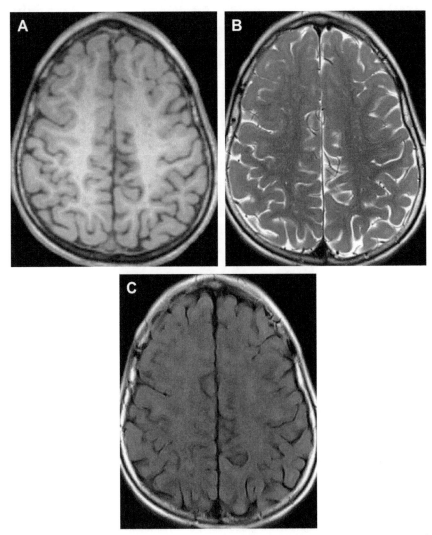

Fig. 9. Eight-year-old girl with galactosemia. Although the axial T1-weighted images suggest normal myelination (*A*), there is poor gray-white matter differentiation on the axial T2-weighted images (*B*) suggesting diffuse poor myelination of the subcortical white matter. These signal abnormalities are more conspicuous on the axial fluid attenuated inversion recovery images (*C*) where there is patchy signal increase.

However, the subcortical white matter often appears slightly heterogeneous on fluid attenuated inversion recovery (FLAIR) images, which is not expected for delayed myelination alone. Hyperintensity on T2-weighted imaging is lower in signal intensity than seen in other leukodystrophies with subcortical white matter predominance. MR spectroscopy can be helpful in securing a diagnosis as untreated patients are reported to have prominent galactitol peaks, a finding that resolves with initiation of a galactose-free diet.[68,69]

Megalencephalic Leukoencephalopathy with Subcortical Cysts

Megalencephalic leukoencephalopathy with subcortical cyst (MLC) is a rare disorder originally characterized as an autosomal recessive disorder secondary to mutations in *MLC1* (22q13), a transmembrane protein involved in regulation of cellular water balance.[70,71] The resulting disorder is interesting for minimal initial symptoms other than large head size when patients present during infancy. However, patients eventually manifest slight delay in achieving motor milestones as well as mild cognitive delay. After a period of several years, there is usually deterioration in motor (ataxia, spasticity) and cognitive function as well as a high incidence of seizures. Imaging findings include expansile T2 signal abnormality in the subcortical and deep white matter, sparing the most central/periventricular white matter and the occipital white matter. There is associated cystic change in the subcortical white matter in the temporal lobes and to a lesser extent, the frontoparietal lobes (**Fig. 10**).[72] Over time, atrophy ensues. Although this scenario accounts for approximately 75% of patients with MLC, a small group of patients with similar imaging findings lack *MLC1* mutations and have milder clinical and imaging phenotypes (eg, fewer or no cysts, abating white matter changes). Recently,

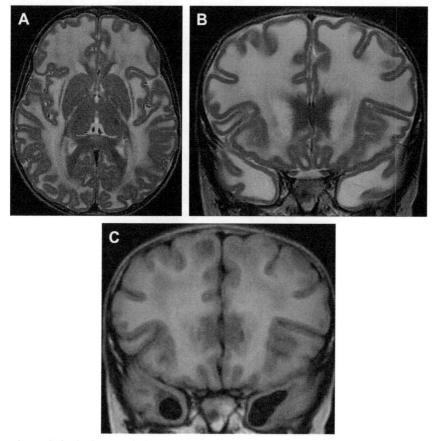

Fig. 10. Megalencephalic leukoencephalopathy with cysts in a 3-year-old child with >97th percentile head circumference and frequent falls/imbalance. Notice the expansile white matter signal abnormality greatest in the frontal lobes on the axial and coronal T2-weighted images (*A, B*). In the temporal lobes there is cystic degeneration best seen on the coronal FLAIR image (*C*).

autosomal dominant mutations in a trafficking protein for MLC1 known as *HEPACAM* were identified as 1 cause for this milder phenotype.[73]

Aicardi-Goutières Syndrome

Aicardi-Goutières syndrome (AGS) was originally described as a pseudo-TORCH syndrome affecting multiple members of a single family without evidence of an inciting infection and has since been recognized in other individuals.[74,75] The patients most often present in early infancy with irritability, sterile pyrexia, truncal hypotonia, extremity spasticity, and cognitive disability proportionate to the progressive microcephaly that is often present.[76] To date, mutations in 6 different genes have been identified that account for approximately 90% of cases of AGS: *TREX1* (3p21),[77] *RNASEH2A-C* (19p13, 13q14, and 11q13),[78] *SAMHD1* (20q11),[79] and *ADAR1*

(1q21).[80] Although there can be some variability in severity of disease for any given AGS mutation,[81] *TREX1* mutations generally have more severe (neonatal) disease, whereas *RNASEH2B* typically have milder phenotypes.[82] Mutations in these genes trigger an activated immune response with increased CSF interferon-α and neopterin levels as well as histopathology suggesting small vessel vasculopathy and leptomeningitis, findings presumed related to the role the AGS gene products play in metabolizing DNA and RNA strands that can trigger an antiviral response.[76,83–85] Imaging evaluation of patients with AGS is notable for subcortical white matter signal abnormality, frontal/temporal pole predominance, and cystic change in patients with early (<3 months) onset of symptoms (**Fig. 11**).[86] All patients with AGS have parenchymal calcifications, primarily in the putamen but also within the dentate nucleus and deep white matter. Although atrophy is almost

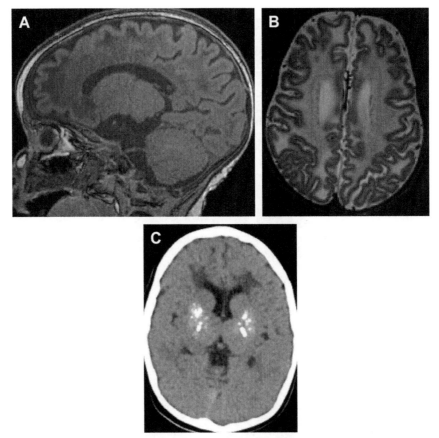

Fig. 11. Presumed case of Aicardi-Goutières syndrome in a patient with microcephaly, hypotonia, developmental delay, and increased CSF neopterin levels. Sagittal T1 (*A*) and axial T2 (*B*) MR imaging images at 5 months demonstrate white matter signal abnormality concentrated in the subcortical region, particularly in the frontal lobes. Computed tomography images from the same patient at 2 years of age (*C*) demonstrate basal ganglia calcifications.

universally present, it was progressive in only a third of the cases from the largest case series so far, possibly reflecting extent of disease at the time of imaging.

PATTERN 3: CENTRAL WHITE MATTER PREDOMINANT SIGNAL ABNORMALITY, WITH OR WITHOUT BRAINSTEM INVOLVEMENT
X-linked Adrenoleukodystrophy

Adrenoleukodystrophy (ALD) is an X-linked recessive disorder caused by mutations of the *ABCD1* gene (Xq28), a peroxisomal membrane transporter required for catabolism of very long chain fatty acids (VLCFA). As a result, there is buildup of VLCFAs detectable in the serum and a related inflammatory demyelination of the brain and atrophy of the adrenal glands.[87,88] In children, the disorder typically manifests in 5- to 10-year-old boys as a mild cognitive (learning) disorder or hyperactivity followed by progressive dementia and loss of motor function leading to quadraparesis. Most children will also have accompanying adrenal insufficiency at some point in their illness including the skin bronzing typical of corticotrophin hypersecretion, and a subset of patients present with adrenal symptoms only.[89,90] These childhood cases have a unique 3-layered pattern of cerebral white matter involvement concentrated in the parietooccipital lobes, classically first involving the splenium: a T2 hyperintense peripheral region of T2 hyperintensity corresponding to zone A where active demyelination occurs; an enhancing and diffusion-restricting rim called zone B where active inflammation occurs; and a central zone C with T2 hyperintensity corresponding only to gliosis at pathology (**Fig. 12**).[91] Although highly characteristic of ALD, a similar imaging appearance can be rarely encountered with mutations in a peroxisomal fatty acid enzyme, acyl-coenzyme A oxidase 1 *ACOX1* (17q25),[92] Recent work has shown that mild mutations in peroxisomal genes other than *ABCD1* can also have similar appearances (T2 hyperintensity of posterior periventricular white matter, splenium, dentate, superior cerebellar peduncle) even in the presence of seemingly normal peroxisomal serum metabolites.[93] Although this pattern is fairly well known for childhood ALD, it is less widely known that half of ALD patients present in adulthood with milder symptoms that typically manifest as lower extremity paresis, bowel/bladder dysfunction, and (in most cases) Addisonian symptoms. Only about half of these adult patients have brain MR imaging abnormalities with greatest signal abnormality in long tracts (including corticospinal tract) of the brainstem (adrenomyeloneuropathy

and portions of the cerebellum.[94,95] Other less common patterns of ALD include a frontal-predominant variant.[96]

Mucopolysaccharidoses

The mucopolysaccharidoses (MPS) are a collection of disorders caused by failed intralysosomal breakdown of various glycosaminoglycan molecules attached to proteoglycans (glycosylated proteins). Currently classified into 6 major subgroups depending on the specific enzyme (I, II, III, IV, VI, and VII), they are all transmitted in a recessive fashion although type II Hunter disease is X-linked. MPS types I, II, III, and VII are notable for their predominance of CNS morbidity, whereas types IV and VI (Morquio and Maroteaux-Lamy, respectively) feature more predominant musculoskeletal abnormalities, including spine abnormalities such as congenital kyphosis or stenosis from dural thickening. Among the CNS-predominant MPS variants, there is a wide spectrum of disability varying from normal intelligence in MPS I-S Scheie disease to severe mental retardation in MPS IH Hurler and MPS IIA Hunter forms of the disease. Associated abnormalities of the different mucopolysaccharidoses include facial dysmorphism, extremity contractures, corneal clouding, airway obstruction, hepatosplenomegaly, dural thickening, and hydrocephalus; these symptoms are attributed to abnormal deposit of glycosaminoglycans in patient tissues.[97,98] On brain imaging, patients with MPS typically have generalized decrease in gray/white matter differentiation, attributed to dysmyelination and faint diffuse increase in the T2 signal of the cerebral white matter.[99–104] This finding, as well as that of more pronounced T2 hyperintensity in the periventricular white matter, is fairly nonspecific. However, cystic enlargement of the perivascular spaces (particularly posteriorly) can be extremely conspicuous in the cerebral white matter and corpus callosum (approximately two-thirds of patients according to available case series[101,102,104]), suggesting the diagnosis of MPS. This spectrum of white matter disease in MPS is illustrated in **Fig. 13**. Intuitively, worsening white matter signal abnormality, volume loss, and nonspecific MR spectroscopy findings are found to correlate with worse cognitive impairment in at least some patients with MPS.[103,105]

Lowe Syndrome (Oculocerebrorenal Syndrome)

Lowe syndrome is a rare disorder caused by X-linked recessive mutation in an inositol polyphosphate 5-phosphatase encoded by *ORCL1*

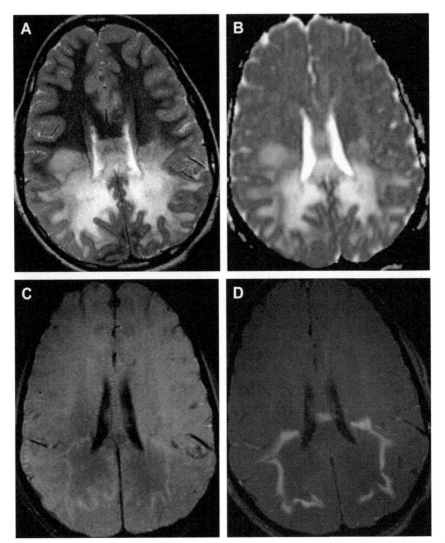

Fig. 12. Childhood X-linked adrenoleukodystrophy in a 10-year-old boy presenting with vomiting. The axial T2 image (A) demonstrates parietooccipital central white matter signal abnormality involving the posterior corpus callosum. Within this signal abnormality, there is a subtle hypointense band of white matter corresponding to faint restricted diffusion on the axial apparent diffusion coefficient diffusion maps (B) and enhancement after contrast injection (C, D precontrast and postcontrast axial T1 with fat saturation). This band of enhancement corresponds histologically to zone B, the inflammatory zone. The demyelinating zone A is peripheral and the gliotic zone C is deep to zone B.

(Xq28).[106,107] Affected patients have congenital cataracts and hypotonia with varying levels of mental retardation. There is eventual development of proteinuria (Fanconi syndrome) and frequently glaucoma also.[108] Although known cases number less than 200, the distinctive clinical findings and MR imaging findings make imaging diagnosis possible. Specifically, there is an unusual combination of periventricular signal increase with interspersed dilated perivascular spaces[109–111] although we have encountered molecularly confirmed instances of this disorder without the latter feature (**Fig. 14**). Elevated peaks at 3.56 ppm have been detected in these patients, possibly representing a phosphatidyl inositol 4,5-biphosphate resonance as opposed to the myoinositol peak normally located at this position.[112,113]

X-linked Charcot-Marie-Tooth

X-linked Charcot-Marie-Tooth (CMTX1) is an X-linked dominant form of Charcot-Marie-Tooth disease, a group of peripheral neuropathies. The

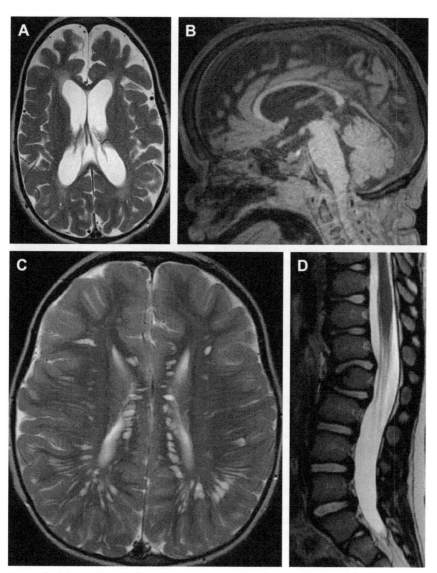

Fig. 13. Spectrum of white matter findings in mucopolysaccharidoses. MPS 1H Hurler in a 6-year-old girl with declining speech production and weakness: Mild ventriculomegaly, poor gray-white differentiation, and nonspecific periventricular white matter signal increase are noted on the axial T2-weighted image (*A*). Sagittal T1 image of the same patient (*B*) demonstrates frontal bossing, J-shaped sella, and crowding of the cervicocranial junction. MPS II Hunter in a 4-year-old boy. Axial T2-weighted image (*C*) demonstrates dilated perivascular spaces and sagittal T2 spine; (*D*) demonstrates a gibbus deformity.

disease is caused by mutations in the *CX32* gene, which encodes a neuronal gap junction protein.[114] Clinical symptoms typically manifest in the first few decades of life as a lower extremity predominant polyneuropathy with symptoms such as sensory loss, ankle drop, pes cavus, and muscle atrophy (eg, calf muscles and intrinsic hand muscles).[115] These symptoms are slowly progressive but do not seem to significantly diminish life expectancy.[116] Patients with CMTX come to

radiologists' attention for occasional periods of focal neurologic deterioration after minor stressors (infection, trauma, high altitude) featuring weakness, ataxia, and even cranial nerve deficits. These symptoms often trigger a stroke evaluation. Symmetric deep white matter and callosal (splenial) T2 hyperintensity and restricted diffusion seen on MR imaging during episodes of acute deterioration suggests a toxic/metabolic cause rather than an infarction. There is spontaneous resolution of the

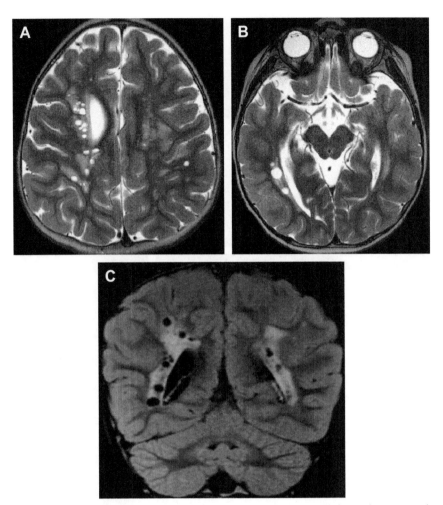

Fig. 14. Four-year-old with Lowe syndrome (seizure, Fanconi syndrome, cataracts). Axial T2 images (*A, B*) and coronal FLAIR (*C*) demonstrate periventricular signal abnormality with interspersed areas of cystic change. Note the lens prostheses in *B* from previous cataract surgery.

clinical symptoms and the MR imaging findings, the latter supporting myelin vacuolization rather than cytotoxic injury as the basis of the observed restricted diffusion (see **Fig. 3**).[117–119] Therefore, radiologists should be aware of this diagnosis because the imaging appearance is highly unusual in patients without toxin exposure, and clinical correlation (eg, symptoms in relatives, pes cavus deformity) can help establish the diagnosis of what is a fairly benign disorder.

Cockayne Syndrome

Cockayne syndrome (CS) is an autosomal recessive disorder resulting from mutations in 1 of 2 nucleotide excision repair genes, *ERCC8* (5q11, CS genetic complementation group A) and *ERCC6* (10q11, CS complementation group B);

these 2 complementation groups account for 35% and 65% of CS cases, respectively. Mutations in either 1 of these genes can present with 1 of the 4 recognized clinical subtypes of CS (in decreasing order of severity): cerebro-oculo-facial syndrome (COFS), type II CS, type I CS, and type III CS. For COFS, there is in utero growth restriction and arthrgryposis with early demise. For the mildest type III CS, the symptoms may not manifest until early childhood and survival to adulthood is reported.[120] Although patient who present later with CS achieve more milestones and may be initially minimally cognitively impaired, all CS subtypes proceed to deterioration/regression with associated sensorimotor disturbances (truncal hypotonia, extremity spasticity, sensorineural hearing loss). Failure to thrive (cachectic dwarfism) is also a universal symptom in these patients. Surprisingly, cancer is not a dominant feature.[121]

Although classified as a disorder of global myelination delay by many investigators, more recent data suggest a wider variation in appearance. Specifically, recent papers suggest that milder forms of CS may have patchy deep and periventricular white matter with sparing of the subcortical white matter.[122] They also suggest that bouts of active demyelination may occur in the subcortical white matter as manifested by restricted diffusion and focal edema.[123] Regardless of the pattern of the white matter abnormality, the degree of parenchymal volume loss is generally more severe in patients with more severe clinical subtypes of CS (eg, affecting the posterior fossa and brainstem in infancy), and it also tends to progress with time as one would expect.[122,124] The calcifications have greatest propensity for the putamen followed by caudate, dentate, and cerebral white matter.[122] In addition to differences in distribution of the white matter signal abnormality, some investigators have noted that AGS-related calcifications have a less homogeneous appearance than seen in CS.[124] A typical case of CS is shown in **Fig. 15.**

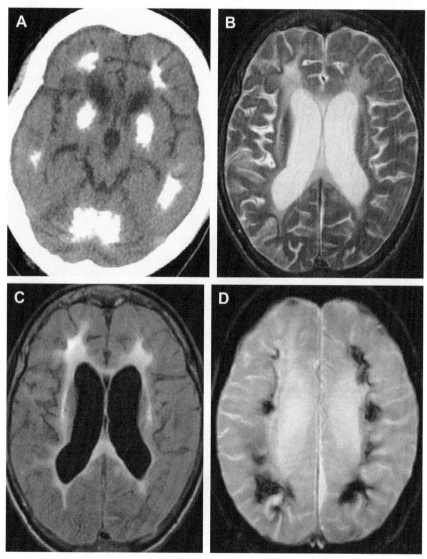

Fig. 15. Twenty-eight year old with Cockayne syndrome. Computed tomography of the head (*A*) demonstrates homogeneous coarse calcification of the basal ganglia, cerebral white matter, and cerebellar white matter. MR imaging of the brain demonstrates volume loss with central white matter signal increase on the axial T2 (*B*) and FLAIR (*C*) sequences. The T2* gradient recalled echo sequence (*D*) also demonstrates white matter calcification.

Leukoencephalopathy with Brainstem and Spinal Cord Involvement and Increased Lactate

Leukoencephalopathy with brainstem and spinal cord involvement and increased lactate (LBSL) is an autosomal recessive disorder caused by mutation in *DARS2*, a mitochondrial aspartyl-tRNA synthetase encoded on chromosome 1 (1q25).[125,126] Clinically, the disease manifests in late childhood with progressive ataxia and spasticity as well as impaired dorsal column function (eg, proprioception). Although exceedingly rare, this disorder does have a highly characteristic pattern of signal abnormality that allows it to be recognized on MR imaging and was used to define the disease entity (Fig. 16): patchy central white matter T2 hyperintensity sparing the subcortical U fibers with involvement of the dorsal/lateral columns of the spinal cord, medullary pyramids, and at least 1 minor location (splenium of the corpus callosum, medial lemniscus, spinocerebellar tracts in medulla, superior and inferior cerebellar peduncles, cerebellar white matter, parenchymal trigeminal nerve, and trigeminal tracts). Lactate on MR spectroscopy is almost always increased.[127] Restricted diffusion has been observed in some of the T2 hyperintense lesions.[128] The pattern of long tract involvement and deep gray structure sparing set this disease apart from leukoencephalopathies such as maple syrup urine disease (MSUD) and Krabbe disease (see later discussion) as well as inflammatory disorders such as acute disseminated encephalomyelitis. However, more severe infantile cases with genetic confirmation have been reported to involve the white matter more extensively and even extend into the globus pallidus, making imaging recognition of the disorder more challenging in this age group.[129] Also, LBSL has similarities to a recently described disorder, hypomyelination with brainstem and spinal cord involvement (HBSL), caused by the cytosolic aspartyl-tRNA synthetase *DARS*.[130] White matter involvement in HBSL appears more homogeneous than LBSL and can extend to the subcortical white matter.

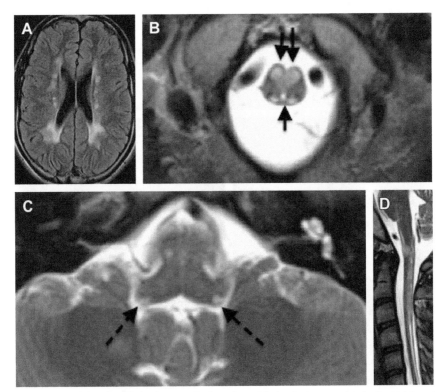

Fig. 16. Seventeen-year-old girl with leukoencephalopathy with brainstem and spinal cord involvement and increased lactate. Axial FLAIR image (*A*) demonstrates patchy central white matter signal increase. Axial T2-weighted images (*B, C*) demonstrate abnormal signal in the dorsal columns (*single arrow*), medullary pyramids (*double arrow*), and inferior cerebellar peduncle (*dashed arrows*). Dorsal column involvement is also visible on the sagittal T2 image of the cervical spine (*D*).

Other Leukodystrophies with Central White Matter Involvement

The pattern 3 diseases discussed thus far have unusual patterns of signal abnormality that make a specific diagnosis feasible. However, it is more common to encounter leukodystrophies with nonspecific periventricular and deep white matter signal increase. Some diseases in this category are illustrated in **Fig. 17**.

Metachromatic leukodystrophy (MLD) is perhaps the most common of these diseases, caused by mutations affecting ARSA or arylsulfatase A (22q13) with similar appearances seen in multiple sulfatase deficiency and saposin B deficiency.[131–134] Late infantile, juvenile, and adult onset forms of the disease are recognized; late infantile presentation is the most common (majority).[135,136] MLD forms all share progressive neurologic deterioration after an initial period of normalcy. In the late infantile form, this manifests as loss of milestones, hypotonia, and eventual cognitive impairment with spastic quadriparesis. The imaging manifestation is confluent signal abnormality in the deep and periventricular white matter with sparing of subcortical U fibers until the end stage of the disease.[137,138] The diagnosis may be suggested by cranial nerve or cauda equina enhancement, which is not commonly seen with other leukodystrophies.[10,139] Although

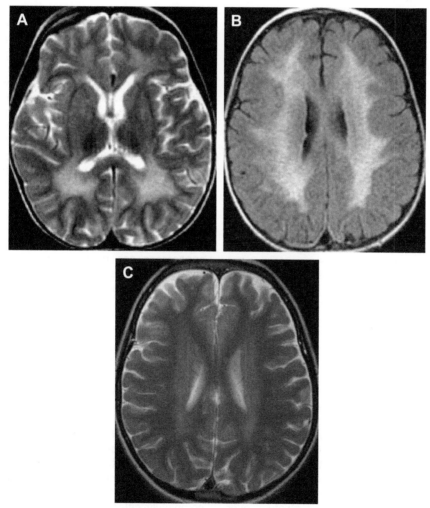

Fig. 17. Additional leukodystrophies with central white matter predominance. Three-year-old with metachromatic leukodystrophy, axial Fluid attenuated inversion recovery (FLAIR) (A) and T2 (B) images. Notice the sparing of the subcortical white matter and confluent appearance of the signal abnormality. Faint tigroid sparing can be seen along the perivascular spaces, particular on the FLAIR image. Neuronal ceroid lipofuscinosis typically presents as gray matter volume loss, but central white matter signal increase can occasionally be detected as in this axial T2 image of a 5-year-old girl with CLN8 (C).

some investigators believe that a tigroid sparing of the perivascular spaces of the affected white matter is characteristic for this disorder, there is pathologic and imaging evidence of such sparing in other leukodystrophies.[140–145]

Other disorders that primarily involve the central white matter include phenylketonuria (deficient phenylalanine hydroxylase, 12q23),[146,147] Sjögren-Larsson syndrome (deficient fatty aldehyde dehydrogenase, 17p11),[148] and hyperhomocysteinemia (multiple responsible enzymatic deficiencies).[149,150] MR spectroscopy can assist with detection of some of these disorders: Sjögren-Larsson has 0.9/1.3 ppm peaks that do not suppress at long TE.[151] Although the neuronal ceroid lipofuscinoses can be classified primarily as disorders of gray matter (cortical atrophy and deep gray hypointensity), deep/periventricular white matter signal abnormalities are seen in some of the 9 neuronal ceroid lipofuscinosis variants, mimicking other diseases discussed in this section.[152,153] Mild forms of vanishing white matter disease (autosomal recessive deficiency in 1 of 5 translation initiation factors, EIFB1-5)[154,155] can initially manifest as nonspecific central white matter signal increase.[156] The evolution to diffuse white matter involvement with cavitation eventually points to vanishing white matter disease, as does the characteristic history of stress-provoked worsening of ataxia/spasticity.

PATTERN 4: COMBINATIONS OF GRAY AND WHITE MATTER SIGNAL ABNORMALITY
Canavan Disease

Canavan disease is an autosomal recessive disorder caused by deficiency of aspartoacylase or *ASPA* (17pter-17p13), an enzyme responsible for degrading NAA.[157–159] The most common presentation is macrocephaly, hypotonia, and irritability before 6 months of age followed by spasticity, blindness, and (in some cases) seizures. The findings are attributed to buildup of NAA (both in the brain and peripherally in urine), a substance believed to cause spongiform changes of white matter as a result of osmotic shifts or impaired myelin synthesis.[160–162] Imaging findings of infantile Canavan disease are distinctive, featuring extensive subcortical white matter signal increase and appearance of mild gyral swelling as well as (almost invariably) globus pallidus T2 signal increase with sparing of the corpus striatum; over time, the white matter signal abnormality becomes more extensive and atrophy ensues (see **Fig. 2**). Occasionally, the brainstem and dentate nucleus may be involved.[163–165] Attenuated severity or atypical imaging patterns (eg, corpus striatum

involvement) have been observed in mild cases of Canavan disease presenting later in childhood.[166–168] Typically, there is some restricted diffusion in the areas of signal abnormality resulting from intramyelinic edema believed to be caused by accumulation of NAA within neurons and increased water migration from the axon into the periaxonal space. Although these findings may resemble some other leukodystrophies (see L-2-hydroxyglutaric aciduria later), the macrocephaly and MR spectroscopy suggest the diagnosis. Specifically, there is a marked increase in NAA in Canavan disease,[169,170] a unique MR spectroscopy finding characteristic of Canavan and Salla diseases.

L-2-Hydroxyglutaric Aciduria

L-2-Hydroxyglutaric aciduria (L2HGA) results from autosomal recessive mutations in the mitochondrial enzyme L-2-hydroxyglutaric acid dehydrogenase (14q22); buildup of L-2-hydroxyglutaric acid results.[171] L2HGA typically presents in early childhood as motor delay and mild to severe mental retardation followed by progressive cerebellar dysfunction (ataxia) and movement disorder (tremor, choreoathetosis); seizure and macrocephaly are present in some patients.[172] MR imaging findings are distinctive if not pathognomonic. According to the largest review of L2HGA cases so far published, virtually all patients had T2 signal increase within the subcortical white matter (multifocal and frontal predominant initially), dentate nucleus, and basal ganglia (initially peripheral in the corpus striatum).[173] Although a similar appearance can be seen in Canavan disease and Kearns-Sayre (a mitochondrial disorder), the consistent presence of dentate signal abnormality and absence of brainstem involvement distinguishes L2HGA from these other possibilities (**Fig. 18**).[171,174] Isocitrate dehydrogenase (*IDH1/2*) mutations in low-grade gliomas, secondary glioblastomas, and leukemia are known to cause buildup of 2-hydroxyglutaric acid enantiomers. Although there does seem to be an association between L2HGA and primary brain tumors,[175] recent evidence suggests that the basis of IDH-related growth dysregulation is actually production of the *R/D*-2-hydroxyglutarate isomer.[176,177] Although similar sounding, D-2-hydroxyglutaric aciduria (deficiency of D-2 hydroxyglutaric acid dehydrogenase, 2q37) has a completely different and somewhat nonspecific imaging pattern: marked lateral ventriculomegaly and germinolytic cysts with delayed gyration and myelination.[178] Because of interest in using 2-hydroxyglutarate as a biomarker for IDH mutation−bearing gliomas, MR spectroscopy

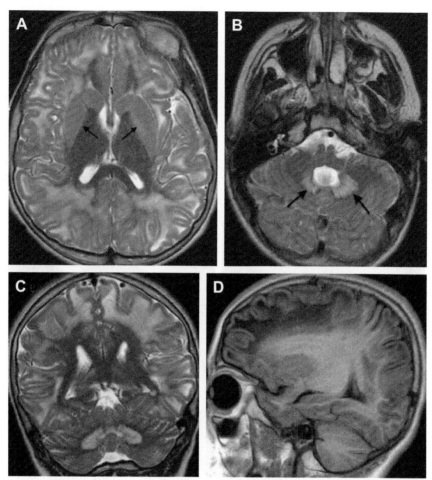

Fig. 18. L-2-hydroxyglutaric aciduria in a 13-year-old boy. Axial T2-weighted (*A, B*), coronal T2-weighted (*C*) and sagittal T1-weighted (*D*) images demonstrate subcortical white matter signal abnormality, frontal predominant and sparing the central white matter. There is also peripheral corpus striatum and dentate nucleus signal increase (*arrows*).

techniques have been developed for the detection of 2-hydroxyglutarate and may eventually become available for analysis of L2HGA also.[179,180]

Alexander Disease

Alexander disease is an autosomal dominant disorder caused by missense mutations in glial fibrillary acidic protein *GFAP* (17q21).[181–183] Mutations in this protein are believed to decrease GFAP solubility and trigger formation of inclusion bodies such as the Rosenthal fibers seen under the microscope in this disorder, leading to accumulation of abnormal astrocytes and myelin pallor throughout affected brain tissue.[184–186] Historically, 3 forms of Alexander disease are recognized: infantile with typical presentation before 6 months of age (51% of cases); juvenile (23% of cases); and adult

(24% of cases).[187] As with the other leukodystrophies discussed, the earlier onset forms are associated with more severe symptoms. The typical infantile form presents with macrocephaly, failure to thrive, difficulty swallowing, loss of intellectual/motor milestones, lower extremity weakness, ataxia, seizures, and occasionally hydrocephalus. The juvenile and adult forms are dominated more by ataxia and bulbar/pseudobulbar symptoms as well as the seizures and lower extremity weakness seen in the infantile form; a small percentage of the juvenile but not adult patients also have macrocephaly.[182,187,188] Typical imaging characteristics include frontal-predominant subcortical to periventricular white matter T2 hyperintensity with swelling of the overlying gyri; swelling of the fornix and optic nerves; periventricular areas of T1/T2 shortening; deep gray matter signal increase or atrophy; dentate hilum signal increase; brainstem (midbrain/medulla) signal increase; and enhancement of involved areas (Fig. 19). Progression to atrophy and occasionally white matter cavitation are common. These findings have been summarized in criteria designed to facilitate diagnosis using MR imaging in infantile and juvenile Alexander disease.[189] However, atypical presentations of Alexander disease (eg, posterior fossa and brainstem-predominant forms including some with tumefactive changes or a ventricular garland) have been recognized, particularly in juvenile forms of the disease.[18,190] Adult cases seem to be distinct in appearance, featuring primarily brainstem and cord atrophy with signal abnormality.[191,192]

GM1/GM2 Gangliosidoses (Tay-Sachs, Sandhoff Disease)

Gangliosides are minor myelin constituents that are composed of a glycosphingolipid (ceramide lipid bound to an oligosaccharide) and at least 1 sialic acid molecule. Autosomal recessive defects

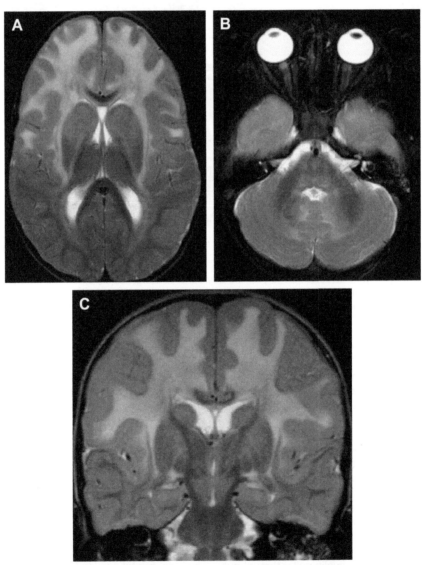

Fig. 19. Five-year-old child with Alexander disease. Axial (A, B) and coronal T2-weighted (C) images of the brain demonstrate expansile frontal subcortical white matter signal abnormality extending to the ventricle and signal increase within the basal ganglia, to a lesser extent also the brainstem. In the setting of macrocephaly, this appearance is virtually pathognomonic of Alexander disease. Other classic features not demonstrated in this case include enhancing areas of white matter T1/T2 shortening.

in the lysosomal enzymes that turn over the gangliosides lead to gangliosidoses.[188,193] GM1 gangliosidosis is caused by mutations in the lysosomal β-galactosidase *GLB1* (3p21),[194–196] the enzyme that degrades GM1 to GM2. GM2 gangliosidosis is caused by mutations in 1 of 3 gene products that control hexomindinase activity necessary to degrade GM2 to GM3: hexominidase A (15q23),[197–199] hexominidase B (5q13),[200,201] and the GM2 activator protein (5q31).[202–204] The GM2 gangliosidosis caused by hexominidase A deficiency is called Tay-Sachs disease, and the GM2 gangliosidosis caused by hexominidase B deficiency is called Sandhoff disease; hexominidase B forms heterodimers with the A isozyme as well as the B homodimers that have different substrates than the A/B heterodimer. The infantile forms of GM1 and GM2 gangliosidoses share similarities in that hypotonia and psychomotor retardation, early blindness, and peculiar startle responses are common. Eventually these infantile cases progress to spastic quadraparesis, seizures, and early death.[188,205,206] However, the GM1 gangliosidoses are somewhat distinct in that they have the hepatomegaly and kyphoscoliosis that resembles a mucopolysaccharidosis (*GLB1* mutations can cause a form of Morquio syndrome). GM2 gangliosidoses are distinctive for their higher incidence of cherry red maculae and macrocephaly although Sandhoff disease also features hepatosplenomegaly. The adult forms of the GM1/GM2 gangliosidoses are dominated by extrapyramidal symptoms (dystonia, choreoathetosis, ataxia); adult-onset GM2 gangliosidoses also have significant cognitive impairment and psychiatric disease.[204,207,208] The juvenile forms fall in between the infantile and adult forms of the disease.

Despite the differences in biochemistry and symptomatology, the neuroimaging features of the gangliosidoses are very similar. Infantile forms present with thalamic T1/T2 shortening attributed to mineralization and T2 hyperintensity of the basal ganglia. There is diffusely delayed white matter myelination, although myelination is preserved in the internal capsules, corpus callosum, and optic radiations (**Fig. 20**).[209,210] In some cases, the white matter T2 hyperintensity is greater than explained by a simple lack of myelination, a finding attributed to abnormal myelin turnover or demyelination.[188] This constellation of findings is characteristic for infantile GM1/GM2 gangliosidosis, but some unusual variant cases have been published (eg, lack of basal ganglia involvement[211]). Krabbe disease can resemble this disease, but the T2 hyperintensities of the basal ganglia and sparing of the corpus callosum are much less common.[188] Also, the thickening and enhancement of the cranial nerves and cauda equina seen in Krabbe disease is not present in the gangliosidoses. Adult forms of the gangliosidoses are notable primarily for faint diffuse cerebral white matter hyperintensity manifesting as poor gray-white matter

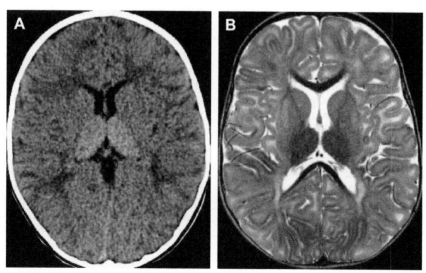

Fig. 20. GM2 gangliosidosis (Sandhoff disease) in a 14-month-old girl with seizures, cherry red macula, and hypotonia. Noncontrast computed tomography of the head (*A*) demonstrates hyperdensity of the thalami and a suggestion of white matter hypodensity. Axial T2 MR imaging of the brain (*B*) demonstrates T2 hypointensity of the thalami corresponding to the computed tomography finding as well as basal ganglia and subcortical white matter signal increase. Note that the internal capsules and corpus callosum remain normal in signal intensity.

differentiation and diffuse brain atrophy.[188] Differences between late-onset GM1 and GM2 include more conspicuous volume loss in the cerebellum for late-onset GM2 gangliosidosis,[207,212,213] and frequent reports of basal ganglia signal increase in late-onset GM1 gangliosidosis.[214,215] Juvenile and late infantile forms of GM1 can have similar appearance to either the infantile or adult onset forms of the disease.[210,216]

Krabbe Disease

Krabbe disease is a disorder caused almost exclusively by autosomal recessive deficiency of the lysosomal enzyme responsible for degrading the myelin constituent cerebroside into galactose and ceramide, β-galactocerebrosidase GALC (14q13).[217–219] The resulting enzyme deficiency leads to buildup of the toxic upstream metabolite psychosine and defective myelin turnover, associated with proliferation of multinucleated giant (globoid) cells and white matter demyelination.[218,220] Most patients (>85%) with Krabbe disease present in infancy, proceeding through 3 recognized stages: irritability, abnormal startle response, temperature dysregulation, and delayed/regressed development (stage I) proceeding to hypertonicity, myoclonus/seizure, and optic atrophy (stage II), then to a vegetative state (stage III).[221] A few patients presenting in childhood or adulthood have milder symptoms (paresis, ataxia, visual loss) with variable progression. Imaging findings are distinctive. On computed tomography, there is increased density in the thalami and more variably in the other deep gray nuclei and other structures of the brain, some of which seem to represent frank calcification.[217,222,223] As the classic presentation occurs at 4 to 6 months of age, affected structures are often normally unmyelinated, which makes it difficult to appreciate signal abnormality on MR imaging.[224] For this reason, some advocate use of quantitative diffusion tensor imaging analysis in early suspected cases.[225,226] However, diagnosis is usually possible through recognition of T2 hypointensity of the thalami and unusual T2 prolongation in the dentate hila, posterior limb of the internal capsules, and the brainstem corticospinal tracts.[217,227] With time, increasing periventricular/central cerebral white matter and cerebellar white matter signal abnormality becomes evident, the former typically involving the corpus callosum.[228] Additional distinctive features include enhancement and thickening of cauda equina nerve roots and the cranial nerves, particularly the optic nerves.[229–233] Typical features of infantile Krabbe are shown in **Fig. 21** and as with most leukodystrophies there

is progression to atrophy with time.[224,227,234] Later presentation forms of Krabbe manifest as signal abnormality confined to the posterior periventricular white matter and corticospinal tracts, resembling MLD or adrenomyeloneuropathy.[227,235]

MSUD

MSUD is an autosomal recessive disorder resulting from deficiency in components of the mitochondrial apparatus responsible for processing branched-chain α-ketoacids, metabolites derived from branched amino acids (eg, leucine, valine, isoleucine): subunit E1α BCKDHA (19q13),[236] subunit E1α BCKDHA (6p21),[237] and subunit E2 DBT (1p21).[238,239] The classic form of MSUD presents in the immediate neonatal period with poor feeding, lethargy, apnea, cerebral edema, and coma with associated ketonuria and maple syrup odor from urine. The intermediate form presents in later infancy or childhood with developmental delay and failure to thrive, reflecting higher residual enzyme activity. However, classic and intermediate MSUD as well as apparently normal children with branched-chain ketoacid deficiency (intermittent MSUD) can all develop metabolic decompensation including cerebral edema and coma when under physiologic stress (eg, mild infection).[240] Subunit E3 deficiency caused by mutations in DLD (7q31) affects additional enzymatic pathways (ie, pyruvate dehydrogenase) causing more complex phenotypes that overlap with other mitochondrial disorders.[241,242] Although the mechanism of brain pathology is incompletely understood, histologic examination of brains of patients with MSUD demonstrates spongiform changes in areas of myelinated nervous tissue.[243] Therefore, abnormal T2 signals in sites of neonatal brain myelination are present in classic MSUD including the posterior limb of the internal capsule as well as the dorsal brainstem, thalami, globus pallidus, and cerebellar white matter (**Fig. 22**)[244]; there are also reports of spinal cord involvement.[245] Intermediate MSUD may have an abnormal deep/periventricular white matter signal in addition to the typical brainstem sites in classic MSUD.[243,246,247] In acute decompensation, there is restricted diffusion in sites of signal abnormality, diffuse cerebral edema, and a characteristic MR spectroscopy peak at 0.9 ppm corresponding to branched-chain amino acid and α-ketoacid in addition to a lactate peak.[248–250] With supportive care and dietary restriction of leucine, there may be near resolution of signal abnormalities or mild residual T2 abnormality in sites of involvement with variable degrees of volume loss including prominent perivascular spaces.

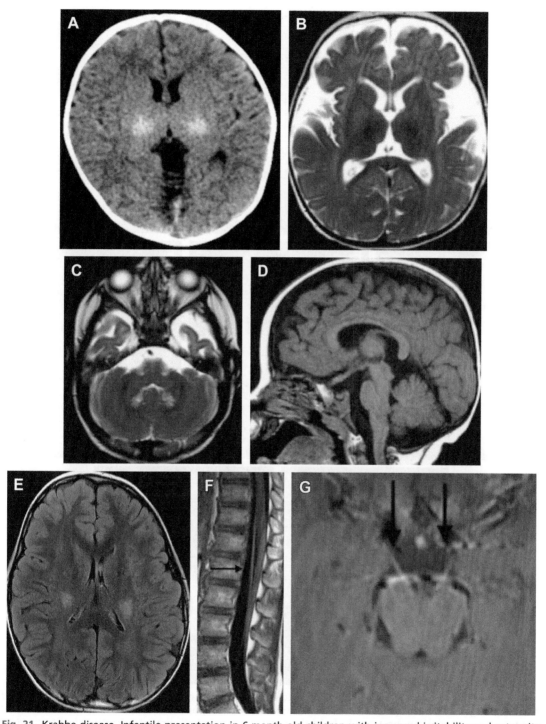

Fig. 21. Krabbe disease. Infantile presentation in 6-month-old children with increased irritability and extremity hypotonia: Axial computed tomography (*A*) demonstrates hyperdensity of the thalami. Axial T2-weighted images (*B, C*) demonstrate hypointensity of the thalamus as well as dentate nucleus signal increase and suggestion of corticospinal tract signal increase. Sagittal T1 (*D*) images demonstrate thickening of the optic nerves. Although the opercula are unusually prominent, the thickening of the optic nerves and the dense appearance of the thalamus suggested Krabbe rather than glutaric aciduria I, which was also considered. Juvenile presentation of Krabbe in a 6-year-old with motor regression: Axial Fluid attenuated inversion recovery images demonstrate signal increase in the corticospinal tracts (*E*). Postcontrast images demonstrate enhancement (*arrows*) of the cauda equina (*F*) and oculomotor nerves (*G*).

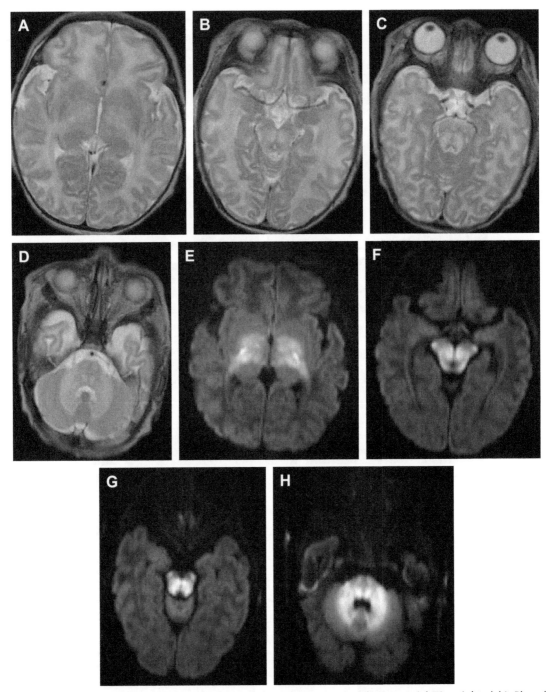

Fig. 22. Eleven-day-old infant with newly diagnosed maple syrup urine disease. Axial T2-weighted (*A–D*) and diffusion-weighted trace images (*E–H*) demonstrate signal abnormality and restricted diffusion in sites of normal neonatal brain myelination: posterior limbs of the internal capsule (*A, E*), brainstem corticospinal tracts (*B–D, F–H*), dorsal brainstem (*B, C, F, G*), and the cerebellar peduncles (*D, H*). The restricted diffusion is typical for patients imaged in acute decompensation.

Gray Matter Diseases with Some Extension into White Matter: Urea Cycle and Mitochondrial Disorders

Although outside the scope of this review, it is important to acknowledge that metabolic disorders primarily affecting gray matter may have resemblance to pattern 4 leukodystrophies (Fig. 23). In the case of urea cycle disorders (caused by recessive mutations in 1 of 6 gene products, the ornithine transcarbamylase gene being on the X chromosome[251]), the insular cortex and deep gray matter are involved similar to non-inherited causes of hyperammonemia (ie, hepatic encephalopathy).[252–255] However, severe cases of urea cycle disorders can present with subcortical white matter edema near these locations or more generalized cerebral edema, often with accompanying restricted diffusion. MR spectroscopy can be of assistance in suggesting hyperammonemia because there is often an increase in glutamine/glutamate.[256] If mitochondrial disorders are defined as disorders of the oxidative phosphorylation pathway regardless of clinical syndrome (eg, Leigh syndrome; mitochondrial encephalomyopathy lactic acidosis, and strokelike episodes or MELAS), there is a strong predisposition for signal abnormalities of the deep gray

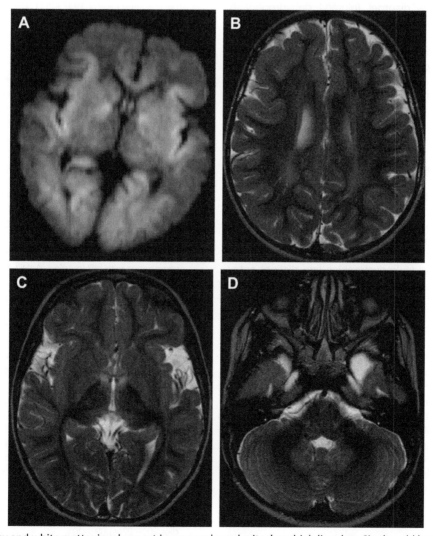

Fig. 23. Gray and white matter involvement in urea cycle and mitochondrial disorders. Six-day-old boy with ornithine transcarbamylase deficiency and seizure: diffusion-weighted image (A) demonstrates insular cortex and globus pallidus signal abnormality as well as areas of subcortical white matter hyperintensity. Three-year-old child with glutaric aciduria type I: axial T2-weighted images (B–D) demonstrate periventricular, basal ganglia, and dentate signal abnormality as well as the characteristic opercular widening seen in this disorder.

matter, brainstem (eg, central tegmental tracts), and (in the case of MELAS) cortical gray matter. However, there can also clearly be white matter involvement associated with these mitochondrial disorders resembling the leukodystrophies discussed in this review.[257] For mutations affecting complex I, white matter lesions were present in roughly a quarter of patients according to a recent review of the topic,[258,259] and for Kearns-Sayre syndrome (progressive external ophthalmoplegia, retinopathy), subcortical white matter signal abnormality usually accompanies the deep gray matter signal increase.[260] A high frequency of periventricular white matter signal abnormality in addition to deep gray signal increase and widened opercula are also seen in glutaric aciduria type I,[261] although this disorder (glutaryl dehydrogenase deficiency) is involved in mitochondrial amino acid catabolism not the respiratory chain directly. The relationships between genomic or mitochondrial DNA defects and specific imaging phenotypes are elusive at present, including for mitochondrial disorders with white matter manifestations.[262]

SUMMARY

As illustrated by the disease entities discussed in this article, leukodystrophies encompass a wide spectrum of imaging manifestations from delay in myelination to complex patterns of signal abnormality involving both white and gray matter. Although the diversity and number of diseases can seem overwhelming, imaging features allow separation of leukodystrophies into distinct categories, 4 of which have been emphasized in this review. With the addition of relevant clinical information and the presence of highly characteristic imaging findings (eg, parenchymal calcifications and photosensitivity in CS; macrocephaly and increased NAA in Canavan disease), a specific diagnosis can often be suggested. But even in cases where fairly generic findings are present (eg, delay in myelination), careful attention to the imaging patterns mentioned in this article can provide a small enough differential to guide an efficient workup. As historical testing strategies transition to an era of whole-genome sequencing, these imaging patterns can be expected to endure as a means of guiding interpretation of genetic data and potentially classifying new disorders.

REFERENCES

1. Seitelberger F. Structural manifestations of leukodystrophies. Neuropediatrics 1984;15(Suppl): 53–61.

2. Menkes JH. The leukodystrophies. N Engl J Med 1990;322(1):54–5.

3. van der Knaap M, Valk J. Classification of myelin disorders. Magnetic resonance of myelination and myelin disorders. Berlin: Springer-Verlag; 2005.

4. Leite CC, Lucato LT, Martin MG, et al. Merosin-deficient congenital muscular dystrophy (CMD): a study of 25 Brazilian patients using MRI. Pediatr Radiol 2005;35(6):572–9.

5. Mercuri E, Topaloglu H, Brockington M, et al. Spectrum of brain changes in patients with congenital muscular dystrophy and FKRP gene mutations. Arch Neurol 2006;63(2):251–7.

6. van der Knaap MS, Smit LM, Barth PG, et al. Magnetic resonance imaging in classification of congenital muscular dystrophies with brain abnormalities. Ann Neurol 1997;42(1):50–9.

7. Poll-The BT, Gartner J. Clinical diagnosis, biochemical findings and MRI spectrum of peroxisomal disorders. Biochim Biophys Acta 2012; 1822(9):1421–9.

8. van der Knaap M, Valk J. Magnetic resonance of myelination and myelin disorders. Berlin: Springer-Verlag; 2005.

9. Patay Z. Metabolic disorders. In: Tortori-Donati P, editor. Pediatric neuroradiology, vol. 1. Berlin: Springer-Verlag; 2005. p. 543–721.

10. Barkovich AJ, Patay Z. Metabolic, toxic, and inflammatory brain disorders. In: Barkovich AJ, editor. Pediatric neuroimaging. Philadelphia: Lippincott Williams & Wilkins; 2012. p. 81–239.

11. Leijser LM, de Vries LS, Rutherford MA, et al. Cranial ultrasound in metabolic disorders presenting in the neonatal period: characteristic features and comparison with MR imaging. AJNR Am J Neuroradiol 2007;28(7):1223–31.

12. Patay Z. Diffusion-weighted MR imaging in leukodystrophies. Eur Radiol 2005;15(11):2284–303.

13. Melhem ER, Loes DJ, Georgiades CS, et al. X-linked adrenoleukodystrophy: the role of contrast-enhanced MR imaging in predicting disease progression. AJNR Am J Neuroradiol 2000; 21(5):839–44.

14. Cecil KM. MR spectroscopy of metabolic disorders. Neuroimaging Clin N Am 2006;16(1):87–116, viii.

15. Cakmakci H, Pekcevik Y, Yis U, et al. Diagnostic value of proton MR spectroscopy and diffusion-weighted MR imaging in childhood inherited neurometabolic brain diseases and review of the literature. Eur J Radiol 2010;74(3):e161–71.

16. Lange T, Dydak U, Roberts TP, et al. Pitfalls in lactate measurements at 3T. AJNR Am J Neuroradiol 2006;27(4):895–901.

17. Afifi AK, Menezes AH, Reed LA, et al. Atypical presentation of X-linked childhood adrenoleukodystrophy with an unusual magnetic resonance imaging pattern. J Child Neurol 1996;11(6):497–9.

18. van der Knaap MS, Salomons GS, Li R, et al. Unusual variants of Alexander's disease. Ann Neurol 2005;57(3):327–38.

19. Barkovich AJ. Concepts of myelin and myelination in neuroradiology. AJNR Am J Neuroradiol 2000; 21(6):1099–109.

20. van der Knaap MS, Breiter SN, Naidu S, et al. Defining and categorizing leukoencephalopathies of unknown origin: MR imaging approach. Radiology 1999;213(1):121–33.

21. Bonkowsky JL, Nelson C, Kingston JL, et al. The burden of inherited leukodystrophies in children. Neurology 2010;75(8):718–25.

22. Vanderver A, Hussey H, Schmidt JL, et al. Relative incidence of inherited white matter disorders in childhood to acquired pediatric demyelinating disorders. Semin Pediatr Neurol 2012;19(4): 219–23.

23. Heim P, Claussen M, Hoffmann B, et al. Leukodystrophy incidence in Germany. Am J Med Genet 1997;71(4):475–8.

24. Kohlschutter A, Eichler F. Childhood leukodystrophies: a clinical perspective. Expert Rev Neurother 2011;11(10):1485–96.

25. Kaye CI, Committee on Genetics, Accurso F, et al. Introduction to the newborn screening fact sheets. Pediatrics 2006;118(3):1304–12.

26. Woodward KJ. The molecular and cellular defects underlying Pelizaeus-Merzbacher disease. Expert Rev Mol Med 2008;10:e14.

27. van der Knaap M, Valk J. Pelizaeus-Merzbacher disease and X-linked spastic paraplegia type 2. Magnetic resonance of myelination and myelin disorders. Berlin: Springer-Verlag; 2005.

28. Southwood CM, Garbern J, Jiang W, et al. The unfolded protein response modulates disease severity in Pelizaeus-Merzbacher disease. Neuron 2002;36(4):585–96.

29. Gow A, Lazzarini RA. A cellular mechanism governing the severity of Pelizaeus-Merzbacher disease. Nat Genet 1996;13(4):422–8.

30. Hobson GM, Garbern JY. Pelizaeus-Merzbacher disease, Pelizaeus-Merzbacher-like disease 1, and related hypomyelinating disorders. Semin Neurol 2012;32(1):62–7.

31. van der Knaap MS, Valk J. The reflection of histology in MR imaging of Pelizaeus-Merzbacher disease. AJNR Am J Neuroradiol 1989;10(1):99–103.

32. Linnankivi T, Tienari P, Somer M, et al. 18q deletions: clinical, molecular, and brain MRI findings of 14 individuals. Am J Med Genet A 2006; 140(4):331–9.

33. Feenstra I, Vissers LE, Orsel M, et al. Genotype-phenotype mapping of chromosome 18q deletions by high-resolution array CGH: an update of the phenotypic map. Am J Med Genet A 2007; 143A(16):1858–67.

34. Lancaster JL, Cody JD, Andrews T, et al. Myelination in children with partial deletions of chromosome 18q. AJNR Am J Neuroradiol 2005;26(3):447–54.

35. Linnankivi TT, Autti TH, Pihko SH, et al. 18q-syndrome: brain MRI shows poor differentiation of gray and white matter on T2-weighted images. J Magn Reson Imaging 2003;18(4):414–9.

36. Tanaka R, Iwasaki N, Hayashi M, et al. Abnormal brain MRI signal in 18q-syndrome not due to dysmyelination. Brain Dev 2012;34(3):234–7.

37. Verheijen FW, Verbeek E, Aula N, et al. A new gene, encoding an anion transporter, is mutated in sialic acid storage diseases. Nat Genet 1999;23(4): 462–5.

38. Adams D, Gahl WA. Free sialic acid storage disorders. GeneReviews 2008. Available at: http://www.ncbi.nlm.nih.gov/books/NBK1470/. Accessed April 2, 2013.

39. Leroy PL. Sialuria. GeneReviews 2012. Available at: http://www.ncbi.nlm.nih.gov/books/NBK1164/. Accessed April 2, 2013.

40. Sonninen P, Autti T, Varho T, et al. Brain involvement in Salla disease. AJNR Am J Neuroradiol 1999; 20(3):433–43.

41. Haataja L, Parkkola R, Sonninen P, et al. Phenotypic variation and magnetic resonance imaging (MRI) in Salla disease, a free sialic acid storage disorder. Neuropediatrics 1994;25(5):238–44.

42. Varho T, Komu M, Sonninen P, et al. A new metabolite contributing to N-acetyl signal in 1H MRS of the brain in Salla disease. Neurology 1999;52(8): 1668–72.

43. Mochel F, Yang B, Barritault J, et al. Free sialic acid storage disease without sialuria. Ann Neurol 2009; 65(6):753–7.

44. van der Knaap M, Valk J. Fucosidosis. Magnetic resonance of myelination and myelin disorders. Berlin: Springer-Verlag; 2005.

45. Steenweg ME, Vanderver A, Blaser S, et al. Magnetic resonance imaging pattern recognition in hypomyelinating disorders. Brain 2010;133(10): 2971–82.

46. Prietsch V, Arnold S, Kraegeloh-Mann I, et al. Severe hypomyelination as the leading neuroradiological sign in a patient with fucosidosis. Neuropediatrics 2008;39(1):51–4.

47. Oner AY, Cansu A, Akpek S, et al. Fucosidosis: MRI and MRS findings. Pediatr Radiol 2007;37(10): 1050–2.

48. Mamourian AC, Hopkin JR, Chawla S, et al. Characteristic MR spectroscopy in fucosidosis: in vitro investigation. Pediatr Radiol 2010;40(8):1446–9.

49. Uhlenberg B, Schuelke M, Ruschendorf F, et al. Mutations in the gene encoding gap junction protein alpha 12 (connexin 46.6) cause Pelizaeus-Merzbacher-like disease. Am J Hum Genet 2004; 75(2):251–60.

50. Bugiani M, Al Shahwan S, Lamantea E, et al. GJA12 mutations in children with recessive hypomyelinating leukoencephalopathy. Neurology 2006;67(2):273–9.

51. Magen D, Georgopoulos C, Bross P, et al. Mitochondrial hsp60 chaperonopathy causes an autosomal-recessive neurodegenerative disorder linked to brain hypomyelination and leukodystrophy. Am J Hum Genet 2008;83(1):30–42.

52. Vaurs-Barriere C, Deville M, Sarret C, et al. Pelizaeus-Merzbacher-Like disease presentation of MCT8 mutated male subjects. Ann Neurol 2009; 65(1):114–8.

53. Feinstein M, Markus B, Noyman I, et al. Pelizaeus-Merzbacher-like disease caused by AIMP1/p43 homozygous mutation. Am J Hum Genet 2010;87(6): 820–8.

54. Tetreault M, Choquet K, Orcesi S, et al. Recessive mutations in POLR3B, encoding the second largest subunit of Pol III, cause a rare hypomyelinating leukodystrophy. Am J Hum Genet 2011;89(5):652–5.

55. Bernard G, Chouery E, Putorti ML, et al. Mutations of POLR3A encoding a catalytic subunit of RNA polymerase Pol III cause a recessive hypomyelinating leukodystrophy. Am J Hum Genet 2011;89(3): 415–23.

56. Harreld JH, Smith EC, Prose NS, et al. Trichothiodystrophy with dysmyelination and central osteosclerosis. AJNR Am J Neuroradiol 2010;31(1): 129–30.

57. Zara F, Biancheri R, Bruno C, et al. Deficiency of hyccin, a newly identified membrane protein, causes hypomyelination and congenital cataract. Nat Genet 2006;38(10):1111–3.

58. van der Knaap MS, Naidu S, Pouwels PJ, et al. New syndrome characterized by hypomyelination with atrophy of the basal ganglia and cerebellum. AJNR Am J Neuroradiol 2002;23(9):1466–74.

59. Simons C, Wolf NI, McNeil N, et al. A de novo mutation in the beta-Tubulin gene TUBB4A results in the leukoencephalopathy hypomyelination with atrophy of the basal ganglia and cerebellum. Am J Hum Genet 2013;92(5):767–73.

60. Hamosh A, Scharer G, Van Hove J. Glycine encephalopathy. In: Pagon RA, Bird TD, Dolan CR, et al, editors. GeneReviews. Seattle (WA): 1993. Available at: http://www.ncbi.nlm.nih.gov/books/NBK1357/.

61. Mourmans J, Majoie CB, Barth PG, et al. Sequential MR imaging changes in nonketotic hyperglycinemia. AJNR Am J Neuroradiol 2006;27(1):208–11.

62. Khong PL, Lam BC, Chung BH, et al. Diffusion-weighted MR imaging in neonatal nonketotic hyperglycinemia. AJNR Am J Neuroradiol 2003;24(6): 1181–3.

63. Viola A, Chabrol B, Nicoli F, et al. Magnetic resonance spectroscopy study of glycine pathways in nonketotic hyperglycinemia. Pediatr Res 2002; 52(2):292–300.

64. Gabis L, Parton P, Roche P, et al. In vivo 1H magnetic resonance spectroscopic measurement of brain glycine levels in nonketotic hyperglycinemia. J Neuroimaging 2001;11(2):209–11.

65. Fridovich-Keil JL. Galactosemia: the good, the bad, and the unknown. J Cell Physiol 2006; 209(3):701–5.

66. Ridel KR, Leslie ND, Gilbert DL. An updated review of the long-term neurological effects of galactosemia. Pediatr Neurol 2005;33(3):153–61.

67. van der Knaap M, Valk J. Galactosemia. Magnetic resonance of myelination and myelin disorders. Berlin: Springer-Verlag; 2005.

68. Otaduy MC, Leite CC, Lacerda MT, et al. Proton MR spectroscopy and imaging of a galactosemic patient before and after dietary treatment. AJNR Am J Neuroradiol 2006;27(1):204–7.

69. Wang ZJ, Berry GT, Dreha SF, et al. Proton magnetic resonance spectroscopy of brain metabolites in galactosemia. Ann Neurol 2001;50(2):266–9.

70. Leegwater PA, Boor PK, Yuan BQ, et al. Identification of novel mutations in MLC1 responsible for megalencephalic leukoencephalopathy with subcortical cysts. Hum Genet 2002;110(3):279–83.

71. van der Knaap MS, Boor I, Estevez R. Megalencephalic leukoencephalopathy with subcortical cysts: chronic white matter oedema due to a defect in brain ion and water homoeostasis. Lancet Neurol 2012;11(11):973–85.

72. van der Knaap MS, Barth PG, Stroink H, et al. Leukoencephalopathy with swelling and a discrepantly mild clinical course in eight children. Ann Neurol 1995;37(3):324–34.

73. Lopez-Hernandez T, Ridder MC, Montolio M, et al. Mutant GlialCAM causes megalencephalic leukoencephalopathy with subcortical cysts, benign familial macrocephaly, and macrocephaly with retardation and autism. Am J Hum Genet 2011;88(4):422–32.

74. Aicardi J, Goutieres F. A progressive familial encephalopathy in infancy with calcifications of the basal ganglia and chronic cerebrospinal fluid lymphocytosis. Ann Neurol 1984;15(1):49–54.

75. Baraitser M, Brett EM, Piesowicz AT. Microcephaly and intracranial calcification in two brothers. J Med Genet 1983;20(3):210–2.

76. Aicardi J, Crow YJ, Stephenson J. Aicardi-Goutieres syndrome. GeneReviews 2012. Available at: http://www.ncbi.nlm.nih.gov/books/NBK1475/. Accessed April 3, 2013.

77. Crow YJ, Hayward BE, Parmar R, et al. Mutations in the gene encoding the 3'-5' DNA exonuclease TREX1 cause Aicardi-Goutieres syndrome at the AGS1 locus. Nat Genet 2006;38(8):917–20.

78. Crow YJ, Leitch A, Hayward BE, et al. Mutations in genes encoding ribonuclease H2 subunits cause

Aicardi-Goutieres syndrome and mimic congenital viral brain infection. Nat Genet 2006;38(8):910–6.

79. Rice GI, Bond J, Asipu A, et al. Mutations involved in Aicardi-Goutieres syndrome implicate SAMHD1 as regulator of the innate immune response. Nat Genet 2009;41(7):829–32.

80. Rice GI, Kasher PR, Forte GM, et al. Mutations in ADAR1 cause Aicardi-Goutieres syndrome associated with a type I interferon signature. Nat Genet 2012;44(11):1243–8.

81. Vogt J, Agrawal S, Ibrahim Z, et al. Striking intrafamilial phenotypic variability in Aicardi-Goutieres syndrome associated with the recurrent Asian founder mutation in RNASEH2C. Am J Med Genet A 2013;161A(2):338–42.

82. Rice G, Patrick T, Parmar R, et al. Clinical and molecular phenotype of Aicardi-Goutieres syndrome. Am J Hum Genet 2007;81(4):713–25.

83. Chahwan C, Chahwan R. Aicardi-Goutieres syndrome: from patients to genes and beyond. Clin Genet 2012;81(5):413–20.

84. Ravenscroft JC, Suri M, Rice GI, et al. Autosomal dominant inheritance of a heterozygous mutation in SAMHD1 causing familial chilblain lupus. Am J Med Genet A 2011;155A(1):235–7.

85. Rice G, Newman WG, Dean J, et al. Heterozygous mutations in TREX1 cause familial chilblain lupus and dominant Aicardi-Goutieres syndrome. Am J Hum Genet 2007;80(4):811–5.

86. Uggetti C, La Piana R, Orcesi S, et al. Aicardi-Goutieres syndrome: neuroradiologic findings and follow-up. AJNR Am J Neuroradiol 2009;30(10):1971–6.

87. Chen X, DeLellis RA, Hoda SA. Adrenoleukodystrophy. Arch Pathol Lab Med 2003;127(1):119–20.

88. Eichler FS, Ren JQ, Cossoy M, et al. Is microglial apoptosis an early pathogenic change in cerebral X-linked adrenoleukodystrophy? Ann Neurol 2008; 63(6):729–42.

89. van der Knaap M, Valk J. X-linked adrenoleukodystrophy. Magnetic resonance of myelination and myelin disorders. Berlin: Springer-Verlag; 2005.

90. Steinberg SJ, Moser AB, Raymond GV. X-linked adrenoleukodystrophy. GeneReviews 2012. Available at: http://www.ncbi.nlm.nih.gov/books/NBK1315/. Accessed April 4, 2013.

91. Ito R, Melhem ER, Mori S, et al. Diffusion tensor brain MR imaging in X-linked cerebral adrenoleukodystrophy. Neurology 2001;56(4):544–7.

92. Carrozzo R, Bellini C, Lucioli S, et al. Peroxisomal acyl-CoA-oxidase deficiency: two new cases. Am J Med Genet A 2008;146A(13):1676–81.

93. van der Knaap MS, Wassmer E, Wolf NI, et al. MRI as diagnostic tool in early-onset peroxisomal disorders. Neurology 2012;78(17):1304–8.

94. Kumar AJ, Kohler W, Kruse B, et al. MR findings in adult-onset adrenoleukodystrophy. AJNR Am J Neuroradiol 1995;16(6):1227–37.

95. Dubey P, Fatemi A, Huang H, et al. Diffusion tensor-based imaging reveals occult abnormalities in adrenomyeloneuropathy. Ann Neurol 2005;58(5):758–66.

96. Loes DJ, Fatemi A, Melhem ER, et al. Analysis of MRI patterns aids prediction of progression in X-linked adrenoleukodystrophy. Neurology 2003; 61(3):369–74.

97. Dekaban AS, Constantopoulos G. Mucopolysaccharidosis type I, II, IIIA and V. Pathological and biochemical abnormalities in the neural and mesenchymal elements of the brain. Acta Neuropathol 1977;39(1):1–7.

98. van der Knaap M, Valk J. Mucopolysaccharidoses. Magnetic resonance of myelination and myelin disorders. Berlin: Springer-Verlag; 2005.

99. Azevedo AC, Artigalas O, Vedolin L, et al. Brain magnetic resonance imaging findings in patients with mucopolysaccharidosis VI. J Inherit Metab Dis 2013;36(2):357–62.

100. Barone R, Nigro F, Triulzi F, et al. Clinical and neuroradiological follow-up in mucopolysaccharidosis type III (Sanfilippo syndrome). Neuropediatrics 1999;30(5):270–4.

101. Manara R, Priante E, Grimaldi M, et al. Brain and spine MRI features of Hunter disease: frequency, natural evolution and response to therapy. J Inherit Metab Dis 2011;34(3):763–80.

102. Matheus MG, Castillo M, Smith JK, et al. Brain MRI findings in patients with mucopolysaccharidosis types I and II and mild clinical presentation. Neuroradiology 2004;46(8):666–72.

103. Vedolin L, Schwartz IV, Komlos M, et al. Correlation of MR imaging and MR spectroscopy findings with cognitive impairment in mucopolysaccharidosis II. AJNR Am J Neuroradiol 2007;28(6):1029–33.

104. Wang RY, Cambray-Forker EJ, Ohanian K, et al. Treatment reduces or stabilizes brain imaging abnormalities in patients with MPS I and II. Mol Genet Metab 2009;98(4):406–11.

105. Fan Z, Styner M, Muenzer J, et al. Correlation of automated volumetric analysis of brain MR imaging with cognitive impairment in a natural history study of mucopolysaccharidosis II. AJNR Am J Neuroradiol 2010;31(7):1319–23.

106. Attree O, Olivos IM, Okabe I, et al. The Lowe's oculocerebrorenal syndrome gene encodes a protein highly homologous to inositol polyphosphate-5-phosphatase. Nature 1992;358(6383):239–42.

107. McPherson PS, Garcia EP, Slepnev VI, et al. A presynaptic inositol-5-phosphatase. Nature 1996;379(6563):353–7.

108. Lewis RA, Nussbaum RL, Brewer ED. Lowe syndrome. In: Pagon RA, Bird TD, Dolan CR, et al, editors. GeneReviews. Seattle (WA): 1993. Available at: http://www.ncbi.nlm.nih.gov/books/NBK1480/.

109. O'Tuama LA, Laster DW. Oculocerebrorenal syndrome: case report with CT and MR correlates. AJNR Am J Neuroradiol 1987;8(3):555–7.

110. Demmer LA, Wippold FJ 2nd, Dowton SB. Periventricular white matter cystic lesions in Lowe (oculocerebrorenal) syndrome. A new MR finding. Pediatr Radiol 1992;22(1):76–7.

111. Carroll WJ, Woodruff WW, Cadman TE. MR findings in oculocerebrorenal syndrome. AJNR Am J Neuroradiol 1993;14(2):449–51.

112. Schneider JF, Boltshauser E, Neuhaus TJ, et al. MRI and proton spectroscopy in Lowe syndrome. Neuropediatrics 2001;32(1):45–8.

113. Yuksel A, Karaca E, Albayram MS. Magnetic resonance imaging, magnetic resonance spectroscopy, and facial dysmorphism in a case of Lowe syndrome with novel OCRL1 gene mutation. J Child Neurol 2009;24(1):93–6.

114. Bergoffen J, Scherer SS, Wang S, et al. Connexin mutations in X-linked Charcot-Marie-Tooth disease. Science 1993;262(5142):2039–42.

115. Bird TD. Charcot-Marie-Tooth neuropathy X type 1. GeneReviews 2012. 2013. Available at: http://www.ncbi.nlm.nih.gov/pubmed/20301548. Accessed April 5, 2013.

116. Shy ME, Siskind C, Swan ER, et al. CMT1X phenotypes represent loss of GJB1 gene function. Neurology 2007;68(11):849–55.

117. Paulson HL, Garbern JY, Hoban TF, et al. Transient central nervous system white matter abnormality in X-linked Charcot-Marie-Tooth disease. Ann Neurol 2002;52(4):429–34.

118. Taylor RA, Simon EM, Marks HG, et al. The CNS phenotype of X-linked Charcot-Marie-Tooth disease: more than a peripheral problem. Neurology 2003;61(11):1475–8.

119. Hanemann CO, Bergmann C, Senderek J, et al. Transient, recurrent, white matter lesions in X-linked Charcot-Marie-Tooth disease with novel connexin 32 mutation. Arch Neurol 2003;60(4):605–9.

120. Laugel V. Cockayne syndrome: the expanding clinical and mutational spectrum. Mech Ageing Dev 2013;134(5–6):161–70.

121. Nance MA, Berry SA. Cockayne syndrome: review of 140 cases. Am J Med Genet 1992;42(1):68–84.

122. Koob M, Laugel V, Durand M, et al. Neuroimaging in Cockayne syndrome. AJNR Am J Neuroradiol 2010;31(9):1623–30.

123. Adachi M, Kawanami T, Ohshima F, et al. MR findings of cerebral white matter in Cockayne syndrome. Magn Reson Med Sci 2006;5(1):41–5.

124. van der Knaap M, Valk J. Cockayne syndrome. Magnetic resonance of myelination and myelin disorders. Berlin: Springer-Verlag; 2005.

125. van Berge L, Kevenaar J, Polder E, et al. Pathogenic mutations causing LBSL affect mitochondrial aspartyl-tRNA synthetase in diverse ways. Biochem J 2013;450(2):345–50.

126. Scheper GC, van der Klok T, van Andel RJ, et al. Mitochondrial aspartyl-tRNA synthetase deficiency causes leukoencephalopathy with brain stem and spinal cord involvement and lactate elevation. Nat Genet 2007;39(4):534–9.

127. van der Knaap MS, van der Voorn P, Barkhof F, et al. A new leukoencephalopathy with brainstem and spinal cord involvement and high lactate. Ann Neurol 2003;53(2):252–8.

128. van der Knaap M, Valk J. Leukoencephalopathy with brain stem and spinal cord involvement and elevated white matter lactate. Magnetic resonance of myelination and myelin disorders. Berlin: Springer-Verlag; 2005.

129. Steenweg ME, van Berge L, van Berkel CG, et al. Early-onset LBSL: how severe does it get? Neuropediatrics 2012;43(6):332–8.

130. Taft RJ, Vanderver A, Leventer RJ, et al. Mutations in DARS cause hypomyelination with brain stem and spinal cord involvement and leg spasticity. Am J Hum Genet 2013;92(5):774–80.

131. Fluharty AL. Arylsulfatase A deficiency. In: Pagon RA, Bird TD, Dolan CR, et al, editors. GeneReviews. Seattle (WA): 1993. Available at: http://www.ncbi.nlm.nih.gov/books/NBK1130/.

132. Al-Hassnan ZN, Al Dhalaan H, Patay Z, et al. Sphingolipid activator protein B deficiency: report of 9 Saudi patients and review of the literature. J Child Neurol 2009;24(12):1513–9.

133. Stevens RL, Fluharty AL, Kihara H, et al. Cerebroside sulfatase activator deficiency induced metachromatic leukodystrophy. Am J Hum Genet 1981;33(6):900–6.

134. Kihara H, Tsay KK, Fluharty AL. Genetic complementation in somatic cell hybrids of cerebroside sulfatase activator deficiency and metachromatic leukodystrophy fibroblasts. Hum Genet 1984;66(4):300–1.

135. MacFaul R, Cavanagh N, Lake BD, et al. Metachromatic leucodystrophy: review of 38 cases. Arch Dis Child 1982;57(3):168–75.

136. Polten A, Fluharty AL, Fluharty CB, et al. Molecular basis of different forms of metachromatic leukodystrophy. N Engl J Med 1991;324(1):18–22.

137. Groeschel S, Kehrer C, Engel C, et al. Metachromatic leukodystrophy: natural course of cerebral MRI changes in relation to clinical course. J Inherit Metab Dis 2011;34(5):1095–102.

138. Eichler F, Grodd W, Grant E, et al. Metachromatic leukodystrophy: a scoring system for brain MR imaging observations. AJNR Am J Neuroradiol 2009;30(10):1893–7.

139. Maia AC Jr, da Rocha AJ, da Silva CJ, et al. Multiple cranial nerve enhancement: a new MR imaging

finding in metachromatic leukodystrophy. AJNR Am J Neuroradiol 2007;28(6):999.

140. Faerber EN, Melvin J, Smergel EM. MRI appearances of metachromatic leukodystrophy. Pediatr Radiol 1999;29(9):669–72.

141. Caro PA, Marks HG. Magnetic resonance imaging and computed tomography in Pelizaeus-Merzbacher disease. Magn Reson Imaging 1990;8(6):791–6.

142. Dziewas R, Stogbauer F, Oelerich M, et al. A case of adrenomyeloneuropathy with unusual lesion pattern in magnetic resonance imaging. J Neurol 2001;248(4):341–2.

143. Nishio H, Kodama S, Matsuo T, et al. Cockayne syndrome: magnetic resonance images of the brain in a severe form with early onset. J Inherit Metab Dis 1988;11(1):88–102.

144. van der Voorn JP, Pouwels PJ, Kamphorst W, et al. Histopathologic correlates of radial stripes on MR images in lysosomal storage disorders. AJNR Am J Neuroradiol 2005;26(3):442–6.

145. Onur MR, Senol U, Mihci E, et al. Tigroid pattern on magnetic resonance imaging in Lowe syndrome. J Clin Neurosci 2009;16(1):112–4.

146. Cleary MA, Walter JH, Wraith JE, et al. Magnetic resonance imaging of the brain in phenylketonuria. Lancet 1994;344(8915):87–90.

147. Leuzzi V, Tosetti M, Montanaro D, et al. The pathogenesis of the white matter abnormalities in phenylketonuria. A multimodal 3.0 tesla MRI and magnetic resonance spectroscopy (1H MRS) study. J Inherit Metab Dis 2007;30(2):209–16.

148. Willemsen MA, Van Der Graaf M, Van Der Knaap MS, et al. MR imaging and proton MR spectroscopic studies in Sjogren-Larsson syndrome: characterization of the leukoencephalopathy. AJNR Am J Neuroradiol 2004;25(4):649–57.

149. van der Knaap M, Valk J. Hyperhomocysteinemias. Magnetic resonance of myelination and myelin disorders. Berlin: Springer-Verlag; 2005.

150. Wilcken B. Leukoencephalopathies associated with disorders of cobalamin and folate metabolism. Semin Neurol 2012;32(1):68–74.

151. Mano T, Ono J, Kaminaga T, et al. Proton MR spectroscopy of Sjogren-Larsson's syndrome. AJNR Am J Neuroradiol 1999;20(9):1671–3.

152. Striano P, Specchio N, Biancheri R, et al. Clinical and electrophysiological features of epilepsy in Italian patients with CLN8 mutations. Epilepsy Behav 2007;10(1):187–91.

153. van der Knaap M, Valk J. Neuronal ceroid lipofuscinoses. Magnetic resonance of myelination and myelin disorders. Berlin: Springer-Verlag; 2005.

154. van der Knaap MS, Pronk JC, Scheper GC. Vanishing white matter disease. Lancet Neurol 2006;5(5):413–23.

155. Leegwater PA, Vermeulen G, Konst AA, et al. Subunits of the translation initiation factor eIF2B are mutant in leukoencephalopathy with vanishing white matter. Nat Genet 2001;29(4):383–8.

156. van der Lei HD, Steenweg ME, Barkhof F, et al. Characteristics of early MRI in children and adolescents with vanishing white matter. Neuropediatrics 2012;43(1):22–6.

157. Kaul R, Gao GP, Aloya M, et al. Canavan disease: mutations among Jewish and non-Jewish patients. Am J Hum Genet 1994;55(1):34–41.

158. Kaul R, Gao GP, Balamurugan K, et al. Cloning of the human aspartoacylase cDNA and a common missense mutation in Canavan disease. Nat Genet 1993;5(2):118–23.

159. Matalon R, Michals K, Sebesta D, et al. Aspartoacylase deficiency and N-acetylaspartic aciduria in patients with Canavan disease. Am J Med Genet 1988;29(2):463–71.

160. Baslow MH. Brain N-acetylaspartate as a molecular water pump and its role in the etiology of Canavan disease: a mechanistic explanation. J Mol Neurosci 2003;21(3):185–90.

161. Matalon RM, Michals-Matalon K. Spongy degeneration of the brain, Canavan disease: biochemical and molecular findings. Front Biosci 2000;5:D307–11.

162. Namboodiri AM, Moffett JR, Arun P, et al. Defective myelin lipid synthesis as a pathogenic mechanism of Canavan disease. Adv Exp Med Biol 2006;576:145–63 [discussion 361–3].

163. van der Knaap M, Valk J. Canavan disease. Magnetic resonance of myelination and myelin disorders. Berlin: Springer-Verlag; 2005.

164. Brismar J, Brismar G, Gascon G, et al. Canavan disease: CT and MR imaging of the brain. AJNR Am J Neuroradiol 1990;11(4):805–10.

165. McAdams HP, Geyer CA, Done SL, et al. CT and MR imaging of Canavan disease. AJNR Am J Neuroradiol 1990;11(2):397–9.

166. Toft PB, Geiss-Holtorff R, Rolland MO, et al. Magnetic resonance imaging in juvenile Canavan disease. Eur J Pediatr 1993;152(9):750–3.

167. Yalcinkaya C, Benbir G, Salomons GS, et al. Atypical MRI findings in Canavan disease: a patient with a mild course. Neuropediatrics 2005;36(5):336–9.

168. Zafeiriou DI, Kleijer WJ, Maroupoulos G, et al. Protracted course of N-acetylaspartic aciduria in two non-Jewish siblings: identical clinical and magnetic resonance imaging findings. Brain Dev 1999;21(3):205–8.

169. Grodd W, Krageloh-Mann I, Klose U, et al. Metabolic and destructive brain disorders in children: findings with localized proton MR spectroscopy. Radiology 1991;181(1):173–81.

170. Janson CG, McPhee SW, Francis J, et al. Natural history of Canavan disease revealed by proton

magnetic resonance spectroscopy (1H-MRS) and diffusion-weighted MRI. Neuropediatrics 2006; 37(4):209–21.

171. Rzem R, Veiga-da-Cunha M, Noel G, et al. A gene encoding a putative FAD-dependent L-2-hydroxy-glutarate dehydrogenase is mutated in L-2-hydroxyglutaric aciduria. Proc Natl Acad Sci U S A 2004; 101(48):16849–54.

172. Kranendijk M, Struys EA, Salomons GS, et al. Progress in understanding 2-hydroxyglutaric acidurias. J Inherit Metab Dis 2012;35(4):571–87.

173. Steenweg ME, Salomons GS, Yapici Z, et al. L-2-Hydroxyglutaric aciduria: pattern of MR imaging abnormalities in 56 patients. Radiology 2009; 251(3):856–65.

174. Topcu M, Erdem G, Saatci I, et al. Clinical and magnetic resonance imaging features of L-2-hydroxyglutaric acidemia: report of three cases in comparison with Canavan disease. J Child Neurol 1996;11(5):373–7.

175. Patay Z, Mills JC, Lobel U, et al. Cerebral neoplasms in L-2 hydroxyglutaric aciduria: 3 new cases and meta-analysis of literature data. AJNR Am J Neuroradiol 2012;33(5):940–3.

176. Ye D, Ma S, Xiong Y, et al. R-2-Hydroxyglutarate as the key effector of IDH mutations promoting oncogenesis. Cancer Cell 2013;23(3):274–6.

177. Losman JA, Looper RE, Koivunen P, et al. (R)-2-hydroxyglutarate is sufficient to promote leukemogenesis and its effects are reversible. Science 2013;339(6127):1621–5.

178. van der Knaap MS, Jakobs C, Hoffmann GF, et al. D-2-hydroxyglutaric aciduria: further clinical delineation. J Inherit Metab Dis 1999;22(4): 404–13.

179. Choi C, Ganji SK, DeBerardinis RJ, et al. 2-hydroxyglutarate detection by magnetic resonance spectroscopy in IDH-mutated patients with gliomas. Nat Med 2012;18(4):624–9.

180. Pope WB, Prins RM, Albert Thomas M, et al. Non-invasive detection of 2-hydroxyglutarate and other metabolites in IDH1 mutant glioma patients using magnetic resonance spectroscopy. J Neurooncol 2012;107(1):197–205.

181. Brenner M, Johnson AB, Boespflug-Tanguy O, et al. Mutations in GFAP, encoding glial fibrillary acidic protein, are associated with Alexander disease. Nat Genet 2001;27(1):117–20.

182. Li R, Johnson AB, Salomons G, et al. Glial fibrillary acidic protein mutations in infantile, juvenile, and adult forms of Alexander disease. Ann Neurol 2005;57(3):310–26.

183. Messing A, Li R, Naidu S, et al. Archetypal and new families with Alexander disease and novel mutations in GFAP. Arch Neurol 2012;69(2):208–14.

184. Hagemann TL, Connor JX, Messing A. Alexander disease-associated glial fibrillary acidic protein mutations in mice induce Rosenthal fiber formation and a white matter stress response. J Neurosci 2006;26(43):11162–73.

185. Hsiao VC, Tian R, Long H, et al. Alexander-disease mutation of GFAP causes filament disorganization and decreased solubility of GFAP. J Cell Sci 2005;118(Pt 9):2057–65.

186. Messing A, Brenner M, Feany MB, et al. Alexander disease. J Neurosci 2012;32(15):5017–23.

187. Gorospe JR. Alexander disease. In: Pagon RA, Bird TD, Dolan CR, et al, editors. GeneReviews. Seattle (WA): 1993. Available at: http://www.ncbi.nlm.nih.gov/books/NBK1172/.

188. van der Knaap M, Valk J. GM1 gangliosidosis and GM2 gangliosidosis. Magnetic resonance of myelination and myelin disorders. Berlin: Springer-Verlag; 2005.

189. van der Knaap MS, Naidu S, Breiter SN, et al. Alexander disease: diagnosis with MR imaging. AJNR Am J Neuroradiol 2001;22(3):541–52.

190. van der Knaap MS, Ramesh V, Schiffmann R, et al. Alexander disease: ventricular garlands and abnormalities of the medulla and spinal cord. Neurology 2006;66(4):494–8.

191. Pareyson D, Fancellu R, Mariotti C, et al. Adult-onset Alexander disease: a series of eleven unrelated cases with review of the literature. Brain 2008;131(Pt 9):2321–31.

192. Stumpf E, Masson H, Duquette A, et al. Adult Alexander disease with autosomal dominant transmission: a distinct entity caused by mutation in the glial fibrillary acid protein gene. Arch Neurol 2003; 60(9):1307–12.

193. Jeyakumar M, Butters TD, Dwek RA, et al. Glycosphingolipid lysosomal storage diseases: therapy and pathogenesis. Neuropathol Appl Neurobiol 2002;28(5):343–57.

194. Okada S, O'Brien JS. Generalized gangliosidosis: beta-galactosidase deficiency. Science 1968; 160(3831):1002–4.

195. Nishimoto J, Nanba E, Inui K, et al. GM1-gangliosidosis (genetic beta-galactosidase deficiency): identification of four mutations in different clinical phenotypes among Japanese patients. Am J Hum Genet 1991;49(3):566–74.

196. Yoshida K, Oshima A, Shimmoto M, et al. Human beta-galactosidase gene mutations in GM1-gangliosidosis: a common mutation among Japanese adult/chronic cases. Am J Hum Genet 1991; 49(2):435–42.

197. Okada S, O'Brien JS. Tay-Sachs disease: generalized absence of a beta-D-N-acetylhexosaminidase component. Science 1969;165(3894):698–700.

198. Lalley PA, Rattazzi MC, Shows TB. Human beta-D-N-acetylhexosaminidases A and B: expression and linkage relationships in somatic cell hybrids. Proc Natl Acad Sci U S A 1974;71(4):1569–73.

199. Myerowitz R, Costigan FC. The major defect in Ashkenazi Jews with Tay-Sachs disease is an insertion in the gene for the alpha-chain of beta-hexosaminidase. J Biol Chem 1988;263(35):18587–9.

200. O'Dowd BF, Klavins MH, Willard HF, et al. Molecular heterogeneity in the infantile and juvenile forms of Sandhoff disease (O-variant GM2 gangliosidosis). J Biol Chem 1986;261(27):12680–5.

201. Gilbert F, Kucherlapati R, Creagan RP, et al. Tay-Sachs' and Sandhoff's diseases: the assignment of genes for hexosaminidase A and B to individual human chromosomes. Proc Natl Acad Sci U S A 1975;72(1):263–7.

202. Sandhoff K, Conzelmann E, Nehrkorn H. Substrate specificity of hexosaminidase A isolated from the liver of a patient with a rare form (AB variant) of infantile GM2 gangliosidosis and control tissues. Adv Exp Med Biol 1978;101:727–30.

203. Chen B, Rigat B, Curry C, et al. Structure of the GM2A gene: identification of an exon 2 nonsense mutation and a naturally occurring transcript with an in-frame deletion of exon 2. Am J Hum Genet 1999;65(1):77–87.

204. Brunetti-Pierri N, Scaglia F. GM1 gangliosidosis: review of clinical, molecular, and therapeutic aspects. Mol Genet Metab 2008;94(4):391–6.

205. Kaback MM, Desnick RJ. Hexosaminidase A deficiency. GeneReviews 1993. 2013. Available at: http://www.ncbi.nlm.nih.gov/pubmed/20301397. Accessed April 21, 2013.

206. Bley AE, Giannikopoulos OA, Hayden D, et al. Natural history of infantile G(M2) gangliosidosis. Pediatrics 2011;128(5):e1233–41.

207. Maegawa GH, Stockley T, Tropak M, et al. The natural history of juvenile or subacute GM2 gangliosidosis: 21 new cases and literature review of 134 previously reported. Pediatrics 2006;118(5):e1550–62.

208. Frey LC, Ringel SP, Filley CM. The natural history of cognitive dysfunction in late-onset GM2 gangliosidosis. Arch Neurol 2005;62(6):989–94.

209. Erol I, Alehan F, Pourbagher MA, et al. Neuroimaging findings in infantile GM1 gangliosidosis. Eur J Paediatr Neurol 2006;10(5–6):245–8.

210. Chen CY, Zimmerman RA, Lee CC, et al. Neuroimaging findings in late infantile GM1 gangliosidosis. AJNR Am J Neuroradiol 1998;19(9):1628–30.

211. Imamura A, Miyajima H, Ito R, et al. Serial MR imaging and 1H-MR spectroscopy in monozygotic twins with Tay-Sachs disease. Neuropediatrics 2008;39(5):259–63.

212. Inglese M, Nusbaum AO, Pastores GM, et al. MR imaging and proton spectroscopy of neuronal injury in late-onset GM2 gangliosidosis. AJNR Am J Neuroradiol 2005;26(8):2037–42.

213. Streifler JY, Gornish M, Hadar H, et al. Brain imaging in late-onset GM2 gangliosidosis. Neurology 1993;43(10):2055–8.

214. Uyama E, Terasaki T, Watanabe S, et al. Type 3 GM1 gangliosidosis: characteristic MRI findings correlated with dystonia. Acta Neurol Scand 1992;86(6):609–15.

215. Roze E, Paschke E, Lopez N, et al. Dystonia and parkinsonism in GM1 type 3 gangliosidosis. Mov Disord 2005;20(10):1366–9.

216. De Grandis E, Di Rocco M, Pessagno A, et al. MR imaging findings in 2 cases of late infantile GM1 gangliosidosis. AJNR Am J Neuroradiol 2009; 30(7):1325–7.

217. van der Knaap M, Valk J. Globoid cell leukodystrophy: Krabbe disease. Magnetic resonance of myelination and myelin disorders. Berlin: Springer-Verlag; 2005.

218. Suzuki K, Suzuki Y. Globoid cell leucodystrophy (Krabbe's disease): deficiency of galactocerebroside beta-galactosidase. Proc Natl Acad Sci U S A 1970;66(2):302–9.

219. Spiegel R, Bach G, Sury V, et al. A mutation in the saposin A coding region of the prosaposin gene in an infant presenting as Krabbe disease: first report of saposin A deficiency in humans. Mol Genet Metab 2005;84(2):160–6.

220. Svennerholm L, Vanier MT, Mansson JE. Krabbe disease: a galactosylsphingosine (psychosine) lipidosis. J Lipid Res 1980;21(1):53–64.

221. Wenger DA. Krabbe disease. GeneReviews. 2013. Available at: http://www.ncbi.nlm.nih.gov/pubmed/20301416. Accessed April 25, 2013.

222. Choi S, Enzmann DR. Infantile Krabbe disease: complementary CT and MR findings. AJNR Am J Neuroradiol 1993;14(5):1164–6.

223. Livingston JH, Graziano C, Pysden K, et al. Intracranial calcification in early infantile Krabbe disease: nothing new under the sun. Dev Med Child Neurol 2012;54(4):376–9.

224. Finelli DA, Tarr RW, Sawyer RN, et al. Deceptively normal MR in early infantile Krabbe disease. AJNR Am J Neuroradiol 1994;15(1):167–71.

225. Escolar ML, Poe MD, Smith JK, et al. Diffusion tensor imaging detects abnormalities in the corticospinal tracts of neonates with infantile Krabbe disease. AJNR Am J Neuroradiol 2009;30(5): 1017–21.

226. Guo AC, Petrella JR, Kurtzberg J, et al. Evaluation of white matter anisotropy in Krabbe disease with diffusion tensor MR imaging: initial experience. Radiology 2001;218(3):809–15.

227. Loes DJ, Peters C, Krivit W. Globoid cell leukodystrophy: distinguishing early-onset from late-onset disease using a brain MR imaging scoring method. AJNR Am J Neuroradiol 1999;20(2): 316–23.

228. Sasaki M, Sakuragawa N, Takashima S, et al. MRI and CT findings in Krabbe disease. Pediatr Neurol 1991;7(4):283–8.

229. Bernal OG, Lenn N. Multiple cranial nerve enhancement in early infantile Krabbe's disease. Neurology 2000;54(12):2348–9.

230. Jones BV, Barron TF, Towfighi J. Optic nerve enlargement in Krabbe's disease. AJNR Am J Neuroradiol 1999;20(7):1228–31.

231. Morana G, Biancheri R, Dirocco M, et al. Enhancing cranial nerves and cauda equina: an emerging magnetic resonance imaging pattern in metachromatic leukodystrophy and krabbe disease. Neuropediatrics 2009;40(6):291–4.

232. Nagar VA, Ursekar MA, Krishnan P, et al. Krabbe disease: unusual MRI findings. Pediatr Radiol 2006;36(1):61–4.

233. Vasconcellos E, Smith M. MRI nerve root enhancement in Krabbe disease. Pediatr Neurol 1998; 19(2):151–2.

234. Zafeiriou DI, Michelakaki EM, Anastasiou AL, et al. Serial MRI and neurophysiological studies in late-infantile Krabbe disease. Pediatr Neurol 1996; 15(3):240–4.

235. Farina L, Bizzi A, Finocchiaro G, et al. MR imaging and proton MR spectroscopy in adult Krabbe disease. AJNR Am J Neuroradiol 2000;21(8):1478–82.

236. Zhang B, Zhao Y, Harris RA, et al. Molecular defects in the E1 alpha subunit of the branched-chain alpha-ketoacid dehydrogenase complex that cause maple syrup urine disease. Mol Biol Med 1991;8(1):39–47.

237. Nobukuni Y, Mitsubuchi H, Akaboshi I, et al. Maple syrup urine disease. Complete defect of the E1 beta subunit of the branched chain alpha-ketoacid dehydrogenase complex due to a deletion of an 11-bp repeat sequence which encodes a mitochondrial targeting leader peptide in a family with the disease. J Clin Invest 1991;87(5):1862–6.

238. Fisher CW, Lau KS, Fisher CR, et al. A 17-bp insertion and a Phe215–Cys missense mutation in the dihydrolipoyl transacylase (E2) mRNA from a thiamine-responsive maple syrup urine disease patient WG-34. Biochem Biophys Res Commun 1991; 174(2):804–9.

239. Herring WJ, Litwer S, Weber JL, et al. Molecular genetic basis of maple syrup urine disease in a family with two defective alleles for branched chain acyltransferase and localization of the gene to human chromosome 1. Am J Hum Genet 1991; 48(2):342–50.

240. Strauss KA, Puffenberger EG, Morton DH. Maple syrup urine disease. GeneReviews. 2013. Available at: http://www.ncbi.nlm.nih.gov/pubmed/20301495. Accessed April 26, 2013.

241. Shaag A, Saada A, Berger I, et al. Molecular basis of lipoamide dehydrogenase deficiency in Ashkenazi Jews. Am J Med Genet 1999;82(2):177–82.

242. Liu TC, Kim H, Arizmendi C, et al. Identification of two missense mutations in a dihydrolipoamide dehydrogenase-deficient patient. Proc Natl Acad Sci U S A 1993;90(11):5186–90.

243. van der Knaap M, Valk J. Maple syrup urine disease. Magnetic resonance of myelination and myelin disorders. Berlin: Springer-Verlag; 2005.

244. Brismar J, Aqeel A, Brismar G, et al. Maple syrup urine disease: findings on CT and MR scans of the brain in 10 infants. AJNR Am J Neuroradiol 1990;11(6):1219–28.

245. Bhat M, Prasad C, Bindu PS, et al. Unusual imaging findings in brain and spinal cord in two siblings with maple syrup urine disease. J Neuroimaging 2013;23(4):540–2.

246. Bindu PS, Shehanaz KE, Christopher R, et al. Intermediate maple syrup urine disease: neuroimaging observations in 3 patients from South India. J Child Neurol 2007;22(7):911–3.

247. Sener RN. Diffusion magnetic resonance imaging in intermediate form of maple syrup urine disease. J Neuroimaging 2002;12(4):368–70.

248. Cavalleri F, Berardi A, Burlina AB, et al. Diffusion-weighted MRI of maple syrup urine disease encephalopathy. Neuroradiology 2002;44(6):499–502.

249. Felber SR, Sperl W, Chemelli A, et al. Maple syrup urine disease: metabolic decompensation monitored by proton magnetic resonance imaging and spectroscopy. Ann Neurol 1993;33(4):396–401.

250. Jan W, Zimmerman RA, Wang ZJ, et al. MR diffusion imaging and MR spectroscopy of maple syrup urine disease during acute metabolic decompensation. Neuroradiology 2003;45(6):393–9.

251. Lanpher BC, Gropman A, Chapman KA, et al. Urea Cycle Disorders Consortium. Urea cycle disorders overview. GeneReviews. 2013. Available at: http://www.ncbi.nlm.nih.gov/pubmed/20301396. Accessed April 30, 2013.

252. Takanashi J, Barkovich AJ, Cheng SF, et al. Brain MR imaging in neonatal hyperammonemic encephalopathy resulting from proximal urea cycle disorders. AJNR Am J Neuroradiol 2003;24(6):1184–7.

253. Majoie CB, Mourmans JM, Akkerman EM, et al. Neonatal citrullinemia: comparison of conventional MR, diffusion-weighted, and diffusion tensor findings. AJNR Am J Neuroradiol 2004;25(1):32–5.

254. McKinney AM, Lohman BD, Sarikaya B, et al. Acute hepatic encephalopathy: diffusion-weighted and fluid-attenuated inversion recovery findings, and correlation with plasma ammonia level and clinical outcome. AJNR Am J Neuroradiol 2010;31(8): 1471–9.

255. Poveda MJ, Bernabeu A, Concepcion L, et al. Brain edema dynamics in patients with overt hepatic encephalopathy A magnetic resonance imaging study. Neuroimage 2010;52(2):481–7.

256. Choi CG, Yoo HW. Localized proton MR spectroscopy in infants with urea cycle defect. AJNR Am J Neuroradiol 2001;22(5):834–7.

257. Finsterer J, Jarius C, Eichberger H. Phenotype variability in 130 adult patients with respiratory chain disorders. J Inherit Metab Dis 2001;24(5):560–76.
258. Koene S, Rodenburg RJ, van der Knaap MS, et al. Natural disease course and genotype-phenotype correlations in Complex I deficiency caused by nuclear gene defects: what we learned from 130 cases. J Inherit Metab Dis 2012;35(5):737–47.
259. Sofou K, Steneryd K, Wiklund LM, et al. MRI of the brain in childhood-onset mitochondrial disorders with central nervous system involvement. Mitochondrion 2013;13(4):364–71.
260. Chu BC, Terae S, Takahashi C, et al. MRI of the brain in the Kearns-Sayre syndrome: report of four cases and a review. Neuroradiology 1999; 41(10):759–64.
261. Twomey EL, Naughten ER, Donoghue VB, et al. Neuroimaging findings in glutaric aciduria type 1. Pediatr Radiol 2003;33(12):823–30.
262. Morava E, Smeitink JA. Mitochondria and mitochondrial disorders. In: van der Knaap M, Valk J, editors. Magnetic resonance of myelination and myelin disorders. Berlin: Springer-Verlag; 2005. p. 195–203.

Advances in Multiple Sclerosis and its Variants
Conventional and Newer Imaging Techniques

Timothy R. Miller, MD[a],*, Suyash Mohan, MD[b],
Asim F. Choudhri, MD[c], Dheeraj Gandhi, MD[a],
Gaurav Jindal, MD[a]

KEYWORDS

- Multiple sclerosis • Conventional MR imaging • Diffusion tensor imaging • MR spectroscopy
- Myelin free water component

KEY POINTS

- Multiple sclerosis (MS) and its variants are inflammatory and neurodegenerative central nervous system (CNS) diseases characterized by white matter plaques, atrophy, and diffuse abnormalities in surrounding gray and white matter.
- Conventional magnetic resonance (MR) imaging is sensitive for focal white matter lesions and atrophy in MS, but correlates poorly with clinical measures of disease.
- Improvements in technology have increased the sensitivity of conventional MR in evaluating MS, and automated techniques have improved accuracy and allowed the quantification of disease.
- Nonconventional MR imaging techniques detect the diffuse CNS changes present outside white matter plaques in MS and may correlate more closely with patients' symptoms.
- Imaging of the spinal cord and optic nerves in MS provides another method for evaluating disease severity and progression, with improved correlations with clinical disease.

INTRODUCTION

Multiple sclerosis (MS) and its variants such as neuromyelitis optica are inflammatory as well as neurodegenerative diseases of the central nervous system (CNS) characterized by demyelination, inflammation, gliosis, and neuronal loss.[1–3] Although MS has traditionally been thought of as a primarily autoimmune disease of white matter with focal demyelinating plaques, diffuse abnormalities are now known to be present throughout the CNS.[3,4] Extensive changes in the normal-appearing white matter (NAWM) have been shown in all MS subtypes and clinically isolated syndromes, with postmortem histopathologic studies showing glial hyperplasia, edema, inflammatory infiltrates, and thinning of myelin.[5,6] In addition, gray matter is not spared by the disease, with focal

Financial Disclosure and Conflict of Interest: The authors have nothing to disclose.
Note: This article has not been previously published in whole or in part. The article is not currently being submitted elsewhere for review.
[a] Neuroradiology Division, Department of Radiology, University of Maryland Medical Center, Baltimore, MD 21201, USA; [b] Neuroradiology Division, Department of Radiology, University of Pennsylvania, Philadelphia, PA 19104, USA; [c] Neuroradiology Division, Department of Radiology, University of Tennessee Health Science Center, Memphis, TN 38163, USA
* Corresponding author. Neuroradiology Division, Department of Radiology, University of Maryland Medical Center, Room N2W78, 22 South Greene Street, Baltimore, MD 21201.
E-mail address: tmiller5@umm.edu

lesions as well as diffuse abnormalities presenting early in cortical and subcortical structures.[5,7,8]

Conventional magnetic resonance (MR) imaging plays an important paraclinical role in the diagnosis of MS by showing dissemination of disease in both space and time.[9] MR imaging also aids in monitoring disease progression, evaluating the efficacy of novel treatments, and providing important prognostic information in patients presenting with clinically isolated syndromes such as transverse myelitis.[2,4,10,11] In transverse myelitis, the demonstration of white matter lesions in the CNS on MR imaging significantly increases the likelihood of the patient subsequently developing clinically definite MS.[11] In addition, in patients with established MS, conventional MR findings such as cerebral atrophy also carry important prognostic implications for the subsequent course of the disease.[1,4]

Although conventional MR remains the mainstay for imaging of MS and variants, several nonconventional MR techniques have been developed that can detect and quantify the full breadth of abnormalities present in the surrounding white and gray matter.[2,12] This article begins by reviewing current conventional MR imaging of MS, highlighting some of the strengths and limitations of the technique. Several recent advances in conventional MR imaging of MS are discussed. The article then explores several of the most promising nonconventional MR methods currently being developed to better characterize inflammatory and neurodegenerative diseases such as MS. In addition, optic nerve imaging is briefly reviewed.

CONVENTIONAL MR IMAGING OF FOCAL WHITE MATTER LESIONS

Conventional MR techniques in MS imaging are based on the delineation of demyelinating white matter plaques in the brain and spinal cord.[4,12] Multiple conventional MR pulse sequences are used in this evaluation, including T2-weighted, proton density–weighted, and fluid-attenuated inversion recovery (FLAIR)–weighted sequences, as well as T1-weighted imaging before and after the administration of gadolinium contrast (Box 1).[4,13] These pulse sequences provide a sensitive method for detecting and quantifying focal white matter disease as well as more acute inflammatory activity in patients with MS (Fig. 1).[14] However, white matter MS lesions shown on conventional MR are not specific to a particular underlying pathologic mechanism, and can reflect various processes including edema, gliosis, inflammation, demyelination, and axonal loss.[12,15]

Certain imaging features of white matter lesions (Box 2) increase the specificity of conventional MR findings for underlying pathologic mechanisms.[14] For example, lesion hypointensity on T1-weighted imaging is correlated with axonal loss, and is found most often in chronic lesions.[4,13,15] Enhancement of white matter lesions on postcontrast T1-weighted imaging is more often associated with acute to subacute inflammation and breakdown of the blood-brain barrier.[4,13,15] Although most of these enhancing MS plaques become permanent T2-hyperintense lesions, only approximately half go on to T1 hypointensity and associated neuronal loss, highlighting the brain's reparative capacity.[15] Restricted diffusion also suggests a more acute process. In addition, hypointensity on T2-weighted imaging in cortical and deep gray matter structures such as the thalamus and basal ganglia is likely caused by excessive iron deposition in patients with MS and may correlate with other imaging findings and patient symptoms.[16–18]

Despite the sensitivity of conventional MR findings for focal white matter disease in MS, as well as the relative pathologic specificity of some imaging features, there remains a discrepancy between the burden of white matter disease as measured

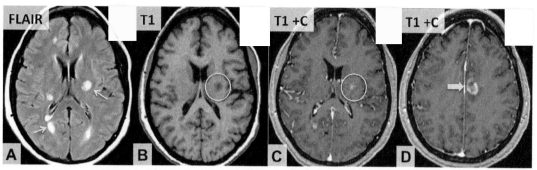

Fig. 1. A 38-year-old woman who presented acutely with dysarthria. Conventional MR imaging shows multiple hyperintense periventricular and subcortical focal white matter lesions on FLAIR-weighted imaging (*arrows in A*). A large lesion in the left centrum semiovale shows hypointensity on T1-weighted imaging, suggesting edema in this setting (*circle in B*), as well as patchy enhancement (*circle in C*) consistent with more acute inflammation. A separate focal white matter lesion more superiorly shows ring enhancement (*arrow in D*).

by conventional MR and clinical disease measures such as physical disability and cognitive impairment.[11,15,19] New white matter lesions on MR are often asymptomatic, whereas a patient may experience worsening symptoms despite stability of conventional MR imaging findings.[1,4,15] Brex and colleagues[11] found only a modest correlation between lesion volume and long-term disability in the first 5 years of follow-up in patients with MS who had originally presented with clinically isolated syndromes. The correlation between conventional MR findings and clinical disease is even weaker with the primary progressive form of MS, in which patients typically develop severe neurologic disability despite having a low white matter

---

Box 2
Conventional MR findings in MS

- Focal cerebral white matter lesions
  - Periventricular and subcortical, often perpendicular to ventricular surface, as well as in posterior fossa
  - T1 hypointensity more often in chronic lesions, or sometimes with excessive edema
  - Diffusion restriction and enhancement more often in acute lesions
- Focal spinal cord white matter lesions
  - Most patients with MS, most often in the cervical cord
- T2 hypointensity in basal ganglia and thalamus
  - Likely caused by iron deposition, progressive
- Atrophy of the brain and spinal cord
  - Progressive, seen in advanced disease

---

plaque burden and activity as measured by gadolinium enhancement.[20–22]

The weak correlation between conventional MR findings in MS and patient symptoms is likely caused, at least in part, by the failure of conventional MR to detect the diffuse structural, metabolic, and functional abnormalities now known to be present in the normal-appearing gray and white matter.[3,7,23] Support for this idea comes from studies that have correlated abnormalities in normal-appearing white and gray matter with clinical measures of disease such as physical disability.[7] In addition, conventional MR remains insensitive in distinguishing focal gray matter lesions because of their small size, poor contrast with surrounding tissue, and partial volume effects with cerebrospinal fluid (CSF) when cortically based.[5] Focal gray matter lesions, along with cerebral atrophy (as discussed later), may correlate more closely with physical disability and cognitive impairment than focal white matter abnormalities.[2,24–26]

CONVENTIONAL MR IMAGING OF CEREBRAL ATROPHY

Cerebral atrophy presents early in the course of MS, is usually progressive, and affects the brain diffusely.[15] As is the case for focal white matter lesions, cerebral atrophy in MS is not specific for an underlying pathologic mechanism, but instead likely reflects the end point of multiple disease processes, including demyelination, inflammation, and gliosis.[15] Although volume loss associated with white matter plaques likely plays a role in the development of cerebral atrophy in MS, disease involving the NAWM and gray matter may be even more important.[1,15] In addition, gray matter atrophy in MS involves both cortical and subcortical structures, and is likely caused by a combination of direct damage from focal lesions as well as indirect damage from white matter disorders, including wallerian degeneration.[15,24]

Cerebral atrophy in MS has been found to correlate strongly with current and future clinical disability as well as cognitive and neuropsychiatric impairment.[15,27,28] For example, Lazeron and colleagues[29] showed that cognitive slowing in patients with MS correlated most strongly with brain volume loss, with a weaker association found with white matter lesion burden. In contrast, Popescu and colleagues[30] found that measurements of cerebral atrophy and lesion volumes were complimentary in predicting long-term disability in MS. In addition, regional variations in gray matter volume loss, particularly in the thalamus, have been associated with MS subtype as well as specific types of functional impairment.[24,31]

Given the correlation between cerebral atrophy and clinical measures of disease, clinical trials are using this finding as a way of measuring the efficacy of novel MS treatments.[1] As a result, accurate and reproducible imaging methods for measuring cerebral volume in patients with MS are essential.[15] Beyond these technical issues, the use of atrophy as a proxy for disease progression is problematic because volume loss in patients with MS can be secondary to other factors.[1,15] For example, reductions in cerebral volume are often seen after treatment of patients with MS with various immunomodulatory therapies, such as interferon beta and corticosteroids, which may reflect alterations in osmotic and inflammatory factors as opposed to tissue loss.[1,15,28]

ADVANCES IN CONVENTIONAL MR IMAGING

Magnets with high field strengths (3.0 T and greater) increase the sensitivity of MR for detecting enhancing and nonenhancing T2-hyperintense white matter lesions compared with 1.5 T, and consequently may improve the early diagnosis of MS (Fig. 2).[32,33] Magnets with high field strengths also detect more focal MS lesions in cortical and subcortical gray matter.[24] In addition,

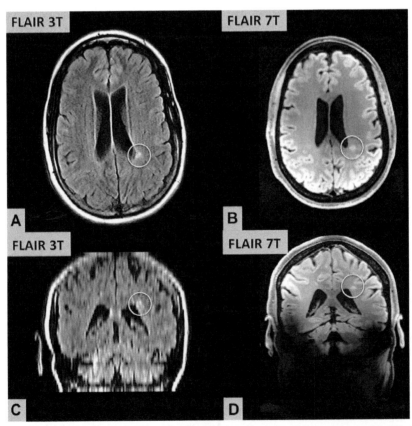

Fig. 2. Comparison of FLAIR imaging performed at 3 T (*A, C*) and 7 T (*B, D*) in a patient with MS. A left periventricular focal white matter lesion (*yellow circles*) is more conspicuous and better delineated on FLAIR imaging performed at 7 T. (*Courtesy of* the Center for Magnetic Resonance and Optical Imaging, University of Pennsylvania, Philadelphia, PA; with permission.)

ultrahigh-field MR imaging (7 T) has begun to help further elucidate understanding of possible pathophysiologic mechanisms in MS, with recent studies showing the presence of a central vein or venule in white matter plaques that may be a distinctive marker of demyelination.[12] Ultrahigh-field MR has also shown the presence of previously unseen small focal white matter lesions that may be responsible, at least in part, for the diffuse abnormalities previously noted in NAWM by other techniques.[1]

Besides increases in field strength, advances in MR pulse sequences have increased the sensitivity of conventional MR for detecting disease-related changes in MS (Fig. 3).[24,34] For example, a double inversion recovery sequence, which suppresses signal from fluid and white matter, is a valuable tool for detecting inflammatory MS lesions in cortical and subcortical gray matter.[24–26] This technique has high specificity, but does not currently detect all cortical lesions as shown on histopathology.[24] Furthermore, gradient echo three-dimensional (3D) FLAIR is another recently developed sequence that has shown improved sensitivity in detecting white matter demyelinating plaques.[34]

Other investigations of conventional MR imaging in MS include the use of new contrast agents, including ultrasmall particles of iron oxide and gadolinium, which may be useful in evaluating inflammatory processes by tracking macrophages that pick up the particles.[35] However, localization of macrophage activity by the use of ultrasmall iron oxide particles does not correlate perfectly with areas of altered blood-brain barrier permeability as shown by gadolinium enhancement.[35] This finding suggests that the two techniques may provide unique and complementary information.[35] Other markers of inflammation and neuronal death are also currently being evaluated, including a myeloperoxide-sensitive molecular probe and gadofluorine, which selectively localizes in axons undergoing wallerian degeneration (Box 3).[1,35]

AUTOMATED IMAGING TECHNIQUES AND QUANTIFICATION OF IMAGING DATA

The expected average annual change in white matter lesion volume in a patient with relapsing-remitting MS is small, on the order of only 10% to 20%.[10] In addition, interobserver variability when manually counting or evaluating white matter lesions can be poor because of differences in MR equipment, protocols, and patient positioning between serial examinations.[36] As a result of these challenges, areas of current research in MS imaging have focused on the use of automated and semiautomated techniques to more accurately and reproducibly detect disease characteristics such as white matter lesion burden and atrophy as well as their progression over time.[1,37] These methods may also allow global and regional quantification of disease features, enhanced comparisons among data sets, and increases in the sensitivity of imaging techniques.[1,31]

Several methods have been developed to process and analyze MR imaging, and require varying degrees of user input.[1] Voxel-based morphometry is an example of an automated technique that quantifies and compares MR data by measuring the signal intensity of individual voxels as well as their change over time on serial examinations.[1,37] The subtraction technique is a semiautomated registration method that highlights interval change in disease by registering, or matching, 2 serial MR examinations and then subtracting the data sets to highlight areas of interval change.[10] More regional measurement of disease parameters may be further analyzed by segmentation of the brain, which involves automated methods for separating gray matter from white matter, as well as identifying individual structures such as the thalamus

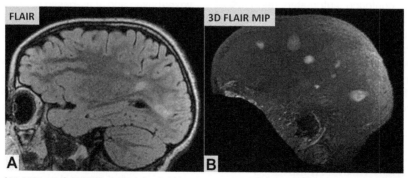

Fig. 3. Sagittal FLAIR-weighted (*A*) and sagittal three-dimensional FLAIR maximum intensity projection (MIP) imaging (*B*) of a patient with MS. The MIP technique, typically used in MR angiography, increases lesion conspicuity compared with conventional FLAIR imaging.

or hippocampus.[15,37] For example, segmentation of voxel-based morphometry data has been used to measure regional variation in cerebral gray matter volume loss and lesion burden.[1]

Challenges remain to this type of the automated or semiautomated imaging analysis. For example, the presence of white matter plaques in patients with MS can confound automated methods of brain segmentation and require manual correction.[24] Furthermore, white matter lesions can vary in their conspicuity on MR and have indistinct borders, making automated methods of detecting and outlining plaques challenging (**Fig. 4**).[4] In addition, it is difficult to determine the accuracy of these methods given the lack of a gold standard for many of the disease features being studied, such as demyelinating plaques (**Box 4**).[4]

MAGNETIZATION TRANSFER IMAGING

Conventional MR imaging detects the signal of free water protons in tissue.[4,13] Protons that are part of cellular macromolecules, which have extremely short relaxation times, usually do not contribute to an MR image.[4,6] However, if an off-frequency pulse is administered to a volume of tissue, a portion of the energy deposited in these cellular macromolecules can be transferred to adjacent free water protons, which then subsequently generates a detectable signal.[12,38] The magnetization transfer ratio (MTR) is obtained by measuring the change in signal intensity between imaging performed with and without the off-frequency pulse and it reflects the structural integrity of tissues by indirectly detecting cellular macromolecules.[4,38] Standardization of MTR data between different scanners and institutions is essential because MTR imaging is sensitive to both variations in acquisition protocols and other independent variables.[39]

Acute as well as chronic focal white matter lesions in MS show reductions in MTR values that correlate with duration of plaque enhancement as well as associated T1 hypointensity.[6] Postmortem as well as animal studies have shown that these reductions in MTR are associated with the degree of underlying tissue structural damage, including demyelination and axonal loss.[38,40,41] The decrease in MTR can vary among white matter lesions, which is likely secondary to variability in both disease severity and underlying pathologic mechanisms.[6,38,40] Reductions in MTR have also been noted in the NAWM and gray matter in patients with MS and seem to be more pronounced in progressive forms of the disease.[5,42,43] Studies have suggested that MTR analysis may have prognostic value for subsequent disease progression, with correlations between MTR values of NAWM and subsequent development of clinical disability.[6] Abnormal MTR values in gray matter have also been associated with clinical disease, including physical disability and cognitive impairment.[6,43]

Areas of active research in MTR imaging include voxel-based and atlas-based approaches for evaluation of regional MTR changes in the brain and their progression over time.[1] In addition, other magnetization transfer parameters, such as the magnetization transfer rate, are currently being evaluated and may provide a more sensitive and specific evaluation of myelin in the CNS.[5] In addition, a more complete characterization of MTR values can be obtained by acquiring a larger data set and extracting information related to the magnetic resonance properties of protons and their local magnetic environment.[39,44,45] This method is called quantitative magnetization transfer imaging and it is less susceptible to variations in acquisition protocols.[39,44,45]

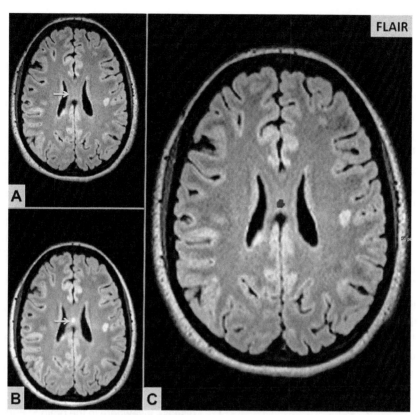

Fig. 4. Computer-aided detection software highlights a new MS lesion in the body of the corpus callosum. Axial FLAIR-weighted imaging shows a new focal white matter lesion developing in the body of the corpus callosum between serial examinations (*yellow arrow in A* and *B*). The automated technique correctly identifies the new lesion (*red dot in C*), and disregards the additional white matter lesions that were already present on the prior study. (*Courtesy of* Dr Michel Bilello, MD, PhD, Perelman School of Medicine at University of Pennsylvania, Philadelphia, PA.)

DIFFUSION TENSOR IMAGING

Diffusion-weighted imaging measures the brownian motion of water molecules in tissues, which is influenced by the presence of various barriers to diffusion such as cell membranes and other macromolecular structures.[4,46] The overall diffusion of water molecules can be measured irrespective of the direction of motion, yielding maps of both mean diffusivity (MD) and apparent diffusion coefficient (ADC).[47,48] Another measure that can be derived from diffusion tensor imaging is the fractional anisotropy (FA), which is a measure of the nonrandomness of water diffusion in a particular region.[4,46] For example, water protons in white matter tracts preferentially follow the direction of the corresponding axons in that region, showing highly anisotropic diffusion along their course.[46,48]

Numerous studies have shown increases in MD and reductions in FA associated with focal white matter lesions, as well as, to a lesser degree, the NAWM of patients with MS (**Fig. 5**).[48,49] These alterations in diffusion parameters vary with the severity, duration, and subtype of MS, and can be detected early in the course of the disease.[47,50,51] The variability in measured MD and FA of MS white matter lesions, as well as their progression over time, suggests considerable heterogeneity of the underlying pathologic mechanisms and their severities.[46] There is also evidence that diffusion abnormalities precede the formation of white matter lesions.[50] For example, Werring and colleagues[52] found that the formation of gadolinium-enhancing white matter plaques was preceded by subtle decreases in ADC, likely reflecting early structural damage.

Increases in MD and decreases in FA correlate with demyelination and axonal loss in patients with MS.[5,46,47,50,53] In addition, these alterations in diffusion parameters have been associated with other imaging findings already linked to cellular damage.[47] For example, white matter plaques with associated T1 hypointensity show

---

Box 4
Summary of nonconventional MR techniques

- Magnetization transfer imaging
  - Detection of damage to macromolecules, including myelin
- Diffusion tensor imaging
  - Detection of damage to highly organized white matter tracts
- Diffusion tensor tractography
  - Detection of damage to specific functional units in the brain
- MR proton spectroscopy
  - Detection of metabolite changers in both acute and chronic white matter lesions as well as in surrounding gray and white matter
- Functional MR imaging
  - Detection of alterations in cortical activation suggesting brain plasticity
- MR perfusion imaging
  - Detections of focal as well as global alterations in cerebral blood flow and volume
- Myelin imaging, multicomponent relaxometry
  - Detection of focal as well as global reductions in myelin

---

higher diffusivity and lower FA than those that do not, likely reflecting the neuronal loss linked to the latter conventional MR finding.[46,48,50] Furthermore, increases in MD are inversely correlated with MTR values, which, as previously discussed, is consistent with processes such as demyelination and loss of axonal integrity.[49] Abnormalities in white matter diffusion parameters have been correlated with clinical measures of disease including physical disability.[50]

Calabrese and colleagues[54] found that gray matter cortical lesions in patients with relapsing-remitting MS showed increased FA compared with normal-appearing gray matter, and that patients' normal-appearing gray matter showed higher FA values relative to healthy controls. Hannoun and colleagues[55] found similar increases in FA in subcortical gray matter structures, including the thalamus and caudate nucleus. These increases in FA may reflect inflammation associated with gray matter lesions as well as changes in the microglia.[54,55] As is the case for findings in white matter, diffusion tensor abnormalities in gray matter structures have also shown correlations with patient symptoms.[54]

DIFFUSION TENSOR TRACTOGRAPHY (DIFFUSION TENSOR IMAGING)

Diffusion tensor tractography, or fiber tracking, uses diffusion tensor imaging data to generate 3D representations of anisotropic diffusion in white matter tracts.[5,46,56] These 3D maps can then be color coded to show the direction of anisotropic diffusion in various regions of the brain.[5,46] Evaluating the distribution of disease in patients with MS on diffusion tensor topographic maps can help to correlate imaging findings with clinical disability by highlighting disruption of white matter tracts that connect various cortical and subcortical gray matter structures.[5,24,46] This type of investigation is designed to evaluate connectivity within the brain, a term that means the degree of confidence that two regions of gray matter are linked.[1]

Various studies have correlated damage to particular white matter tracts on diffusion tensor tractography with specific patient symptoms in MS (**Fig. 6**).[1,50] For example, lesions in white matter tracts associated with cognition seem to correlate more closely with cognitive impairment than disease elsewhere in the brain.[24] Furthermore, patients early in the course of the disease with motor impairment show increased MD and T2 lesion volume in the corticospinal tracts compared with patients without pyramidal symptoms.[46] However, numerous challenges remain in the evaluation of connectivity on diffusion tractography, including tracking through MS plaques caused by tissue disruption as well as the complexity of white matter connections in subcortical regions.[1,5] In addition, it is still uncertain to what extent damage to regional white matter tracts predicts clinical disability when accounting for other imaging variables (**Box 5**).[24]

MR PROTON SPECTROSCOPY

Metabolite abnormalities on MR proton spectroscopy with short and long echo times have been noted early in the course of MS in both demyelinating plaques and in surrounding NAWM and gray matter (**Box 6**).[1,57] Alterations in various metabolites have been shown, including N-acetyl aspartate (NAA), choline, myo-inositol, glutamate, lactate, and creatine.[1,58] Choline, a metabolite associated with cell membrane phospholipids, is thought to be a marker of cell turnover as well as myelin breakdown and repair.[13,58] Increases in myo-inositol and creatine suggest gliosis, increases of lactate can be seen secondary to the

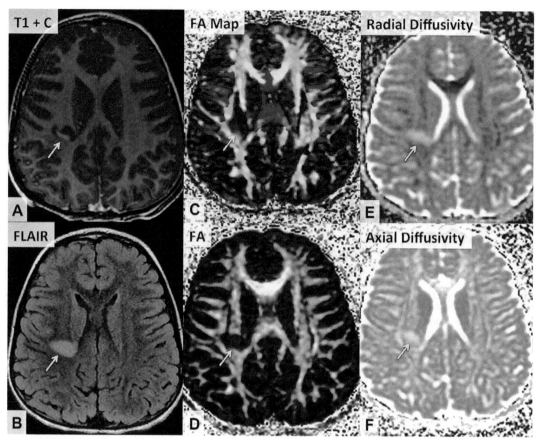

Fig. 5. Conventional MR imaging shows an enhancing focal white matter lesion in the right centrum semiovale on both enhanced T1-weighted and FLAIR-weighted imaging (*arrows in A and B*). On diffusion tensor imaging, the lesion shows a reduction in FA (*arrows in C and D*) and an increase in diffusivity (*arrows in E and F*).

metabolism of inflammatory cells, and increases in the excitatory neurotransmitter glutamate have been associated with glutamate excitotoxicity and neuronal damage.[5,13,58] In addition, decreases in the concentration of NAA, a neuronal marker, have been correlated with neuronal death and loss of axon integrity.[58]

In active enhancing MS white matter lesions, increases in choline, myo-inositol, lactate and glutamate, and decreases in NAA, have been identified (**Fig. 7**).[1,58] Creatine is often also increased in acute demyelinating plaques, but can be decreased in large lesions.[58] Metabolite alterations in acute lesions may subsequently resolve, including normalization of lactate, creatine, and NAA; normalization of NAA possibly reflects resolution of edema as well as increases in axonal diameter following remyelination.[58] In chronic, nonenhancing MS plaques, NAA is markedly reduced, myo-inositol remains increased, and glutamate levels are often normal.[1] The further reductions in NAA in chronic plaques are consistent with progression of neuronal loss.[58]

Progressive decreases in NAA have also been shown in the NAWM of patients with MS and these reductions seem to vary with distance from focal white matter lesions.[58–60] Furthermore, decreases in the NAA/creatine ratio, particularly in NAWM, have been correlated with clinical disability in patients with clinically isolated syndromes and early relapsing-remitting MS.[58] Additional metabolic abnormalities in the NAWM include increases of glutamate and myo-inositol.[59–61] In addition, focal increases of lipids and choline in NAWM have been shown before the development of a focal white matter lesions on conventional MR, indicating that MR spectroscopy may be a sensitive indicator of early myelin disorders and acute inflammation.[58]

Metabolite abnormalities have also been shown in the gray matter of patients with MS, including reductions in NAA, choline, and glutamate, which are more pronounced in progressive forms of MS.[3] Reductions of NAA in subcortical gray matter have been shown early in the course of MS, whereas cortical involvement is found only in later

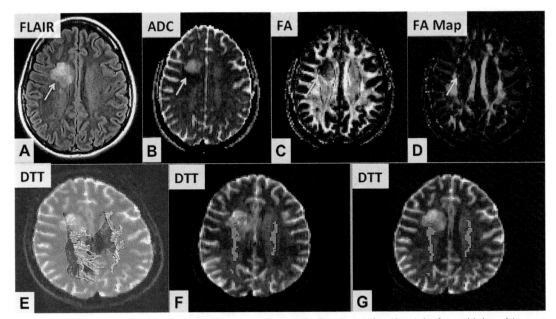

Fig. 6. Conventional MR imaging shows a focal hyperintense lesion situated in the right frontal lobe white matter on FLAIR imaging (*arrow in A*), with an area of restricted diffusion along its posterior margin (*arrow in B*). There is a corresponding reduction in FA associated with the lesion (*arrows in C and D*). On diffusion tensor tractography, the lesion is noted to partially involve a portion of the right anterior corticospinal tract (*E–G*).

stages of the disease.[58] More global analyses of MR spectroscopy data have shown reductions in whole-brain NAA in both MS and clinically isolated syndromes.[5] This latter finding suggests that MR spectroscopy may be a useful marker of generalized neurodegeneration.[5]

Current challenges to the widespread use of MR proton spectroscopy in the clinical evaluation of MS include the limited spatial coverage associated with voxel-based techniques, as well as the lack of spatial localization when whole-brain approaches are used.[58] In addition, measurements of absolute concentrations of metabolites can be affected by multiple acquisition variables, making the reproducibility of MR spectroscopy challenging.[5,58] Although measuring relative concentrations of metabolites can help to overcome the issue of reproducibility, the validity of the approach can be compromised if the reference metabolite is altered by disease.[1,58] Areas of active research in MR spectroscopy include the use of MR magnets with high field strengths with corresponding improvement in signal/noise ratio, improvements in methods of metabolite quantification, and the investigation of the role of additional metabolites associated with myelin, including valine, alanine, and leucine.[1]

FUNCTIONAL MR IMAGING

Function MR (fMR) imaging is a noninvasive method of measuring neuronal activity in vivo.[1,5] When an area of the brain becomes activated while performing a task, the metabolic demand of that region increases and results in changes in the concentration of deoxyhemoglobin, which provides the contrast for fMR imaging.[62] Numerous studies have shown a correlation between structural damage in the brain of patients with MS and changes in activation patterns on fMR imaging, suggesting cortical reorganization.[5,63] Changes in activation patterns on fMR imaging have been shown in patients with clinically isolated

---

Box 5
Diffusion tensor abnormalities in MS

- Focal white matter lesions
  - Varying degrees of increased MD and reduced FA
  - Restricted diffusion can be seen associated with acute plaques
- NAWM
  - More mild increases in MD and reductions in FA
- Gray matter
  - Focal lesions may show increased FA, possibly secondary to inflammation

---

Box 6
Metabolite abnormalities in MS

- *N*-acetyl aspartate (NAA), a neuronal marker
  - Reductions in focal lesions, NAWM, gray matter
  - More pronounced in chronic disease
  - Global reductions in whole-brain NAA also noted
- Choline, a marker of cell turnover
  - Increased in acute white matter lesions
  - Can be decreased in gray matter
- Myo-inositol, marker of gliosis
  - Increased in both acute and chronic white matter lesions and NAWM
- Creatine, marker of gliosis
  - Often increased in acute white matter lesions, but can be decreased
- Glutamate, excitatory neurotransmitter
  - Increases in focal white matter lesions and NAWM may indicate glutamate excitotoxicity and neuronal damage
- Lactate, marker for inflammation
  - Can be increased in acute white matter lesions
- Valine, alanine, and leucine
  - Potential markers of myelin

---

syndromes, suggesting that functional abnormalities are an early feature of MS.[5]

Cortical reorganization in patients with MS as shown by fMR imaging varies with the stage of the disease and seems to correlate with specific symptoms.[1,63] For example, increased activation of both ipsilateral and contralateral classic motor networks has been shown in patients with MS undergoing simple motor tasks and this finding has been strongly correlated with the extent of white matter disorder as shown by other imaging techniques.[5,63] Furthermore, reductions in the activation of movement-associated subcortical networks, including the thalamus, have been linked to fatigue in patients with MS.[1,5] In addition, there is increased recruitment of cognitive-related networks in patients with primary progressive MS with cognitive impairment compared with those who remain cognitively intact.[64] These studies indicate that brain plasticity as shown on fMR imaging may compensate for the clinical consequences of structural MS lesions such as white

matter plaques and may help explain the discordance between conventional MR findings and patient symptoms.[1,5,63] Eventual progression of clinical disability in patients with more advanced disease may occur once damage to the brain is severe enough that it overcomes the brain's plasticity reservoir.[62,63]

MR PERFUSION IMAGING

There is evidence that vascular inflammation plays a role in the pathogenesis of MS, including the periventricular distribution of white matter plaques, hypoxia-like tissue injury on histopathology, and blood vessel abnormalities such as wall hyalinization and lymphocytic cuffing.[65,66] Various MR perfusion techniques have been applied in the evaluation of MS, using both exogenous tracers such as gadolinium chelates and endogenous agents as in arterial spin labeling.[1,65] These methods have shown increased cerebral perfusion associated with acute, enhancing MS plaques, and decreased perfusion in normal-appearing white and gray matter.[65] Nonenhancing white matter plaques can show either increased or decreased perfusion, suggesting heterogeneity in the underlying pathophysiology of these lesions, including microvascular impairment and inflammatory vasodilatation.[65]

Given the increasing recognition of the role of gray matter disorders in MS, as well as the high metabolic demand of the tissue, attention has been turned to MR perfusion imaging to evaluate for changes in cerebral blood flow (CBF) and cerebral blood volume (CBV) in cortical and subcortical structures.[66] Aviv and colleagues[66] used a new dynamic susceptibility contrast method to show a correlation between cognitive impairment in patients with MS and global reductions in relative CBF and CBV in gray and white matter.[66] Another study found that reductions in cortical and subcortical gray matter CBF and CBV correlated with cognitive test scores in secondary progressive MS.[67] The results of these studies suggest that alterations in cerebral perfusion may have a role in the development of cognitive impairment in MS, although further work is needed to better characterize these findings.

MYELIN IMAGING

Both in vitro and in vivo studies have shown that T2 relaxation times measured by conventional MR imaging of the CNS represent a composite of individual relaxation times corresponding with discrete biological compartments.[4,68,69] These compartments include a long T2 relaxation

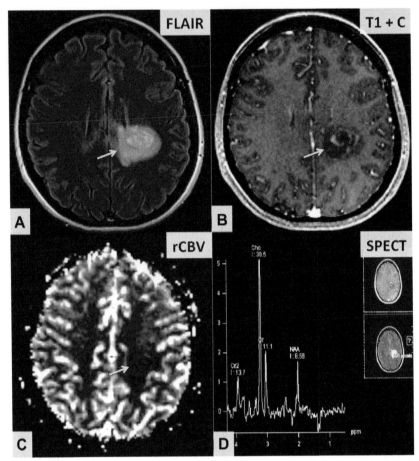

Fig. 7. Conventional MR imaging shows a focal hyperintense white matter lesion on FLAIR imaging in the left periventricular region, which extends into the centrum semiovale and shows rimlike enhancement (*arrows in A and B*). Dynamic susceptibility contrast MR perfusion imaging shows no appreciable increase in relative cerebral blood volume associated with the lesion (*arrow in C*). MR spectroscopy shows mildly increased choline/creatine and choline/NAA ratios within the lesion, as well as a small amount of lactate (*D*).

component corresponding with CSF, an intermediate component corresponding with intracellular and extracellular water, and a short T2 relaxation component that is thought to be caused by water within the lipid bilayer of myelin.[68,69] The analysis and quantification of these individual T2 relaxation time components is called multicomponent relaxometry and it has proved to be a useful tool in evaluating MS and its variants (**Box 7**).[70] The summation of the three components is the composite T2 relaxation time, which is measured by conventional MR, whereas the ratio of the short myelin component to the composite time is the myelin water fraction (MWF).[68,69]

Reductions in MWF in NAWM have been shown to be primarily a result of loss of myelin integrity as opposed to inflammation or edema, thus offering increased specificity for demyelination compared with other nonconventional MR techniques.[12,68] For example, Moore and colleagues[71] showed

> **Box 7**
> **Multicomponent relaxometry: myelin imaging**
>
> - Long T2 relaxation component
>   - ○ Corresponds with CSF
> - Intermediate T2 relaxation component
>   - ○ Corresponds with intracellular and extracellular water
> - Short T2 relaxation component
>   - ○ Corresponds with water within myelin
> - Composite T2 relaxation time
>   - ○ Summation of long, intermediate, and short components
> - Myelin water fraction
>   - ○ Ratio of short myelin component to composite relaxation time

that the MWF correlates closely with the distribution of myelin in the brain and that MS plaques on postmortem studies were associated with reductions in the short T2 myelin component. In vivo studies have shown decreases in the MWF in white matter lesions, as well as, to a lesser extent, the NAWM of patients with MS compared with healthy controls.[68,72] Furthermore, reductions in the MWF of NAWM have been correlated with disease duration and severity.[72] However, technical challenges to myelin imaging remain, including poor image quality, longer scan times, and limited spatial coverage of the brain.[1,24]

SPINAL CORD IMAGING

More than 90% of patients with MS have involvement of the spinal cord at autopsy, with most showing focal cord lesions on conventional MR, most often in the cervical spine.[73,74] In patients who do not have a definite diagnosis of MS, such as in the setting of a clinically isolated syndrome, the visualization of disease in the spinal cord on conventional MR imaging can help make the diagnosis by showing distribution of disease in space.[9] Furthermore, spinal cord lesions show a robust correlation with clinical disability, making them useful makers of disease.[75] Spinal cord atrophy is also common in MS, with reductions in cervical spinal cord volume also correlating strongly with clinical disability.[12,73,76,77]

Nonconventional MR techniques have shown widespread abnormalities in the spinal cord, including in focal lesions as well as in normal-appearing gray and white matter.[1,5,6,73] For example, Agosta and colleagues[8] found lower average MTR in cervical spinal cord gray matter in patients with relapsing-remitting MS compared with healthy controls, whereas reductions in cord T1 relaxations times suggesting expansion of the extracellular space have also been noted.[73] In addition, abnormalities in spinal cord diffusion metrics such as MD and FA have been identified and associated with both demyelination and axonal injury.[46,56,78] In addition, MR spectroscopy has revealed reductions in spinal cord NAA.[79] The diffuse structural and metabolic abnormalities noted in the spinal cord by these advanced imaging techniques have been correlated with various measures of clinical disease.[8,46,56,78,79]

Continued challenges to spinal cord imaging in patients with MS include the small size of the target structure, which makes evaluation of regional changes difficult, as well as the mobility of the cord, which leads to motion artifact from respiratory and cardiac cycles.[8,56,73,74] However, improvements in conventional MR imaging of the

spinal cord have been realized with advances in receiver coils, faster imaging techniques, and magnets with higher field strengths.[4,24,73,80] In addition, newer MR pulse sequences as well as semiautomated methods for outlining the cervical spinal cord have improved lesion detection and quantification of cord atrophy.[73,75] Higher resolution imaging of the spinal cord may allow a more regional analysis of damage in patients with MS, helping to further clarify the relationship between structural lesions and clinical disability.[8]

OPTIC NERVE IMAGING

The small size of the optic nerves makes imaging evaluation of these structures a challenge.[1,46] However, increasing field strength of clinical MR magnets allows evaluation of lesion size and distribution in optic neuritis as well as measurements and quantification of optic nerve cross-sectional area.[1] These imaging findings can then be correlated with physiologic measures such as nerve block.[1] MTR and diffusion imaging have provided evidence of myelin damage and repair in the optic nerves, as well as reduction in structural integrity of the underlying axons.[1,6] Non-MR techniques are also being used to investigate the optic nerves, including optic coherence tomography, which uses near-infrared light to measure the thickness of the retinal nerve fiber layer (RNFL).[81,82] Reductions in the RNFL have been shown in patients with MS relative to controls and may provide another noninvasive method for evaluating the disease.[81,82]

SUMMARY

Conventional MR imaging continues to play an important role in the diagnosis and follow-up of patients with MS and its variants. However, despite advances in technique, findings on conventional MR still show only a modest correlation with clinical measures of disease including physical disability and cognitive impairment. Nonconventional MR imaging methods have show greater success at linking patient symptoms with imaging findings by more accurately characterizing the full extent of structural, metabolic, and functional changes present throughout the CNS. These advanced imaging techniques have also led to new areas of research by better characterizing the pathophysiology of MS as well as the adaptive capabilities of the brain. However, additional work is needed to further clarify what role, if any, advanced imaging should play in the evaluation of MS and variants in clinical practice.

REFERENCES

1. Bakshi R, Thompson AJ, Rocca MA, et al. MRI in multiple sclerosis: current status and future prospects. Lancet Neurol 2008;7(7):615–25.
2. Derfuss T. Personalized medicine in multiple sclerosis: hope or reality? BMC Med 2012;10:116.
3. Filippi M, Rocca MA. MRI evidence for multiple sclerosis as a diffuse disease of the central nervous system. J Neurol 2005;252(Suppl 5):v16–24.
4. Miller DH, Grossman RI, Reingold SC, et al. The role of magnetic resonance techniques in understanding and managing multiple sclerosis. Brain 1998;121(Pt 1):3–24.
5. Miller DH, Thompson AJ, Filippi M. Magnetic resonance studies of abnormalities in the normal appearing white matter and grey matter in multiple sclerosis. J Neurol 2003;250(12):1407–19.
6. Filippi M, Rocca MA. Magnetization transfer magnetic resonance imaging of the brain, spinal cord, and optic nerve. Neurotherapeutics 2007;4(3):401–13.
7. Geurts JJ, Calabrese M, Fisher E, et al. Measurement and clinical effect of grey matter pathology in multiple sclerosis. Lancet Neurol 2012;11(12):1082–92.
8. Agosta F, Pagani E, Caputo D, et al. Associations between cervical cord gray matter damage and disability in patients with multiple sclerosis. Arch Neurol 2007;64(9):1302–5.
9. Polman CH, Reingold SC, Banwell B, et al. Diagnostic criteria for multiple sclerosis: 2010 revisions to the McDonald criteria. Ann Neurol 2011;69(2):292–302.
10. Duan Y, Hildenbrand PG, Sampat MP, et al. Segmentation of subtraction images for the measurement of lesion change in multiple sclerosis. AJNR Am J Neuroradiol 2008;29(2):340–6.
11. Brex PA, Ciccarelli O, O'Riordan JI, et al. A longitudinal study of abnormalities on MRI and disability from multiple sclerosis. N Engl J Med 2002;346(3):158–64.
12. Ciccarelli O, Wheeler-Kingshott CA, McLean MA, et al. Spinal cord spectroscopy and diffusion-based tractography to assess acute disability in multiple sclerosis. Brain 2007;130(Pt 8):2220–31.
13. Moore GR, Laule C. Neuropathologic correlates of magnetic resonance imaging in multiple sclerosis. J Neuropathol Exp Neurol 2012;71(9):762–78.
14. Rovira A, Leon A. MR in the diagnosis and monitoring of multiple sclerosis: an overview. Eur J Radiol 2008;67(3):409–14.
15. Bermel RA, Bakshi R. The measurement and clinical relevance of brain atrophy in multiple sclerosis. Lancet Neurol 2006;5(2):158–70.
16. Stankiewicz J, Panter SS, Neema M, et al. Iron in chronic brain disorders: imaging and neurotherapeutic implications. Neurotherapeutics 2007;4(3):371–86.
17. Sicotte NL. Neuroimaging in multiple sclerosis: neurotherapeutic implications. Neurotherapeutics 2011;8(1):54–62.
18. Bermel RA, Puli SR, Rudick RA, et al. Prediction of longitudinal brain atrophy in multiple sclerosis by gray matter magnetic resonance imaging T2 hypointensity. Arch Neurol 2005;62(9):1371–6.
19. Rovaris M, Comi G, Filippi M. MRI markers of destructive pathology in multiple sclerosis-related cognitive dysfunction. J Neurol Sci 2006;245(1–2):111–6.
20. Rocca MA, Absinta M, Filippi M. The role of advanced magnetic resonance imaging techniques in primary progressive MS. J Neurol 2012;259(4):611–21.
21. Filippi M, Rovaris M, Rocca MA. Imaging primary progressive multiple sclerosis: the contribution of structural, metabolic, and functional MRI techniques. Mult Scler 2004;10(Suppl 1):S36–44 [discussion: S44–5].
22. Thompson AJ, Montalban X, Barkhof F, et al. Diagnostic criteria for primary progressive multiple sclerosis: a position paper. Ann Neurol 2000;47(6):831–5.
23. Pirko I, Lucchinetti CF, Sriram S, et al. Gray matter involvement in multiple sclerosis. Neurology 2007;68(9):634–42.
24. Ceccarelli A, Bakshi R, Neema M. MRI in multiple sclerosis: a review of the current literature. Curr Opin Neurol 2012;25(4):402–9.
25. Filippi M, Rocca MA, Comi G. The use of quantitative magnetic-resonance-based techniques to monitor the evolution of multiple sclerosis. Lancet Neurol 2003;2(6):337–46.
26. Wattjes MP, Lutterbey GG, Gieseke J, et al. Double inversion recovery brain imaging at 3T: diagnostic value in the detection of multiple sclerosis lesions. AJNR Am J Neuroradiol 2007;28(1):54–9.
27. Bakshi R, Dandamudi VS, Neema M, et al. Measurement of brain and spinal cord atrophy by magnetic resonance imaging as a tool to monitor multiple sclerosis. J Neuroimaging 2005;15(Suppl 4):30S–45S.
28. Chen JT, Collins DL, Atkins HL, et al. Brain atrophy after immunoablation and stem cell transplantation in multiple sclerosis. Neurology 2006;66(12):1935–7.
29. Lazeron RH, de Sonneville LM, Scheltens P, et al. Cognitive slowing in multiple sclerosis is strongly associated with brain volume reduction. Mult Scler 2006;12(6):760–8.
30. Popescu V, Agosta F, Hulst HE, et al. Brain atrophy and lesion load predict long term disability in multiple sclerosis. J Neurol Neurosurg Psychiatry 2013;84(10):1082–91.

31. Duan Y, Liu Y, Liang P, et al. Comparison of grey matter atrophy between patients with neuromyelitis optica and multiple sclerosis: a voxel-based morphometry study. Eur J Radiol 2012;81(2): e110–4.

32. Sicotte NL, Voskuhl RR, Bouvier S, et al. Comparison of multiple sclerosis lesions at 1.5 and 3.0 Tesla. Invest Radiol 2003;38(7):423–7.

33. Wattjes MP, Harzheim M, Kuhl CK, et al. Does high-field MR imaging have an influence on the classification of patients with clinically isolated syndromes according to current diagnostic MR imaging criteria for multiple sclerosis? AJNR Am J Neuroradiol 2006;27(8):1794–8.

34. Pagani E, Bammer R, Horsfield MA, et al. Diffusion MR imaging in multiple sclerosis: technical aspects and challenges. AJNR Am J Neuroradiol 2007; 28(3):411–20.

35. Dousset V, Brochet B, Deloire MS, et al. MR imaging of relapsing multiple sclerosis patients using ultra-small-particle iron oxide and compared with gadolinium. AJNR Am J Neuroradiol 2006;27(5): 1000–5.

36. Erbayat Altay E, Fisher E, Jones SE, et al. Reliability of classifying multiple sclerosis disease activity using magnetic resonance imaging in a multiple sclerosis clinic. JAMA Neurol 2013;70(3):338–44.

37. Grassiot B, Desgranges B, Eustache F, et al. Quantification and clinical relevance of brain atrophy in multiple sclerosis: a review. J Neurol 2009;256(9): 1397–412.

38. Brochet B, Dousset V. Pathological correlates of magnetization transfer imaging abnormalities in animal models and humans with multiple sclerosis. Neurology 1999;53(5 Suppl 3):S12–7.

39. Janve VA, Zu Z, Yao SY, et al. The radial diffusivity and magnetization transfer pool size ratio are sensitive markers for demyelination in a rat model of type III multiple sclerosis (MS) lesions. Neuroimage 2013;74:298–305.

40. Schmierer K, Scaravilli F, Altmann DR, et al. Magnetization transfer ratio and myelin in postmortem multiple sclerosis brain. Ann Neurol 2004; 56(3):407–15.

41. van Waesberghe JH, Barkhof F. Magnetization transfer imaging of the spinal cord and the optic nerve in patients with multiple sclerosis. Neurology 1999;53(5 Suppl 3):S46–8.

42. Filippi M, Iannucci G, Tortorella C, et al. Comparison of MS clinical phenotypes using conventional and magnetization transfer MRI. Neurology 1999; 52(3):588–94.

43. Vrenken H, Pouwels PJ, Geurts JJ, et al. Altered diffusion tensor in multiple sclerosis normal-appearing brain tissue: cortical diffusion changes seem related to clinical deterioration. J Magn Reson Imaging 2006;23(5):628–36.

44. Rausch M, Tofts P, Lervik P, et al. Characterization of white matter damage in animal models of multiple sclerosis by magnetization transfer ratio and quantitative mapping of the apparent bound proton fraction f. Mult Scler 2009;15(1):16–27.

45. Tozer D, Ramani A, Barker GJ, et al. Quantitative magnetization transfer mapping of bound protons in multiple sclerosis. Magn Reson Med 2003; 50(1):83–91.

46. Inglese M, Bester M. Diffusion imaging in multiple sclerosis: research and clinical implications. NMR Biomed 2010;23(7):865–72.

47. Horsfield MA, Jones DK. Applications of diffusion-weighted and diffusion tensor MRI to white matter diseases – a review. NMR Biomed 2002;15(7–8): 570–7.

48. Filippi M, Cercignani M, Inglese M, et al. Diffusion tensor magnetic resonance imaging in multiple sclerosis. Neurology 2001;56(3):304–11.

49. Cercignani M, Iannucci G, Rocca MA, et al. Pathologic damage in MS assessed by diffusion-weighted and magnetization transfer MRI. Neurology 2000;54(5):1139–44.

50. Rovaris M, Filippi M. Diffusion tensor MRI in multiple sclerosis. J Neuroimaging 2007;17(Suppl 1): 27S–30S.

51. Preziosa P, Rocca MA, Mesaros S, et al. Intrinsic damage to the major white matter tracts in patients with different clinical phenotypes of multiple sclerosis: a voxelwise diffusion-tensor MR study. Radiology 2011;260(2):541–50.

52. Werring DJ, Brassat D, Droogan AG, et al. The pathogenesis of lesions and normal-appearing white matter changes in multiple sclerosis: a serial diffusion MRI study. Brain 2000;123(Pt 8):1667–76.

53. Schmierer K, Wheeler-Kingshott CA, Boulby PA, et al. Diffusion tensor imaging of post mortem multiple sclerosis brain. Neuroimage 2007;35(2): 467–77.

54. Calabrese M, Rinaldi F, Seppi D, et al. Cortical diffusion-tensor imaging abnormalities in multiple sclerosis: a 3-year longitudinal study. Radiology 2011;261(3):891–8.

55. Hannoun S, Durand-Dubief F, Confavreux C, et al. Diffusion tensor-MRI evidence for extra-axonal neuronal degeneration in caudate and thalamic nuclei of patients with multiple sclerosis. AJNR Am J Neuroradiol 2012;33(7):1363–8.

56. Sasiadek MJ, Szewczyk P, Bladowska J. Application of diffusion tensor imaging (DTI) in pathological changes of the spinal cord. Med Sci Monit 2012;18(6):RA73–9.

57. Chard DT, Griffin CM, McLean MA, et al. Brain metabolite changes in cortical grey and normal-appearing white matter in clinically early relapsing-remitting multiple sclerosis. Brain 2002; 125(Pt 10):2342–52.

58. De Stefano N, Filippi M. MR spectroscopy in multiple sclerosis. J Neuroimaging 2007;17(Suppl 1):31S–5S.

59. Kirov II, Tal A, Babb JS, et al. Serial proton MR spectroscopy of gray and white matter in relapsing-remitting MS. Neurology 2013;80(1):39–46.

60. Tisell A, Leinhard OD, Warntjes JB, et al. Increased concentrations of glutamate and glutamine in normal-appearing white matter of patients with multiple sclerosis and normal MR imaging brain scans. PLoS One 2013;8(4):e61817.

61. Srinivasan R, Sailasuta N, Hurd R, et al. Evidence of elevated glutamate in multiple sclerosis using magnetic resonance spectroscopy at 3 T. Brain 2005;128(Pt 5):1016–25.

62. Tedeschi G, Gallo A. Multiple sclerosis patients and immunomodulation therapies: the potential role of new MRI techniques to assess responders versus non-responders. Neurol Sci 2005;26(Suppl 4):S209–12.

63. Rocca MA, Absinta M, Moiola L, et al. Functional and structural connectivity of the motor network in pediatric and adult-onset relapsing-remitting multiple sclerosis. Radiology 2010;254(2):541–50.

64. Rocca MA, Riccitelli G, Rodegher M, et al. Functional MR imaging correlates of neuropsychological impairment in primary-progressive multiple sclerosis. AJNR Am J Neuroradiol 2010;31(7):1240–6.

65. Ge Y, Law M, Johnson G, et al. Dynamic susceptibility contrast perfusion MR imaging of multiple sclerosis lesions: characterizing hemodynamic impairment and inflammatory activity. AJNR Am J Neuroradiol 2005;26(6):1539–47.

66. Aviv RI, Francis PL, Tenenbein R, et al. Decreased frontal lobe gray matter perfusion in cognitively impaired patients with secondary-progressive multiple sclerosis detected by the bookend technique. AJNR Am J Neuroradiol 2012;33(9):1779–85.

67. Francis PL, Jakubovic R, O'Connor P, et al. Robust perfusion deficits in cognitively impaired patients with secondary-progressive multiple sclerosis. AJNR Am J Neuroradiol 2013;34(1):62–7.

68. Laule C, Vavasour IM, Moore GR, et al. Water content and myelin water fraction in multiple sclerosis. A T2 relaxation study. J Neurol 2004;251(3):284–93.

69. Beaulieu C, Fenrich FR, Allen PS. Multicomponent water proton transverse relaxation and T2-discriminated water diffusion in myelinated and nonmyelinated nerve. Magn Reson Imaging 1998;16(10):1201–10.

70. Spader HS, Ellermeier A, O'Muircheartaigh J, et al. Advances in myelin imaging with potential clinical application to pediatric imaging. Neurosurg Focus 2013;34(4):E9.

71. Moore GR, Leung E, MacKay AL, et al. A pathology-MRI study of the short-T2 component in formalin-fixed multiple sclerosis brain. Neurology 2000;55(10):1506–10.

72. Oh J, Han ET, Lee MC, et al. Multislice brain myelin water fractions at 3T in multiple sclerosis. J Neuroimaging 2007;17(2):156–63.

73. Tench CR, Morgan PS, Jaspan T, et al. Spinal cord imaging in multiple sclerosis. J Neuroimaging 2005;15(Suppl 4):94S–102S.

74. Ozturk A, Aygun N, Smith SA, et al. Axial 3D gradient-echo imaging for improved multiple sclerosis lesion detection in the cervical spinal cord at 3T. Neuroradiology 2013;55(4):431–9.

75. Kearney H, Yiannakas MC, Abdel-Aziz K, et al. Improved MRI quantification of spinal cord atrophy in multiple sclerosis. J Magn Reson Imaging 2013. [Epub ahead of print].

76. Cohen AB, Neema M, Arora A, et al. The relationships among MRI-defined spinal cord involvement, brain involvement, and disability in multiple sclerosis. J Neuroimaging 2012;22(2):122–8.

77. Gilmore CP, DeLuca GC, Bo L, et al. Spinal cord atrophy in multiple sclerosis caused by white matter volume loss. Arch Neurol 2005;62(12):1859–62.

78. Klawiter EC, Schmidt RE, Trinkaus K, et al. Radial diffusivity predicts demyelination in ex vivo multiple sclerosis spinal cords. Neuroimage 2011;55(4):1454–60.

79. Inglese M, Oesingmann N, Casaccia P, et al. Progressive multiple sclerosis and gray matter pathology: an MRI perspective. Mt Sinai J Med 2011;78(2):258–67.

80. Martin N, Malfair D, Zhao Y, et al. Comparison of MERGE and axial T2-weighted fast spin-echo sequences for detection of multiple sclerosis lesions in the cervical spinal cord. AJR Am J Roentgenol 2012;199(1):157–62.

81. Kallenbach K, Frederiksen J. Optical coherence tomography in optic neuritis and multiple sclerosis: a review. Eur J Neurol 2007;14(8):841–9.

82. Fisher JB, Jacobs DA, Markowitz CE, et al. Relation of visual function to retinal nerve fiber layer thickness in multiple sclerosis. Ophthalmology 2006;113(2):324–32.

Secondary Demyelination Disorders and Destruction of White Matter

Michael Ryan, MD, Mohannad Ibrahim, MD,
Hemant A. Parmar, MD*

KEYWORDS

- Secondary demyelinating disorders • White matter • Destruction • Central nervous system

KEY POINTS

- Secondary demyelinating disorders are a group of diseases defined by damage to neurons and axons with subsequent myelin breakdown.
- Disorders of secondary demyelination are a heterogeneous mix of conditions, including infections, nutritional/vitamin deficiencies, vascular diseases, chemical agents, and genetic disorders.
- Imaging of secondary demyelinating diseases is characterized by white matter damage in various patterns. Although some of the imaging findings of secondary demyelinating diseases are nonspecific, many diseases have specific imaging patterns that, in correlation with clinical history, aid in diagnosis.

INTRODUCTION

Demyelinating disorders of the central nervous system (CNS) are classically characterized by the breakdown of myelin, with or without the preservation of the associated axons.[1] Primary demyelinating diseases, including multiple sclerosis (MS), typically involve the loss of myelin with relative sparing of axons.[1] In contrast, secondary demyelinating disorders represent a spectrum of white matter disease characterized by damage to neurons or axons with the resultant breakdown of myelin.[1] The pathologic changes seen in secondary demyelinating disorders are varied, ranging from pure demyelination to necrosis with subsequent demyelination.[1] Secondary demyelinating diseases are associated with a wide variety of conditions, including infections/vaccinations, nutritional/vitamin deficiencies, chemical agents, genetic abnormalities, and vascular insult. Demyelinating diseases are usually diagnosed using a combination of cerebrospinal fluid (CSF) analysis,

neuroimaging, patient history, and neurologic examination. Many disorders of secondary demyelination have nonspecific imaging findings with signal abnormalities seen within the white matter. However, some diseases of secondary demyelination have characteristic imaging features; recognition of these characteristic features is crucial to make a prompt and correct diagnosis.

Associated with Infection/Vaccination

Acute disseminated encephalomyelitis

Acute disseminated encephalomyelitis (ADEM) is an inflammatory demyelinating disorder of the CNS typically preceded by a viral infection or vaccination.[2] ADEM most commonly affects the cerebral hemisphere, brainstem, and spinal cord. The incidence of ADEM is 0.4 per 100,000 per year in patients less than 20 years old.[3] ADEM is predominantly a disease of children, with a mean age at presentation of 5 to 8 years and an equal presentation among females and males.[4]

Department of Radiology, University of Michigan Health System, 1500 E Medical Center Drive, Ann Arbor, MI 48109-5030, USA
* Corresponding author. Department of Radiology, University of Michigan, Taubman Center/B1/132 F, 1500 East Medical Center Drive, Ann Arbor, MI 48105.
E-mail addresses: hparmar@umich.edu; parurad@hotmail.com

Consistent with the pathogenesis of a preceding infection, ADEM has a winter and spring predominance.[3] ADEM typically occurs within 2 to 4 weeks of viral infection or vaccination, with up to 90% of patients reporting an identifiable preceding infection.[3] Patients with ADEM present with acute multifocal neurologic symptoms and encephalopathy. CSF analysis often shows a mild increase in total protein without bacterial growth or positive viral polymerase chain reaction (PCR). Clinical symptoms are varied and include pyramidal signs, hemiplegia, ataxia, cranial nerve palsies, optic neuritis, seizures, spinal cord involvement, speech impairment, and change in mental status.[2] Treatment involves corticosteroids and/or other immunomodulating agents along with supportive care.

Complete recovery has been reported in 53% to 94% of cases, and mortality is rare.[2]

Magnetic resonance (MR) imaging is the most valuable imaging tool in the diagnosis of ADEM. It is characterized by T2-weighted and fluid-attenuated inversion-recovery (FLAIR) sequence signal abnormalities. The signal abnormalities seen in ADEM are large, multiple, and patchy with an asymmetric distribution. The most commonly affected site is the subcortical white matter, seen in up to 90% of cases (**Fig. 1**A).[5] Lesions of ADEM can also be seen in the deep nuclei, cerebellum, brainstem, and spinal cord (see **Fig. 1**B–D).[5] Although the periventricular white matter can also be involved, it has been suggested that it is less commonly involved as compared with

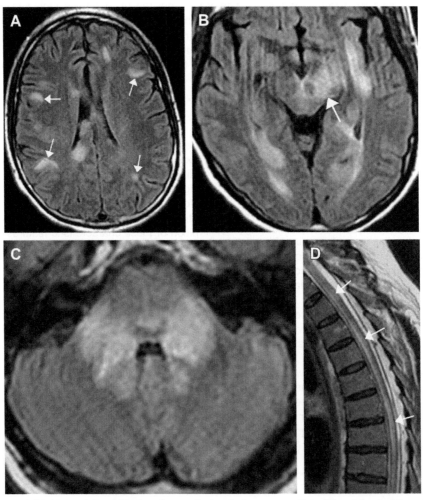

Fig. 1. ADEM. Axial FLAIR-weighted MR imaging at the level of corona radiate (*A*), midbrain (*B*), and cerebellum (*C*) in a 38-year-old man with ADEM. Multiple areas of signal abnormality are noted in the subcortical white matter (*arrows*) and also in the periventricular region. Lesions are seen in the midbrain (*B*) (*arrow*) and in bilateral middle cerebellar peduncles (*C*). Sagittal T2-weighted MR imaging (*D*) shows hyperintensity involving the cervicothoracic cord (*arrows*).

MS.[6] Gadolinium enhancement of lesions is variable.[2,5] MR imaging of the spinal cord can show large intramedullary signal abnormalities extending across multiple spinal levels with variable post-contrast enhancement and associated cord swelling.[2]

Four MR imaging patterns of cerebral involvement in ADEM have been described: (1) ADEM with small lesions (less than 5 mm); (2) ADEM with large, confluent, tumefactive lesions; (3) ADEM with symmetric thalamic involvement; and (4) acute hemorrhagic encephalomyelitis characterized by evidence of hemorrhage within some of the lesions.[7] Although these patterns do not seem to have prognostic value, they may be useful in classification. The differential diagnosis of ADEM includes MS, posterior reversible encephalopathy syndrome (PRES), vasculitis, and Bechet disease. Complete resolution of ADEM lesions is seen in 37% to 75% of patients on follow-up MR imaging, with partial resolution seen in up to 50% of cases.[5]

Progressive multifocal leukoencephalopathy

Progressive multifocal leukoencephalopathy (PML) is a demyelinating disorder caused by the JC virus. PML is seen almost exclusively in immunocompromised patients. PML was initially described in immunocompromised patients, including patients with cancer, transplants, sarcoidosis, and tuberculosis.[8] More recently, there has been an increase in the incidence of PML associated with the human immunodeficiency virus (HIV)/AIDS epidemic of the 1980s.[9] Although the incidence of PML has decreased in patients with AIDS because of retroviral therapy, AIDS remains the most common cause (79%) of PML today. Other causes include hematological malignancies (13%), organ transplantation (5%), and immunosuppressant medications (3%).[9] PML is rarely seen in immunocompetent patients, with less than 50 total cases reported in the literature.[10] The clinical presentation of PML is varied. PML typically begins as a subacute illness evolving into more focal neurologic symptoms over days to weeks.[11] Neurologic symptoms reflect the affected areas of the brain and can mimic stroke. PML is a progressive disease with symptoms increasing over weeks to months, eventually resulting in severe disability and death.[11] The diagnosis of PML is made with a combination of clinical symptoms, laboratory data, and neuroimaging features. CSF-PCR analysis for the JC virus is the diagnostic method of choice, with a reported sensitivity ranging from 74% to 92% and a specificity of 92% to 100%.[11] Biopsy is occasionally required in patients with the JC virus who are PCR negative.

MR imaging is the imaging modality of choice in evaluating PML. The classic appearance of PML on MR imaging is characterized by single or multifocal T2-weighted/FLAIR signal abnormalities that begin as round to oval and become more confluent as the disease progresses.[9] Lesions of PML are typically asymmetric and involve the periventricular and subcortical white matter (Fig. 2).[12,13] In addition, lesions do not tend to demonstrate

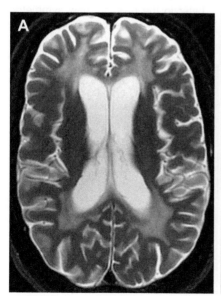
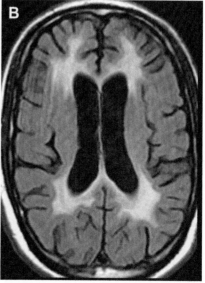

Fig. 2. PML. Axial T2 (A) and FLAIR (B) in a 45-year-old patient with proven PML shows increased T2 and FLAIR hyperintensity in bilateral periventricular white matter. There is no mass effect, and no contrast enhancement was noted (not shown).

mass effect or significant postcontrast enhancement.[9] PML most frequently involves the parietal-occipital junction, thalamus, basal ganglia, and corpus callosum, although posterior fossa involvement can be seen, frequently in the middle cerebellar peduncles and cerebellum.[9,14] Gray matter involvement can be seen in up to 50% of patients.[15] Spinal cord involvement in PML is rare.[9] Newer lesions can demonstrate high signal on diffusion-weighted imaging (DWI), with corresponding normal to low signal on apparent diffusion coefficient (ADC) sequences consistent with restricted diffusion.[9] On follow-up imaging, the MR imaging findings of PML are usually worse with increased size and confluence of lesions, interval development of new lesions, and resultant cortical atrophy.[14] However, reports have shown stabilization or a decrease in the size of the lesions in patients on retroviral therapy.[16] The main imaging differential diagnoses of PML include HIV encephalitis, MS, mitochondrial encephalopathies, and vasculitis. The overall prognosis is poor, with 1-year survival rates ranging from 38% to 58% in patients on retroviral therapy.[9]

Subacute sclerosing panencephalitis

Subacute sclerosing panencephalitis (SSPE) is a progressive neurodegenerative disorder of the CNS caused by persistent infection by a form of the measles virus known as the SSPE virus.[17] As with ADEM, SSPE is primarily a disease of children, specifically children infected with measles at a young age. Infection in patients younger than 1 year carries a significantly higher risk of subsequent SSPE when compared with older children.[18] SSPE is rare in developed countries because of the widespread immunization programs. For example, the most recent incidence in Canada was reported as 0.06 million children per year.[19] However, SSPE remains a problem in less-developed countries. The incidence of SSPE in patients infected with measles is estimated at 4 to 11 cases per 100,000 cases of measles.[17] No association has been proven between the measles vaccine and subsequent development of SSPE.[20]

The age of presentation is typically 8 to 18 years, with disease onset occurring, on average, 6 years after measles infection.[21] The clinical manifestations of SSPE include behavioral abnormalities, cognitive decline, myoclonic jerks, seizures, and vision abnormalities.[17] The clinical presentation of SSPE typically begins with subtle behavioral changes and progresses to more severe symptoms, including characteristic myoclonic jerks, autonomic disturbances, and visual impairment.[17] Diagnosis is made using a combination of clinical features, antimeasles virus antibodies within the CSF, electroencephalography, and MR imaging findings.[21]

MR imaging remains the best imaging modality in the evaluation of SSPE. Early in the course of the disease, MR imaging demonstrates increased T2-weighted signal abnormalities in the cortical and subcortical white matter (Fig. 3).[22] Lesions of SSPE typically involve the posterior parts of the brain including the occipital lobes.[21] The basal ganglia, thalami, and corpus callosum are also frequently involved after the development of white matter lesions.[23] Contrast enhancement and mass effect are not common but have been reported.[24] Later in the disease, new symmetric lesions are seen in the periventricular white matter with

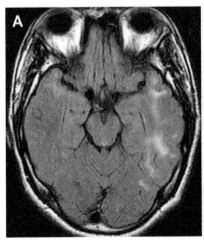
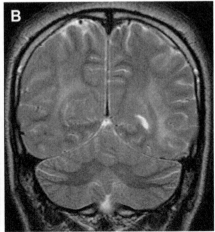

Fig. 3. SSPE. Axial (A) FLAIR and coronal T2-weighted (B) MR imaging in a 12-year-old with SSPE shows multifocal areas of signal abnormalities in the white matter, especially in left temporal lobe and within bilateral peritrigonal regions.

associated cortical atrophy.[21] Lesions of SSPE can demonstrate a high DWI signal consistent with restricted diffusion.[25] MR spectroscopy has been shown to demonstrate decreased N-acetlyaspartate and increased choline consistent with demyelination.[23] The differential diagnosis of SSPE includes ADEM, MS, acute viral encephalitis, tumors, and metabolic white matter disease.[20] Therapy for SSPE remains limited, with a modest benefit seen in 30% to 35% of patients.[26,27] The most common treatment involves a combination of interferon-alpha and isoprinosine.[26,27] Despite these therapies, the prognosis of SSPE is extremely poor, with a mortality of up to 95%.[28] The mean survival ranges from 1 year 9 months to 3 years.[28]

Associated with Nutritional/Vitamin Deficiency

Central pontine myelinosis

Central pontine myelinosis (CPM) was originally described in 1959 as a disease of alcoholics and the chronically malnourished.[29] Currently, CPM is associated with many diseases, including alcoholism, chronic malnutrition, and electrolyte abnormalities, as well as many systemic conditions, including postdiuretic therapy, postliver transplantation, and postpituitary surgery. CPM has been most frequently associated with the rapid correction of hyponatremia leading to the proposed name *osmotic demyelination syndrome*.[30] In addition, lesions have been demonstrated to occur outside the pons, the so-called *extrapontine myelinosis*.[31] The clinical manifestations of CPM usually begin with dysarthria and dysphagia, followed by flaccid (and later spastic) quadriparesis, changing levels of consciousness (locked-in syndrome), and coma.[31]

CPM has a characteristic appearance on imaging. MR imaging shows lesions within the central pons with sparing of the peripheral rim. Lesions of CPM are typically T2-weighted and FLAIR hyperintense (**Fig.** 4A).[32] Increased diffusion-weighted signal is often seen, reflecting restricted diffusion caused by cytotoxic edema (see **Fig.** 4B).[32] In addition, postcontrast enhancement can be seen along the periphery of the lesions.[1] Extrapontine lesions typically involve the deep white matter and the deep gray matter (**Fig.** 5).[33] Findings on MR imaging can be delayed, and repeat imaging in 10 to 14 days can be useful to detect lesions occult on initial imaging.[31] The lesions of CPM may improve slightly but rarely completely resolve.[34] Patients who survive may have persistent MR imaging signal abnormalities within the pons.[35]

The differential diagnosis of CPM includes ischemia, MS, encephalitis, toxic encephalopathy, and brainstem glioma. The imaging appearance of CPM must be correlated with the clinical picture and specifically associated electrolyte abnormalities. There is no accepted treatment of CPM other than supportive care. Crucial in the avoidance of CPM is proper correction of hyponatremia, specifically chronic hyponatremia.[31] The prognosis of CPM was originally bleak; but with improved detection on MR imaging, more patients are surviving. A large case series reported a mortality of 6%, with approximately 30% of patients left completely dependent.[35] Thirty-two percent of patients had deficits but remained independent, and another 32% of patients had complete resolution.[35] Although the MR imaging findings are characteristic, MR imaging has been shown to have little or no prognostic value.[35] In addition, MR imaging has increased the detection of clinically silent lesions of uncertain clinical significance.

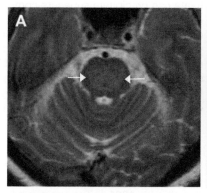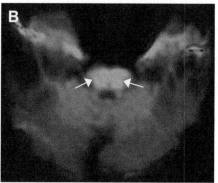

Fig. 4. CPM. Axial T2-weighted MR imaging (*A*) in 65-year-old man with prolonged stay in intensive care unit shows lesions within the central pons with sparing of the peripheral rim (*arrows*). (*B*) There is increased diffusion-weighted signal in the involved area on the DWI (*arrows*).

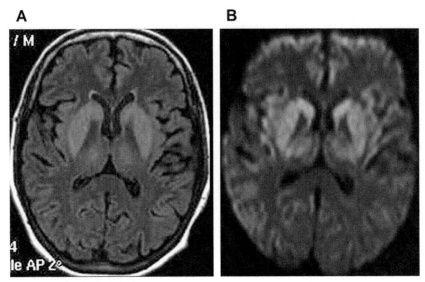

A   **B**

Fig. 5. Extrapontine CPM. Axial FLAIR-weighted MR imaging (*A*) in a 72-year-old woman with known electrolyte imbalance shows FLAIR hyperintense lesions within bilateral corpus striatum and thalami. The abnormality is bilateral and symmetric. (*B*) Increased diffusion-weighted signal is noted on the DWI.

Subacute combined degeneration (vitamin B12 deficiency)

Subacute combined degeneration refers to a deficiency of vitamin B12, which can affect the central or peripheral nervous system. Subacute combined degeneration typically involves the spinal cord, specifically the posterior and lateral columns.[36] The most common cause of vitamin B12 deficiency in the Western world is pernicious anemia, an autoimmune gastritis.[36] Other common causes of vitamin B12 deficiency include gastric surgery, malabsorption syndromes, alcoholism, and rarely vegetarianism.[1] Additionally, an increasing prevalence of vitamin B12 deficiency has been reported in patients infected with HIV.[37] The symptoms of vitamin B12 deficiency include areflexia and paresthesias, reflecting damage to peripheral nerves.[38] Later in the course of the disease, symptoms include weakness, stiffness, and ataxia. Impairment in position and vibratory sense is seen, reflecting damage to the posterior columns of the spinal cord.[39] The pathology of vitamin B12 deficiency is not completely understood, although vitamin B12 is required as a cofactor in the conversion of methylmalonyl coenzyme A (CoA) to succinyl CoA.[39]

The imaging findings of subacute combined degeneration are best seen on spinal MR imaging. Findings include increased T2-weighted signal within the dorsal columns of the cervical and thoracic spinal cord (**Fig. 6**A).[39] Lesions often involve a long continuous segment of the dorsal columns.[1] T1-weighted images are often unremarkable; postcontrast enhancement is not typical, although it has been reported.[39] Edema and mild expansion of the involved spinal cord segment are often seen.[38] MR imaging of the brain may show focal areas of high T2-weighted signal within the cerebral white matter, which typically resolve after treatment (see **Fig. 6**B).[40]

The differential diagnosis of the MR imaging findings of subacute combined degeneration includes infectious myelitis, peripheral neuropathy, radiation myelitis, MS, ischemia, traumatic cord injury, other metabolic diseases, and transverse myelitis. The diagnosis of subacute combined degeneration is made by measuring vitamin B12 and folic acid levels. Treatment involves lifetime intramuscular injections of vitamin B12.[1] In patients with folic acid deficiency, care must be made to correctly diagnosis coexisting vitamin B12 deficiency because isolated treatment with folate can precipitate subacute combined degeneration in patients with undiagnosed vitamin B12 deficiency. Most patients show clinical improvement or resolution of symptoms following treatment with vitamin B12.[41] Spinal cord MR imaging signal abnormalities can resolve completely after treatment with vitamin B12, and radiographic resolution may even precede clinical improvement by several months.[42]

Wernicke encephalopathy

Wernicke encephalopathy is an acute neurologic disorder caused by thiamine deficiency, first described in 1881.[43] The exact incidence of Wernicke encephalopathy is unknown, with reports ranging from 0.5% up to 3.0%.[44,45] Wernicke

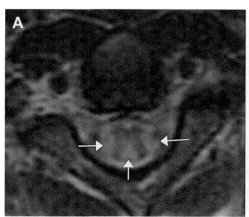
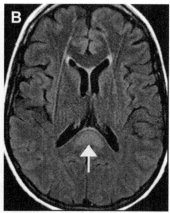

Fig. 6. Vitamin B12 deficiency. Axial T2-weighted MR imaging (*A*) in a 61-year-old man with pernicious anemia and vitamin B12 deficiency shows increased T2 signal in the dorsal and lateral columns of the cervical cord (*arrows*). (*B*) FLAIR-weighted MR imaging of the brain shows focal areas of high FLAIR signal within the splenium of the corpus callosum (*arrow*).

encephalopathy has been most frequently associated with alcoholism, although it can be seen in many other conditions, including postgastrointestinal surgery, prolonged vomiting, systemic infections, and in patients on chemotherapy.[43] Classically, Wernicke was defined by a triad of clinical symptoms, including ocular signs, altered consciousness, and ataxia.[43] The ocular signs of Wernicke include nystagmus, lateral rectus muscle palsies, and conjugate gaze palsies.[43] However, newer studies have shown that the classic triad occurs in only 16% to 38% of patients.[44,46] Newer criteria involve documented dietary deficiencies, ocular signs, cerebellar dysfunction, and altered mental status.[47]

MR imaging remains the mainstay of imaging in the evaluation of Wernicke encephalopathy. Like many disorders of demyelination, MR imaging findings of Wernicke include high T2-weighted/FLAIR and low T1-weighted signal abnormalities within characteristic locations.[46] Lesions of acute Wernicke encephalopathy symmetrically involve the thalami, mammillary bodies, tectal plate, and periaqueductal area (**Fig. 7**).[43] These areas have a higher oxidative metabolism and may be more susceptible to deficiencies in thiamine.[43] Atypical MR imaging findings include involvement of the cerebellum, cerebellar vermis, cranial nerve nuclei, and caudate nuclei.[43] Atypical findings are seen more frequently in nonalcoholic patients.[43] Postcontrast enhancement can be seen, most commonly, in the mammillary bodies.[46,48] Lesions of Wernicke encephalopathy can have high DWI and low ADC signal intensity consistent with restricted diffusion caused by ischemia.[49] These DWI signal abnormalities have been shown to normalize with appropriate therapy.[49] In chronic

disease, atrophy of the mammillary bodies, cerebellum, and corpus callosum is frequently seen with resultant dilatation of the third ventricle.[50]

The differential diagnosis of Wernicke encephalopathy includes toxic poisoning (including carbon monoxide, methanol, and cyanide), liver disease, hypoglycemia, hypoxic ischemic encephalopathy, Wilson disease, central pontine myelinosis, and infection.[51] Wernicke encephalopathy has a varied prognosis ranging from complete resolution of clinical symptoms to irreversible neurologic damage.[50] In the most advanced form of disease, patients develop psychosis with classic antegrade amnesia, referred to as *Wernicke-Korsakoff syndrome*.[50] MR imaging findings typically resolve completely after thiamine treatment.[50] Clinical symptoms also tend to improve dramatically after thiamine treatment, although ataxia may persist in up to 25% of patients.[51] Wernicke-Korsakoff syndrome has been reported to develop in up to 75% of patients.[52]

Associated with Physical/Chemical Agents and Medical Therapy

Radiation changes

Radiation therapy to the CNS typically causes vascular injury, specifically to the small vessels, with resultant small vessel arteritis and ischemia.[1] The effects of radiation therapy on the CNS include focal CNS necrosis, white matter injury, CNS atrophy, microangiopathic changes, and large vessel vasculopathy.[53] Other effects include secondary osseous changes and delayed development of secondary malignancies.[53] Radiation-induced white matter damage is characterized by radiation-induced demyelination in the periventricular white

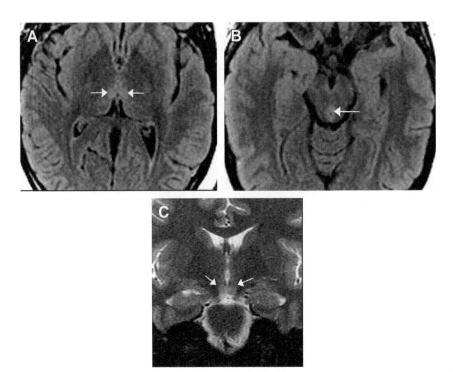

Fig. 7. Wernicke encephalopathy. Axial FLAIR-weighted MR imaging at the level of thalamus (*A*), midbrain (*B*), coronal T2-weighted MR imaging at the level of third ventricle (*C*) in a 26-year-old pregnant woman with malnutrition and acute worsening of mental status. Bilateral symmetric areas of increased signal is noted in the medial thalami (*arrows*) (*A*), periaqueductal gray (*arrow*) (*B*), and in the mammillary bodies (*arrows*) (*C*). Intravenous contrast agent was not given.

matter.[53] These changes can be seen in up 50% of patients treated with radiation, although many cases are subclinical.[53] White matter disease is more commonly seen after whole brain radiation compared with more targeted radiotherapy. Symptoms of radiation-induced CNS damage include seizures, headaches, and focal neurologic deficits and are often difficult to distinguish from recurrent or progressive CNS tumor.[1]

Radiation-related CNS injury is often classified into acute, early delayed, and late delayed effects.[54] This article focuses on acute and early delayed effects because they relate to secondary demyelination. Acute effects typically occur during radiation therapy and are postulated to reflect transient edema within the white matter caused by underlying vascular injury.[1] MR imaging findings of acute white matter injury related to radiation therapy include high T2-weighted/FLAIR signal abnormalities within the white matter.[55] These lesions may show localized mass effect but do not generally demonstrate postcontrast enhancement (Fig. 8).[55] Early delayed effects can occur within weeks to months after radiation therapy and are thought to reflect demyelination.[56] Early delayed effects on MR imaging are characterized by multiple or focal high T2-weighted/

FLAIR signal abnormalities within the deep white matter (see Fig. 8C, D).[57] Lesions of early delayed radiation change are usually symmetric with associated edema and variable patchy postcontrast enhancement.[53] However, a more recent study did not demonstrate a statistically significant difference between white matter signal abnormalities in patients treated with radiotherapy versus those not treated with radiotherapy within the early delayed postradiation period.[56] This distinction remains an important imaging distinction because the prevalence of periventricular and deep white matter signal abnormalities increases with increasing age likely because of the underlying chronic small vessel ischemic disease.

The differential diagnosis of radiation therapy–related CNS changes includes recurrent neoplasm, chronic small vessel ischemic disease, MS, PML, and vasculitis. The resolution of MR imaging abnormalities and clinical symptoms is extremely variable and depends on the severity of the radiation changes, patient age at treatment, and radiation therapy dosage.[57] More chronic or late delayed effects are characterized by areas of diffuse white matter injury, radiation necrosis, and brain atrophy with variable degrees of postcontrast enhancement, which can be difficult to

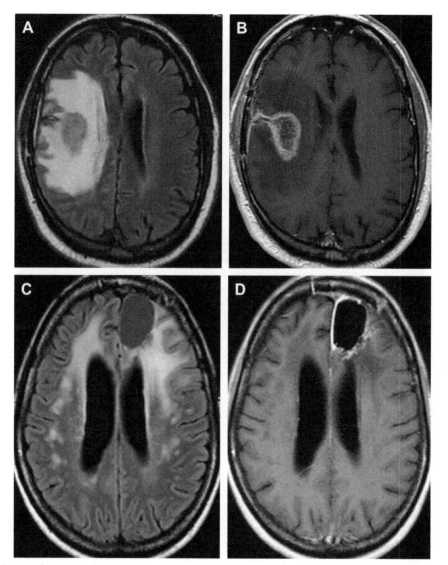

Fig. 8. Radiation changes. Axial FLAIR (*A*) and contrast-enhanced T1-weighted MR imaging (*B*) in a patient with right frontal glioblastoma shows extensive FLAIR hyperintensity with mass effect in the right frontal lobe/corona radiate surrounding the surgical site. This image was 6 weeks after initiation of radiation and was thought to represent acute postradiation changes. Follow-up at 3 months (not shown) showed near-complete resolution of the FLAIR signal changes and mass effect. Axial FLAIR (*C*) and contrast-enhanced T1-weighted MR imaging (*D*) in another patient with left frontal glioblastoma with radiation 8 months ago. There is FLAIR hyperintensity in the left frontal lobe white matter (posterior to the surgical site), which also involves the right frontal lobe white matter and the genus of the corpus callosum (not shown). There was no contrast enhancement in the areas of FLAIR signal abnormality.

differentiate from recurrent tumor.[57] Chemotherapy is also well known to potentiate the effects of radiation on the brain, specifically causing a subacute leukoencephalopathy, which is not discussed in this article.

Toxic drug exposure
Related to drug use Drug abuse is a serious problem in the United States. Because most drugs target the CNS, much toxicity associated with these drugs affects the CNS. Although many common drugs can potentially affect the CNS, the most common are alcohol, cocaine, heroin, and methadone (**Fig. 9**). Heroin is a drug derived from opium that can be ingested, injected, or even inhaled. Heroin acts on multiple subtypes of opioid receptors causing analgesia and euphoria. In the acute setting, heroin, like cocaine, can cause

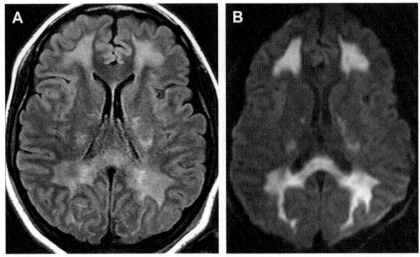

Fig. 9. Methadone-induced leukoencephalopathy. (A) Axial FLAIR-weighted MR imaging in an 18-year-old girl with history of methadone ingestion show bilateral, near symmetric areas of signal abnormality in the white matter of frontal and parietal lobes. (B) Axial DWI shows extensive diffusion hyperintensity in the involved areas suggestive for acute cytotoxic edema.

ischemia and stroke related to vasospasm and emboli from impurities in the heroin.[58] Heroin can also cause chronic microvascular ischemia, which manifests as nonspecific symmetric foci of T2-weighted/FLAIR hyperintensity within the subcortical and periventricular white matter.[58–60] Heroin is also classically associated with a leukoencephalopathy specifically seen in patients who inhale the drug, a practice known as "chasing the dragon."[59] Characteristic imaging findings of heroin-related leukoencephalopathy include increased T2-weighted/FLAIR signal within the cerebellar white matter and posterior internal capsule with sparing of the dentate nuclei.[61,62]

Cocaine is an alkaloid drug that is easily absorbed across mucous membranes. Cocaine can be administered by inhalation or intranasal means. Inhalation of cocaine has a rapid onset of action, ranging from 8 to 10 seconds, significantly faster than intranasal administration.[63] Cocaine acts by blocking monoamine reuptake causing the classic symptoms of vasoconstriction, hypertension, and tachycardia.[63] In the acute setting, cocaine is well known to cause a wide variety of neurologic complications, including ischemia and subarachnoid and intraparenchymal hemorrhage related to the effects of vasoconstriction (Fig. 10).[58] In addition, because of the impaired vascular relaxation,

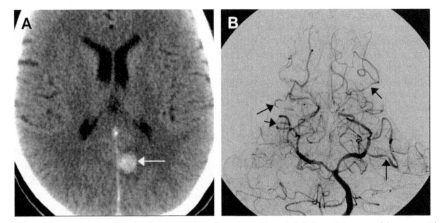

Fig. 10. Cocaine exposure. Axial computed tomography of the head (A) in a 25-year-old man with history of cocaine abuse and presenting with acute mental status change, shows focal acute parenchymal hemorrhage in the left occipital lobe (arrow). (B) Catheter angiogram done after 2 days reveals multiple areas of narrowing (arrows) suggestive for diffuse vasoconstriction associated with cocaine exposure.

cocaine is also associated with PRES and chronic leukoencephalopathy.[58] Cocaine can cause a PRES-type effect because of its vasoconstriction properties, which results in impaired autoregulation of cerebral pressures leading to hyperperfusion and edema.[64] The imaging features of cocaine-induced PRES are indistinguishable from other causes of PRES, and a good clinical history is crucial to the diagnosis. In the more chronic setting, cocaine usage is associated with a chronic ischemic leukoencephalopathy. Cocaine-induced leukoencephalopathy is characterized by nonspecific T2-weighted/FLAIR hyperintensity within the cerebral and periventricular white matter. Although nonspecific, these changes are often seen out of proportion to the patients' age, suggesting an alternative diagnosis to normal age-related chronic microvascular changes.[64] Cocaine is also associated with brain atrophy with specific involvement of the white matter. These atrophic changes can be magnified by multidrug use.[65]

Neurologic complications can also be seen with iatrogenic drug exposure. Intrathecal methotrexate being are fairly common, with recent estimates of the incidence of transient motor paralysis or seizures ranging up to 10% of patients receiving this therapy.[66] It has been associated with intrathecal as well as intermediate- to high-dose intravenous administration.[66] The most common neuropathologic abnormality associated with methotrexate use is multifocal necrotizing leukoencephalopathy (**Fig. 11**).[1,3]

Marchiafava Bignami

A rare disorder associated with alcohol usage is Marchiafava-Bignami disease (MBD). MBD typically affects the corpus callosum causing a characteristic demyelination and necrosis.[58] MBD is divided into 2 subtypes, type A and type B, which are defined by imaging findings and the degree of clinical symptoms. Type A is defined by impaired consciousness with extensive edema of the corpus callosum manifested in T2-weighted high signal and enlargement of the entire corpus callosum.[58] Type A MBD typically has a very poor outcome. In contrast, type B disease is characterized by milder clinical symptoms with only partial involvement of the corpus callosum.[67] In the more chronic form of MBD, atrophy and cystic changes are seen within the corpus callosum (**Fig. 12**).[67] Signal changes can also be seen in the white matter and cerebral cortex in up to 40% of cases with associated edema and, in some cases, restricted diffusion.[68,69] The differential diagnosis of T2-weighted callosal hyperintensity includes status epilepticus, drug toxicity, encephalitis, and hypoglycemia. However, in the appropriate clinical setting, diffuse swelling of the corpus callosum is nearly pathognomonic for MBD.

Vascular

PRES

PRES is a neurotoxic syndrome characterized by vasogenic edema seen in the setting of a wide

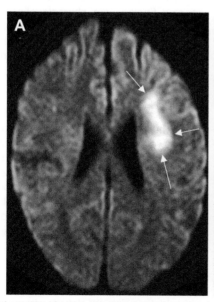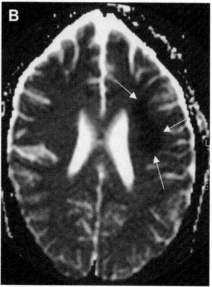

Fig. 11. Methotrexate-induced leukoencephalopathy. (*A*) Axial DWI shows restricted diffusion in the left corona radiata (*arrows*), which showed hypointensity on the ADC map (*B*). There was no abnormality on the FLAIR-weighted images (not shown).

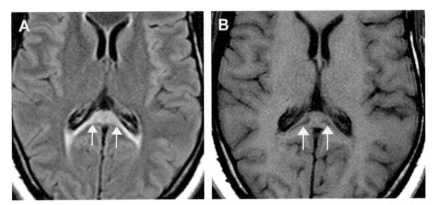

Fig. 12. Marchiafava Bignami. Axial FLAIR (*A*) and T1-weighted MR imaging (*B*) in a 68-year-old man with long history of alcohol abuse and presenting with confusion shows increased FLAIR signal hyperintensity within the splenium of corpus callosum (*arrows*). There is cystic necrosis seen on the T1-weighted image (*arrows*).

variety of systemic conditions. It is thought that PRES is caused by hypertension and failed autoregulation leading to hyperperfusion with resultant endothelial damage, ischemia, and demyelination.[1] The clinical symptoms of PRES are variable, including headache, vision changes, paresis, hemianopsia, nausea, and altered mental status.[70] In advanced cases, seizures and coma can be seen.[70] Hypertension is seen in up to 80% of cases, although normal blood pressure can be seen, especially in eclampsia and after bone marrow transplant.[70] PRES has been associated with many clinical conditions, including most commonly hypertension and toxemia of pregnancy as well as infection/sepsis/shock, autoimmune diseases, chemotherapy, and after transplantation. By definition, reversible, early diagnosis of PRES is crucial because severe complications can develop, including status epilepticus, hemorrhage, and infarction.[71]

PRES has a classic computed tomography (CT) and MR imaging appearance. Lesions are characterized by symmetric edema (low attenuation on CT, high T2-weighted/FLAIR signal) within the hemispheres.[70] Lesions are seen most commonly in the parietal and occipital lobes (Fig. 13A, B) and less commonly in the frontal lobes (see Fig. 11B), temporal-occipital junction, and cerebellum (see Fig. 13C).[70] This distribution is thought to reflect watershed areas related to the vascular nature of PRES.[70] Lesions typically begin as patchy but may become more confluent as edema progresses.[70] Edema can also be seen within atypical locations, including the basal ganglia, brainstem, and deep white matter, which can confounds the diagnosis.[72] Lesions of PRES typically do not demonstrate high diffusion-weighted signal in the reversible stage. However, in the more advanced (nonreversible) stage, lesions may show high

diffusion-weighted signal with pseudonormalized ADC values reflecting cerebral infarction.[73] Focal parenchymal hemorrhage, seen as blooming artifact on T2-weighted gradient echo sequences, has been described in up to 15% of patients.[70] Lesions of PRES do not typically show postcontrast enhancement, although patchy enhancement is seen occasionally.[74]

The differential diagnosis of PRES includes acute ischemia, status epilepticus, hypoglycemia, and microangiopathic disease. The clinical and imaging findings of PRES are typically reversible after controlling blood pressure or correction of the underlying condition (see Fig. 13D). However, residual encephalomalacia can be seen in cases of hemorrhage and infarction.[74] Although the imaging findings are characteristic, a history of antecedent hypertension or seizures is not always present. Therefore, recognition of the imaging pattern is crucial because prompt treatment is necessary to prevent irreversible neurologic damage.

Subcortical arteriosclerotic encephalopathy
Subcortical arteriosclerotic encephalopathy (SAE), or Binswanger encephalopathy, is a clinical syndrome characterized by dementia caused by chronic hypertension with small vessel ischemic changes. The term *SAE* was first proposed in 1962 by Olszewski to describe a cerebral arteriosclerosis affecting the small vessels of the deep white matter and basal ganglia with resultant small areas of ischemia and demyelination.[75] The pathologic changes of SAE include gliosis, loss of myelinated axons, and ischemia.[76] The clinical symptoms of SAE include mental deterioration, pyramidal neurologic deficits, frequent transient ischemic attacks, psuedobulbar disturbances, and cerebellar and extrapyramidal defects.[75]

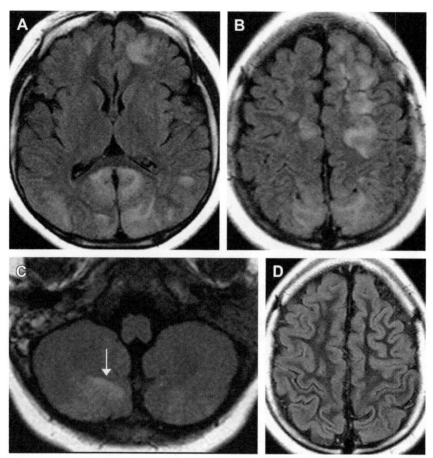

Fig. 13. PRES. A 28-year-old pregnant woman presented with acute onset of confusion, seizures, and vision disturbances. Axial FLAIR-weighted MR imaging at the level of basal ganglia (*A*) and centrum semiovale (*B*) show multiple foci of FLAIR hyperintensity within the parieto-occipital lobes and also in the frontal lobes suggestive for PRES. (*C*) There was also FLAIR hyperintensity noted within cerebellum (*arrow*). (*D*) Follow-up MR imaging after 4 weeks showed complete normalization of the signal abnormality seen before.

Patients typically demonstrate hypertension. SAE has a classically stepwise progression of symptoms reflecting the underlying ischemic cause of the disease. The onset of SAE is seen in middle-aged patients or elderly patients and is insidious over a period of 5 to 10 years.[75] Many patients never experience an acute ischemic event, although an acute stroke is the inciting event in up to one-third of patients.[75]

The diagnosis of SAE is based on classic CT/MR imaging findings with associated characteristic clinical symptoms. CT findings of SAE include multifocal areas of low attenuation within the periventricular and deep white matter as well as more distinct areas of prior lacunar infarction.[75] MR imaging of SAE demonstrates patchy, multifocal, high T2-weighted/FLAIR signal abnormalities in the periventricular and deep white matter of the centrum semiovale (**Fig. 14**). Focal T2 and FLAIR signal abnormalities can also be seen in the basal ganglia. Lesions are typically less conspicuous on T1-weighted imaging and do not generally demonstrate postcontrast enhancement. Multifocal low-signal-intensity abnormalities are frequently seen on T2-weighted gradient echo sequences, reflecting microhemorrhage. Lesions of SAE do not typically demonstrate high diffusion-weighted signal, although restricted diffusion is seen with acute infarcts.

The differential diagnosis of SAE includes changes related to chronic small vessel disease, amyloid angiopathy, cerebral autosomal dominant arteriopathy with subcortical infarcts and leukoencephalopathy (CADASIL), MS, and vasculitis. The MR imaging findings of SAE, specifically signal abnormalities within the periventricular and deep white matter with associated atrophy or so-called leukoaraiosis, are seen frequently in the elderly in the absence of neurologic deficits.[77] This point illustrates the need for clinical correlation because

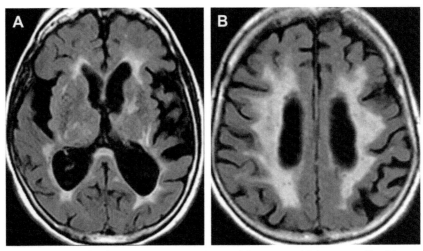

Fig. 14. SAE. Axial FLAIR-weighted MR imaging in a 76-year-old woman with long-standing history of hypertension and dementia and transient ischemic attacks reveals multiple focal and confluent areas of hyperintensity in
the basal ganglia and thalamus (A) and bilateral periventricular and deep white matter (B).

these MR imaging findings are extremely common
in patients without a clinical diagnosis of SAE. The
definitive diagnosis of SAE is, unfortunately, made
only by pathologic examination.[75]

CADASIL

CADASIL is an inherited disorder caused by
mutations on the NOTCH3 gene.[78] Histologically,
CADASIL is characterized by luminal narrowing
or obliteration of small- and medium-sized leptomeningeal arteries and perforating vessels caused
by the deposition of granular material adjacent to
vascular smooth muscle.[79] Clinical symptoms
include frequent subcortical ischemic events,
progressive dementia with psuedobulbar palsy,
migraines, and severe mood disorders.[80] Symptoms generally present within the third decade of
life and are progressive, with death occurring typically in the sixth decade.[80] Although imaging features may be suggestive, the definitive diagnosis
of CADAIL is made by the detection of NOTCH3
mutations. However, NOTCH3 testing is not common and is generally only considered in patients
with unexplained neurologic symptoms with suggestive family history and imaging findings.[81]

The imaging modality of choice in the evaluation
of CADASIL remains MR imaging. MR imaging findings include confluent, diffuse, symmetric white
matter changes characterized by T2-weighted/
FLAIR high signal.[82] These lesions involve the
periventricular and subcortical white matter with
predilection for the frontal and temporal lobes
(Fig. 15A).[82] Also characteristic are high
T2-weighted punctate signal abnormalities in the
periventricular and subcortical white matter,
external capsule, basal ganglia, thalamus, and

pons (see Fig. 15B, C).[82] Another characteristic
MR imaging finding of CADASIL is the so-called
subcortical lacunar lesions (SLL), which are linear
groups of round lesions seen at the gray-white
matter junction that demonstrate signal intensity
matching CSF on all sequences (see Fig. 15D).[83]
Cerebral microbleeds are also commonly seen in
CADASIL. Microbleeds are defined as focal areas
of signal loss on T2-weighted sequences that
increase in size, so-called blooming, on
T2-weighted gradient echo sequences.[84] In one
study, microbleeds were commonly seen in the
thalami, occipital, and temporal lobes.[84] Restricted
diffusion can be seen with acute lacunar infarcts.
van den Boom and colleagues[81] characterized the
pattern of MR imaging findings in CADASIL based
on patient age, noting early white matter changes
and SLLs in younger patients with later development of focal lacunar infarcts and microbleeds in
more advanced patients. In addition, MR imaging
findings can precede the development of clinical
symptoms.[85]

The average age of the first stroke is earlier for
men, and disease progression is typically faster
in men compared with women. CADASIL is an
invariably progressive disease, with most patients
dying between 60 and 70 years of age. There is no
specific treatment of CADASIL at this time. The
imaging differential diagnosis of CADASIL includes
sporadic subcortical arteriosclerotic encephalopathy, mitochondrial encephalomyopathy with
lactic acidosis and stroke, primary angiitis, and
multiple infarcts. Many of the early MR imaging
findings of CADASIL, specifically white matter
changes, lacunar infarcts, and microbleeds, are
not specific and are difficult to differentiate from

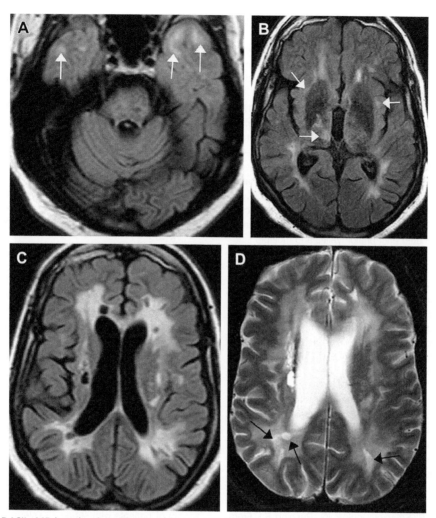

Fig. 15. CADASIL. MR imaging in a 39-year-old man with known CADASIL. Axial FLAIR-weighted MR imaging at the level of temporal lobes (*A*), thalamus (*B*), and corona radiate (*C*) shows hyperintense signal abnormality involving the anterior temporal white matter (*arrows*) (*A*), thalami and external capsules (*arrows*) (*B*), and corona radiate. (*D*) Axial T2-weighted MR imaging at the level of corona radiata shows high T2-weighted signal abnormalities in the subcortical lacunar lesions (*arrows*).

other small vessel CNS diseases. However, involvement of certain areas with white matter changes (anterior temporal lobe and external capsule) combined with SLL can suggest the diagnosis of CADASIL in the appropriate clinical setting.[83] The recognition of the more characteristic imaging features combined with the appropriate clinical history may allow for early diagnosis.

SUMMARY

Disorders of secondary myelination are a varied group of diseases characterized by damage to neurons and/or axons with the resultant breakdown of myelin. Although the disorders of secondary myelination have a wide range of imaging features, they are linked by signal changes in white matter reflecting the underlying pathologic condition of white matter damage. Although many diseases of secondary demyelination have nonspecific imaging findings, they also have certain characteristic imaging and clinical features. The recognition of specific imaging patterns of individual demyelinating diseases is crucial to make a prompt diagnosis.

REFERENCES

1. Atlas S. 4th edition. Magnetic resonance imaging of the brain and spine, vol. 1. Philadelphia: Lippincott, Williams & Wilkins; 2008.

2. Alper G. Acute disseminated encephalomyelitis. J Child Neurol 2012;27(11):1408–25.

3. Leake JA, Albani S, Kao AS, et al. Acute disseminated encephalomyelitis in childhood: epidemiologic, clinical and laboratory features. Pediatr Infect Dis J 2004;23:756–64.

4. Torisu H, Kira R, Ishizaki Y, et al. Clinical study of childhood acute disseminated encephalomyelitis, multiple sclerosis, and acute transverse myelitis in fukuoka prefecture, Japan. Brain Dev 2010;32:454–62.

5. Tenembaum S, Chitnis T, Ness J, et al, International Pediatric MS Study Group. Acute disseminated encephalomyelitis. Neurology 2007;68:S23–36.

6. Dale RC, de Sousa C, Chong WK, et al. Acute disseminated encephalomyelitis, multiphasic disseminated encephalomyelitis and multiple sclerosis in children. Brain 2000;123:2407–22.

7. Tenembaum S, Chamoles N, Fejerman N. Acute disseminated encephalomyelitis: a long-term follow-up study of 84 pediatric patients. Neurology 2002;59:1224–31.

8. Richardson EP Jr. Progressive multifocal leukoencephalopathy. N Engl J Med 1961;265:815–23.

9. Shah R, Bag AK, Chapman PR, et al. Imaging manifestations of progressive multifocal leukoencephalopathy. Clin Radiol 2010;65:431–9.

10. Gheuens S, Pierone G, Peeters P, et al. Progressive multifocal leukoencephalopathy in individuals with minimal or occult immunosuppression. J Neurol Neurosurg Psychiatry 2010;81:247–54.

11. Sahraian MA, Radue EW, Eshaghi A, et al. Progressive multifocal leukoencephalopathy: a review of the neuroimaging features and differential diagnosis. Eur J Neurol 2012;19:1060–9.

12. Smith AB, Smirniotopoulos JG, Rushing EJ. From the archives of the AFIP: central nervous system infections associated with human immunodeficiency virus infection: radiologic-pathologic correlation. Radiographics 2008;28:2033–58.

13. Offiah CE, Turnbull IW. The imaging appearances of intracranial CNS infections in adult HIV and AIDS patients. Clin Radiol 2006;61:393–401.

14. Post MJ, Yiannoutsos C, Simpson D, et al. Progressive multifocal leukoencephalopathy in AIDS: are there any MR findings useful to patient management and predictive of patient survival? AIDS clinical trials group, 243 team. AJNR Am J Neuroradiol 1999;20:1896–906.

15. Mark AS, Atlas SW. Progressive multifocal leukoencephalopathy in patients with AIDS: appearance on MR images. Radiology 1989;173:517–20.

16. Garrels K, Kucharczyk W, Wortzman G, et al. Progressive multifocal leukoencephalopathy: clinical and MR response to treatment. AJNR Am J Neuroradiol 1996;17:597–600.

17. Garg RK. Subacute sclerosing panencephalitis. J Neurol 2008;255:1861–71.

18. Garg RK. Subacute sclerosing panencephalitis. Postgrad Med J 2002;78:63–70.

19. Campbell C, Levin S, Humphreys P, et al. Subacute sclerosing panencephalitis: results of the canadian paediatric surveillance program and review of the literature. BMC Pediatr 2005;5:47.

20. Gutierrez J, Issacson RS, Koppel BS. Subacute sclerosing panencephalitis: an update. Dev Med Child Neurol 2010;52:901–7.

21. Tuncay R, Akman-Demir G, Gokyigit A, et al. MRI in subacute sclerosing panencephalitis. Neuroradiology 1996;38:636–40.

22. Brismar J, Gascon GG, von Steyern KV, et al. Subacute sclerosing panencephalitis: evaluation with CT and MR. AJNR Am J Neuroradiol 1996;17:761–72.

23. Oguz KK, Celebi A, Anlar B. MR imaging, diffusion-weighted imaging and MR spectroscopy findings in acute rapidly progressive subacute sclerosing panencephalitis. Brain Dev 2007;29:306–11.

24. Anlar B, Saatci I, Kose G, et al. MRI findings in subacute sclerosing panencephalitis. Neurology 1996;47:1278–83.

25. Abuhandan M, Cece H, Calik M, et al. An evaluation of subacute sclerosing panencephalitis patients with diffusion-weighted magnetic resonance imaging. Clin Neuroradiol 2013;23:25–30.

26. Gascon GG. International consortium on subacute sclerosing panencephalitis. Randomized treatment study of inosiplex versus combined inosiplex and intraventricular interferon-alpha in subacute sclerosing panencephalitis (SSPE): international multicenter study. J Child Neurol 2003;18:819–27.

27. Dyken PR, Swift A, DuRant RH. Long-term follow-up of patients with subacute sclerosing panencephalitis treated with inosiplex. Ann Neurol 1982;11:359–64.

28. Risk WS, Haddad FS. The variable natural history of subacute sclerosing panencephalitis: a study of 118 cases from the middle east. Arch Neurol 1979;36:610–4.

29. Adams RD, Victor M, Mancall EL. Central pontine myelinolysis: a hitherto undescribed disease occurring in alcoholic and malnourished patients. AMA Arch Neurol Psychiatry 1959;81:154–72.

30. Gerard E, Healy ME, Hesselink JR. MR demonstration of mesencephalic lesions in osmotic demyelination syndrome (central pontine myelinolysis). Neuroradiology 1987;29:582–4.

31. Martin RJ. Central pontine and extrapontine myelinolysis: the osmotic demyelination syndromes. J Neurol Neurosurg Psychiatry 2004;75:22–8.

32. Sharma P, Eesa M, Scott JN. Toxic and acquired metabolic encephalopathies: MRI appearance. AJR Am J Roentgenol 2009;193:879–86.

33. Dickoff DJ, Raps M, Yahr MD. Striatal syndrome following hyponatremia and its rapid correction.

A manifestation of extrapontine myelinolysis confirmed by magnetic resonance imaging. Arch Neurol 1988;45:112–4.

34. McGraw P, Edwards-Brown MK. Reversal of MR findings of central pontine myelinolysis. J Comput Assist Tomogr 1998;22:989–91.

35. Menger H, Jorg J. Outcome of central pontine and extrapontine myelinolysis (n = 44). J Neurol 1999; 246:700–5.

36. Srikanth SG, Jayakumar PN, Vasudev MK, et al. MRI in subacute combined degeneration of spinal cord: a case report and review of literature. Neurol India 2002;50:310–2.

37. Kieburtz KD, Giang DW, Schiffer RB, et al. Abnormal vitamin B12 metabolism in human immunodeficiency virus infection. Association with neurological dysfunction. Arch Neurol 1991;48: 312–4.

38. Yamada K, Shrier DA, Tanaka H, et al. A case of subacute combined degeneration: MRI findings. Neuroradiology 1998;40:398–400.

39. Hemmer B, Glocker FX, Schumacher M, et al. Subacute combined degeneration: clinical, electrophysiological, and magnetic resonance imaging findings. J Neurol Neurosurg Psychiatry 1998;65: 822–7.

40. Stojsavljevic N, Levic Z, Drulovic J, et al. 44-month clinical-brain MRI follow-up in a patient with B12 deficiency. Neurology 1997;49:878–81.

41. Vasconcelos OM, Poehm EH, McCarter RJ, et al. Potential outcome factors in subacute combined degeneration: review of observational studies. J Gen Intern Med 2006;21:1063–8.

42. Berlit P, Ringelstein A, Liebig T. Spinal MRI precedes clinical improvement in subacute combined degeneration with B12 deficiency. Neurology 2004; 63:592.

43. Zuccoli G, Pipitone N. Neuroimaging findings in acute Wernicke's encephalopathy: review of the literature. AJR Am J Roentgenol 2009;192:501–8.

44. Harper C. The incidence of Wernicke's encephalopathy in Australia–a neuropathological study of 131 cases. J Neurol Neurosurg Psychiatry 1983; 46:593–8.

45. Harper CG, Giles M, Finlay-Jones R. Clinical signs in the wernicke-korsakoff complex: a retrospective analysis of 131 cases diagnosed at necropsy. J Neurol Neurosurg Psychiatry 1986;49:341–5.

46. Zuccoli G, Gallucci M, Capellades J, et al. Wernicke encephalopathy: MR findings at clinical presentation in twenty-six alcoholic and nonalcoholic patients. AJNR Am J Neuroradiol 2007;28: 1328–31.

47. Caine D, Halliday GM, Kril JJ, et al. Operational criteria for the classification of chronic alcoholics: identification of wernicke's encephalopathy. J Neurol Neurosurg Psychiatry 1997;62:51–60.

48. Shogry ME, Curnes JT. Mamillary body enhancement on MR as the only sign of acute wernicke encephalopathy. AJNR Am J Neuroradiol 1994; 15:172–4.

49. Chu K, Kang DW, Kim HJ, et al. Diffusion-weighted imaging abnormalities in wernicke encephalopathy: reversible cytotoxic edema? Arch Neurol 2002;59:123–7.

50. Cerase A, Rubenni E, Rufa A, et al. CT and MRI of wernicke's encephalopathy. Radiol Med 2011;116: 319–33.

51. Hegde AN, Mohan S, Lath N, et al. Differential diagnosis for bilateral abnormalities of the basal ganglia and thalamus. Radiographics 2011;31: 5–30.

52. Thomson AD, Marshall EJ. The natural history and pathophysiology of Wernicke's encephalopathy and Korsakoff's psychosis. Alcohol 2006;41:151–8.

53. Rabin BM, Meyer JR, Berlin JW, et al. Radiation-induced changes in the central nervous system and head and neck. Radiographics 1996;16: 1055–72.

54. Lampert PW, Davis RL. Delayed effects of radiation on the human central nervous system; "early" and "late" delayed reactions. Neurology 1964;14:912–7.

55. Ball WS Jr, Prenger EC, Ballard ET. Neurotoxicity of radio/chemotherapy in children: pathologic and MR correlation. AJNR Am J Neuroradiol 1992;13: 761–76.

56. Armstrong CL, Hunter JV, Hackney D, et al. MRI changes due to early-delayed conformal radiotherapy and postsurgical effects in patients with brain tumors. Int J Radiat Oncol Biol Phys 2005; 63:56–63.

57. Tsuruda JS, Kortman KE, Bradley WG, et al. Radiation effects on cerebral white matter: MR evaluation. AJR Am J Roentgenol 1987;149:165–71.

58. Tamrazi B, Almast J. Your brain on drugs: imaging of drug-related changes in the central nervous system. Radiographics 2012;32:701–19.

59. Bartlett E, Mikulis DJ. Chasing "chasing the dragon" with MRI: leukoencephalopathy in drug abuse. Br J Radiol 2005;78:997–1004.

60. Offiah C, Hall E. Heroin-induced leukoencephalopathy: characterization using MRI, diffusion-weighted imaging, and MR spectroscopy. Clin Radiol 2008; 63:146–52.

61. Borne J, Riascos R, Cuellar H, et al. Neuroimaging in drug and substance abuse part II: opioids and solvents. Top Magn Reson Imaging 2005;16: 239–45.

62. Geibprasert S, Gallucci M, Krings T. Addictive illegal drugs: structural neuroimaging. AJNR Am J Neuroradiol 2010;31:803–8.

63. Fessler RD, Esshaki CM, Stankewitz RC, et al. The neurovascular complications of cocaine. Surg Neurol 1997;47:339–45.

64. Hagan IG, Burney K. Radiology of recreational drug abuse. Radiographics 2007;27:919–40.

65. Bjork JM, Grant SJ, Hommer DW. Cross-sectional volumetric analysis of brain atrophy in alcohol dependence: effects of drinking history and comorbid substance use disorder. Am J Psychiatry 2003; 160:2038–45.

66. Rollins N, Winick NM, Bash R, et al. Acute methotrexate neurotoxicity: findings on diffusion-weighted imaging and correlation with clinical outcome. AJNR Am J Neuroradiol 2004;25:1688–95.

67. Heinrich A, Runge U, Khaw AV. Clinicoradiologic subtypes of Marchiafava-Bignami disease. J Neurol 2004;251:1050–9.

68. Ruiz-Martinez J, Martinez Perez-Balsa A, Ruibal M, et al. Marchiafava-Bignami disease with widespread extracallosal lesions and favourable course. Neuroradiology 1999;41:40–3.

69. Johkura K, Naito M, Naka T. Cortical involvement in Marchiafava-Bignami disease. AJNR Am J Neuroradiol 2005;26:670–3.

70. Bartynski WS. Posterior reversible encephalopathy syndrome, part 1: fundamental imaging and clinical features. AJNR Am J Neuroradiol 2008;29:1036–42.

71. Fugate JE, Claassen DO, Cloft HJ, et al. Posterior reversible encephalopathy syndrome: associated clinical and radiologic findings. Mayo Clin Proc 2010;85:427–32.

72. McKinney AM, Short J, Truwit CL, et al. Posterior reversible encephalopathy syndrome: incidence of atypical regions of involvement and imaging findings. AJR Am J Roentgenol 2007;189:904–12.

73. Covarrubias DJ, Luetmer PH, Campeau NG. Posterior reversible encephalopathy syndrome: prognostic utility of quantitative diffusion-weighted MR images. AJNR Am J Neuroradiol 2002;23:1038–48.

74. Bartynski WS, Boardman JF. Distinct imaging patterns and lesion distribution in posterior reversible encephalopathy syndrome. AJNR Am J Neuroradiol 2007;28:1320–7.

75. Loeb C. Binswanger's disease is not a single entity. Neurol Sci 2000;21:343–8.

76. Scheltens P, Barkhof F, Leys D, et al. Histopathologic correlates of white matter changes on MRI in Alzheimer's disease and normal aging. Neurology 1995;45:883–8.

77. Boone KB, Miller BL, Lesser IM, et al. Neuropsychological correlates of white-matter lesions in healthy elderly subjects. A threshold effect. Arch Neurol 1992;49:549–54.

78. Joutel A, Corpechot C, Ducros A, et al. Notch3 mutations in CADASIL, a hereditary adult-onset condition causing stroke and dementia. Nature 1996; 383:707–10.

79. Baudrimont M, Dubas F, Joutel A, et al. Autosomal dominant leukoencephalopathy and subcortical ischemic stroke. A clinicopathological study. Stroke 1993;24:122–5.

80. Chabriat H, Vahedi K, Iba-Zizen MT, et al. Clinical spectrum of CADASIL: a study of 7 families. Cerebral autosomal dominant arteriopathy with subcortical infarcts and leukoencephalopathy. Lancet 1995;346:934–9.

81. van den Boom R, Lesnik Oberstein SA, Ferrari MD, et al. Cerebral autosomal dominant arteriopathy with subcortical infarcts and leukoencephalopathy: MR imaging findings at different ages–3rd-6th decades. Radiology 2003;229:683–90.

82. Skehan SJ, Hutchinson M, MacErlaine DP. Cerebral autosomal dominant arteriopathy with subcortical infarcts and leukoencephalopathy: MR findings. AJNR Am J Neuroradiol 1995;16:2115–9.

83. van Den Boom R, Lesnik Oberstein SA, van Duinen SG, et al. Subcortical lacunar lesions: an MR imaging finding in patients with cerebral autosomal dominant arteriopathy with subcortical infarcts and leukoencephalopathy. Radiology 2002; 224:791–6.

84. Lesnik Oberstein SA, van den Boom R, van Buchem MA, et al. Cerebral microbleeds in CADASIL. Neurology 2001;57(6):1066–70.

85. Coulthard A, Blank SC, Bushby K, et al. Distribution of cranial MRI abnormalities in patients with symptomatic and subclinical CADASIL. Br J Radiol 2000;73(867):256–65.

Viral Infections and White Matter Lesions

Toshio Moritani, MD, PhD[a],*, Aristides Capizzano, MD[a],
Patricia Kirby, MD[b], Bruno Policeni, MD[a]

KEYWORDS

- Viral infection • White matter • Magnetic resonance • Diffusion weighted • Brain • Pathology

KEY POINTS

- Viral infections with white matter involvement are mainly divided into viral infectious and noninfectious diseases.
- Magnetic resonance imaging provides many clues for the specific diagnosis and differential diagnosis in infectious and noninfectious encephalitis/encephalopathy.
- Understanding the underlying disorder and pathophysiology is useful for the image interpretation and treatment.

INTRODUCTION

White matter diseases related to viral infections are divided into 2 major types: (1) infectious encephalitis/encephalopathy caused by direct viral infection to the central nervous system (CNS), and (2) noninfectious encephalitis/encephalopathy mainly caused by an autoimmune-mediated mechanism.[1,2]

Although viruses are the most common causes of infectious encephalitis/encephalopathy, the causative virus can be unknown in up to 60% of cases.[1] There are many known viral CNS infections involving white matter.[1–7] Herpes simplex virus (HSV) and varicella-zoster virus (VZV) are the most common causes of acute infectious encephalitis. Human immunodeficiency virus (HIV) can cause either leukoencephalopathy or encephalitis. In immunocompromised patients, there are many types of viral infection involving the white matter, including VZV vasculitis/vasculopathy, cytomegalovirus (CMV) infection, John Cunningham virus (JCV) producing progressive multifocal leukoencephalopathy (PML), human herpes virus

(HHV) 6 encephalitis, and Epstein-Barr virus (EBV) encephalitis/encephalopathy and EBV-associated neoplastic conditions. Subacute sclerosing panencephalitis (SSPE) is a slow virus infection caused by the measles virus. Newer viral encephalitides such as West Nile virus (WNV) encephalitis and HHV6 encephalitis are emerging because of human host modification of viral agents,[1,8,9] which potentially increases the ability to infect the CNS.

Noninfectious encephalitis/encephalopathy includes acute disseminated encephalomyelitis (ADEM), acute hemorrhagic leukoencephalopathy (AHLE), Bickerstaff brainstem encephalitis (BBE), acute necrotizing encephalopathy, and mild encephalitis/encephalopathy with a reversible splenial lesion (MERS).[1,2,8,10]

Acute viral encephalitis is a medical emergency. It requires prompt diagnosis and specific antiviral treatment or symptomatic treatment.[2,11] Thus, differentiating between infectious and noninfectious CNS involvement is imperative because noninfectious immune-mediated CNS involvement

No disclosures.
[a] Department of Radiology, University of Iowa Hospitals & Clinics, 200 Hawkins Drive, Iowa City, IA 52242, USA;
[b] Department of Pathology, University of Iowa Hospitals & Clinics, 200 Hawkins Drive, Iowa City, IA 52242, USA
* Corresponding author. Department of Radiology, University of Iowa Hospitals & Clinics, 200 Hawkins Drive, 0426 JCP, Iowa City, IA 52242.
E-mail address: moritani2001@yahoo.com

is mainly treated with corticosteroids. Symptoms are often nonspecific, including an acute onset of altered mental status, fever, headache, focal neurologic deficit, and possible seizures. Cerebrospinal fluid (CSF) findings of acute viral encephalitis usually show lymphocytic pleocytosis, with increased protein and normal glucose. However, CSF findings can be similar in noninfectious virus-associated CNS diseases. Prompt introduction of treatment has a significant influence on survival and the extent of permanent brain injury. Although the confirmation of the diagnosis often needs the detection of specific viral antigen or serologic markers in CSF, neuroimaging, especially magnetic resonance (MR) imaging, provides many clues for the specific diagnosis and differentiation from noninfectious encephalitis/encephalopathy.

This article discusses neuroimaging findings with the emphasis on MR imaging, including diffusion-weighted imaging (DWI) of infectious and noninfectious white matter lesions associated with various viral infections. It discusses the characteristic distribution and underlying disorder and pathophysiology.

INFECTIOUS VIRAL WHITE MATTER DISEASES
HIV Infection

Initial case reports of what would later become known as acquired immunodeficiency syndrome (AIDS) first appeared in 1981.[12] HIV was first described as the putative cause for AIDS in 1983.[13] HIV is a single-stranded ribonucleic acid (RNA) retrovirus that is lymphotropic and neurotropic. CNS is a primary target for HIV. Between 20% and 30% of patients with AIDS progress into AIDS dementia complex, characterized by neurocognitive impairment, emotional disturbance, and motor abnormalities.[14] The diagnosis

of HIV infection is made through detection of HIV antibody using enzyme-linked immunosorbent assay (ELISA) and Western blot, which are usually detectable within 4 weeks of inoculation. Polymerase chain reaction (PCR)–based tests measure the load of replicating HIV virus within the blood stream, which is useful both for testing for HIV before seroconversion and as a quantitative estimate of viral load. CD4 count is used to stage HIV infection. Circulating monocytes carry the virus across the blood-brain barrier. In the CNS, HIV-infected or activated monocytes differentiate into HIV-infected or activated macrophages and microglia, which produce neurotoxic viral proteins and increased concentration of excitotoxic glutamate via astrocyte activation, resulting in neurodegeneration.[14]

The pathologic hallmark of HIV encephalopathy/encephalitis is multinucleated giant cells of macrophage/microglia origin. HIV encephalopathy is characterized pathologically by diffuse myelin breakdown, astrogliosis, multinucleated giant cells, and little inflammation. The corpus callosum can be spared. HIV encephalitis is identified in 26% in neuropathologic AIDS autopsies and is characterized by perivascular inflammation, microglial nodules, and multinucleated giant cells. Brains frequently show overlap of encephalopathy and encephalitis.[15–17]

MR imaging shows parenchymal volume loss and diffuse periventricular white matter lesions (Fig. 1). T2-weighted and fluid-attenuated inversion recovery (FLAIR) images show diffuse periventricular hyperintensity, with no mass effect or contrast enhancement.[18] DWI shows high signal with increased apparent diffusion coefficient (ADC) (T2 shine-through). In some cases, brainstem, basal ganglia, and corpus callosum are involved, which suggests the presence of HIV encephalitis (Fig. 2). Patients with HIV have a small

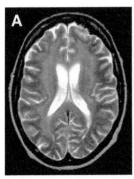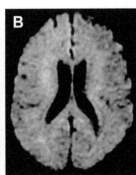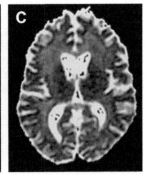

Fig. 1. HIV encephalopathy. A 46-year-old man with AIDS dementia complex. T2-weighted image (A) shows diffuse periventricular hyperintense lesions. U fibers are spared. DWI reveals these lesions as mild hyperintensity (B). Apparent diffusion coefficient (ADC) map shows these lesions as increased ADC (C). Mild hyperintensity on DWI is caused by a T2 shine-through effect.

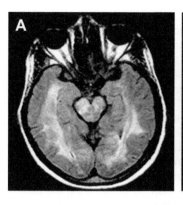
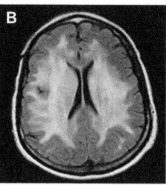

Fig. 2. HIV encephalitis. A 39-year-old man with AIDS dementia complex. FLAIR images (A, B) reveal extensive white matter changes with vasogenic edema involving basal ganglia and brain stem, which suggests the presence of HIV encephalitis.

increased incidence of stroke (6%–12%), mainly caused by opportunistic VZV infection or HIV vasculopathy.[19] HIV vasculopathy was found in 5.5% of an autopsy cohort of patients infected with HIV.[20] MR imaging with DWI is useful to detect infarctions. HIV infection is associated with many other opportunistic CNS infections, including viral infections such as VZV, CMV, PML, EBV, HHV6, and HSV, as well as bacterial, fungal, and parasitic infections. Multiple coexistent CNS infections sometimes make the interpretation of MR imaging findings complicated. Highly active antiretroviral therapy (HAART) can result in deterioration by a paradoxic activation of an inflammatory response causing fulminant leukoencephalitis, known as immune reconstitution inflammatory syndrome (IRIS) (Fig. 3).[21–23] IRIS can be responsive to steroid therapy.

Eighty-five percent of AIDS in children is vertically transmitted from an infected mother.[7] The onset of neurologic disease is between 2 months and 5 years. The prevalence of CNS disease in children infected with HIV ranges from 20% to 60%. The most common abnormalities are brain atrophy and white matter disease (Fig. 4).[7,24,25] Intracranial calcifications can be detected in 33% of children infected with HIV, which is usually not seen before 10 months of age. An annual risk of cerebrovascular accident in HIV-positive children is 1.3%.[26]

HHV Infections

Herpes virus infections are responsible for a wide spectrum of diseases in humans.[27] Herpes virus infections range from being asymptomatic to producing life-threatening CNS disease. HHVs are classified into 8 double-stranded deoxyribonucleic acid (DNA) viruses. The primary sites of HHV infection are skin, conjunctiva, and mucosa of oropharynx or genitalia where virus replicates and spreads hematogenously.

- HHV1. HSV1: Oral more commonly than genital herpes
- HHV2. HSV2: Genital more commonly than oral herpes
- HHV3. VZV: Chickenpox, shingles
- HHV4. EBV: Infectious mononucleosis, lymphoma, nasopharyngeal carcinoma
- HHV5. CMV: Infectious mononucleosislike syndrome, retinitis
- HHV6. Roseolovirus: Exanthem subitum/roseola infantum
- HHV7. Pityriasis rosea
- HHV8. Kaposi sarcoma–associated herpes virus

HSV Infection

Herpes simplex encephalitis (HSE) is the most common cause of sporadic fatal encephalitis, accounting for 10% to 20% of encephalitic viral

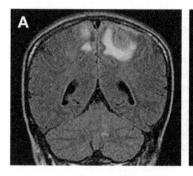
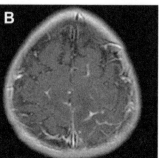

Fig. 3. IRIS related to cryptococcal meningitis in a patient with HIV. FLAIR image (A) shows a progression of bilateral parietal white matter edema. Postcontrast axial T1-weighted image (B) reveals leptomeningeal enhancement.

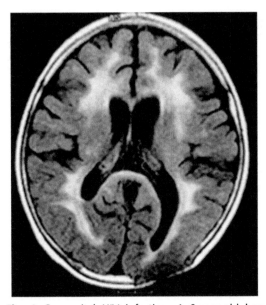

Fig. 4. Congenital HIV infection. A 9-year-old boy with a remote history of CNS lymphoma. FLAIR image shows characteristic white matter hyperintensity with diffuse brain atrophy consistent with HIV encephalopathy. Postbiopsy changes for CNS lymphoma are seen in the left occipital region.

infections.[28,29] HSE is nonepidemic and shows no seasonal predilection. HSE can occur in either immunocompetent or immunocompromised patients, such as HIV-positive subjects.[30,31] Prompt recognition of HSE is paramount, because early treatment with acyclovir has been shown to decrease both morbidity and mortality. Because the clinical findings are nonspecific, the diagnosis must be focused on the CSF analysis along with neuroimaging studies, specifically computed tomography (CT) and MR imaging. PCR analysis of viral DNA in the CSF is both sensitive and specific for the diagnosis of HSE (sensitivity 95%, specificity 100%).[32] The pathogenesis of HSV infection remains unclear. The virus consists of 2 different morphologically identical but antigenically distinct agents: type 1 (HSV1) and type 2 (HSV2). Although HSV1 usually causes oral lesions and HSV2 typically genital lesions, either virus can be found at either site. Most patients develop HSE as a result of secondary reactivation of latent HSV in the trigeminal or sacral ganglia, but the primary infection can occur in neonates and children.[28,29]

On pathology, HSE shows both cytotoxic and vasogenic edema associated with congestion and later evolving to tissue necrosis, perivascular and subarachnoid mononuclear cell infiltrate, and petechial or confluent hemorrhage.[17,28,29] In adults, the medial temporal lobes, inferior frontal lobes, and insula, encompassing limbic and paralimbic areas, are commonly involved (Fig. 5). Predominantly cortical involvement may extend into the white matter. In infants and young children, the lesions tend to extend into frontoparietal lobes (Fig. 6).[33] In neonatal HSE, cerebral cortex and white matter are involved in a more global fashion (Fig. 7).[34]

CT shows a region of hypodensity consistent with cerebral edema in the lesions, usually with subtle mass effect. The end stage of HSE is characterized by encephalomalacia, atrophy, and cystic necrosis of the involved area. MR imaging is more sensitive than CT in detecting the parenchymal abnormalities of HSE. MR imaging shows asymmetric T2 and FLAIR hyperintensity in the lesions, often associated with leptomeningeal and gyral enhancement. Petechial or confluent hemorrhages can be seen on T1-weighted or T2* gradient echo (GRE) images. DWI is more sensitive than conventional MR imaging in detecting early changes of herpes encephalitis.[34–38] Postictal changes may show unilateral diffuse reduced diffusion in the hippocampal formation and amygdaloid complex, often with ipsilateral thalamic pulvinar lesion.

HHV6 Infection

HHV6 is a ubiquitous neurotropic virus that is latent in most adults. Primary infection usually occurs in the first 2 years of life and is also known to cause exanthem subitum or roseola infantum. HHV6-associated encephalitis has been increasingly recognized as a serious complication in immunocompromised patients, such as patients with HIV and bone marrow or stem cell transplant recipients.[39–41] The virus is classified into 2 subtypes: HHV6A and HHV6B. HHV6B is mainly responsible for primary infection and reactivation. In transplantation, acyclovir is routinely administered but is not effective against HHV6 because of the lack of virus-specific thymidine kinase. Ganciclovir and foscarnet are the treatment of choice of HHV6 encephalitis. The diagnosis of HHV6 encephalitis is performed by PCR analysis for viral DNA in the CSF. However, the specificity is not high because chromosomal integration of viral DNA from primary infection causes false-positives.[42]

MR imaging usually shows a pattern of T2 and FLAIR hyperintensity in the medial temporal lobe, which has been seen in adult patients (Fig. 8). HHV6 infection typically involves a smaller portion of the medial temporal lobe than that seen in HSV infection. Intraparenchymal hemorrhage is rare. More extensive changes have been reported in infants and young children. Extrahippocampal

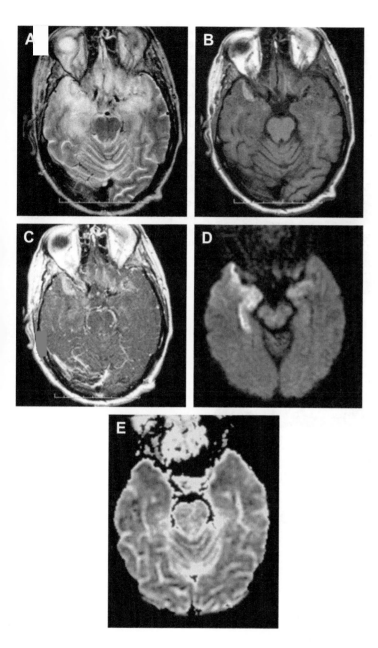

Fig. 5. Herpes encephalitis. A 56-year-old woman with mental status changes. T2-weighted image (*A*) shows hyperintense lesions in bilateral medial temporal lobes and inferior frontal lobes. T1-weighted image (*B*) reveals hemorrhage. Postcontrast T1-weighted image (*C*) shows leptomeningeal enhancement. DWI (*D*) shows the lesions as hyperintense. ADC map shows decreased ADC of the lesions (*E*).

involvement (basal ganglia, other cortical and white matter structures) has also been reported (Fig. 9).[39] DWI high signal intensity with ADC reduction consistent with cytotoxic edema is observed.

VZV Infection

VZV is a ubiquitous human DNA virus. Primary infection occurs via respiratory aerosols or contact with vesicles from an infected individual and results in the disseminated rash of chickenpox.[3,7] A parainfectious, immune-mediated syndrome with cerebellar ataxia is the most common CNS manifestation of chickenpox (0.1%). Acute varicella encephalitis is rare (0.05%). VZV becomes latent in the cranial nerve ganglia, spinal dorsal root ganglia, and autonomic ganglia. VZV reactivation commonly manifests as herpes zoster (shingles). Herpes zoster meningoencephalitis, myelitis, or polyradiculopathy usually occurs in elderly and immunocompromised patients. The diagnostic value of anti-VZV immunoglobulin G in CSF (93% sensitivity) is greater than that of VZV DNA by PCR in CSF (30% sensitivity).[19] Negative results for both tests tend to exclude VZV

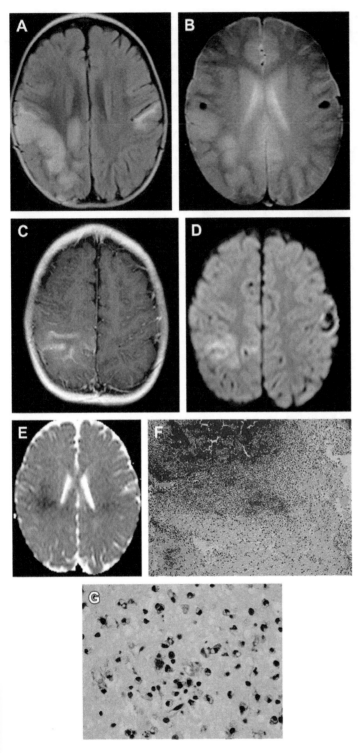

Fig. 6. Herpes simplex type 1 and 2 encephalitis in a 2-year-old girl with seizures. FLAIR image shows bilateral frontoparietal cortical lesions (*A*). Gradient echo (GRE) reveals hemorrhage in the lesions (*B*). Postcontrast T1-weighted image reveals leptomeningeal and gyral enhancement (*C*). DWI (*D*) shows hyperintensity in the cortical lesions extending into the white matter associated with decreased ADC (*E*). Brain biopsy shows petechial hemorrhage, cytotoxic edema, and necrosis (*F*). (*G*) HSV stain was positive ([*F*] hematoxylin-eosin, original magnification ×100; [*G*] original magnification ×1000).

infection. Pathologic findings in herpes zoster encephalitis include perivascular lymphocytic cuffing and focal demyelination with intranuclear inclusion bodies in endothelial cells, neurons, and glial cells.[19] Granulomatous angiitis can be seen.

MR imaging of herpes zoster meningoencephalitis shows multifocal cortical and white matter lesions with leptomeningeal enhancement. VZV vasculopathy results from productive viral infection of arteries. VZV can affect both large and small

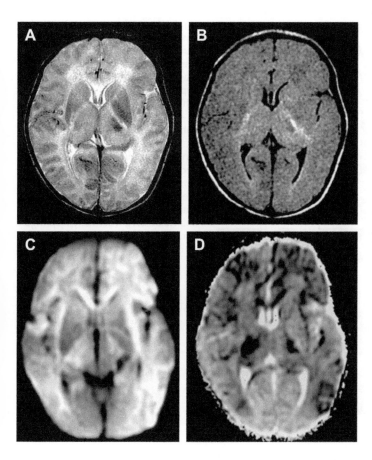

Fig. 7. Neonatal herpes simplex type 2 encephalitis in a 2-week-old girl. T2-weighted (*A*) and FLAIR (*B*) images show asymmetric hyperintense lesions in the gray and white matter including thalami and right basal ganglia. However, the precise extent of the lesions is difficult to determine. DWI (*C*) shows asymmetric and extensive hyperintense lesions in the gray and white matter in both hemispheres in a more global fashion associated with decreased ADC (*D*). (*From* Moritani T, Ekholm SE, Westesson PL. Diffusion-weighted MR imaging of the brain. 2nd edition. Berlin, Heidelberg (Germany): Springer-Verlag; 2009. p. 312; with permission.)

arteries, which results in aneurysm formation, arterial ectasia, dissection, subarachnoid hemorrhage, infarction, and hemorrhage.[19,43,44] Thirty-seven percent of VZV vasculopathy cases do not have the characteristic varicella or zoster rash.[19] VZV vasculopathy occurs more frequently late in the course of AIDS, especially when there is significant CD4+ depletion (see Fig. 9). MR imaging with DWI is useful to detect ischemic stroke, which often involves gray matter–white matter junctions (Fig. 10). MR or CT angiogram is useful to detect vascular abnormalities (Fig. 11). Treatment of VZV vasculopathy is intravenous acyclovir and oral steroids.

CMV Infection

CMV is the most common cause of serious neonatal brain infection and infection is caused by transplacental spread.

The mechanisms of CNS injury in congenital CMV infection are thought to be the affinity of the virus for the rapid-growing germinal matrix cells and lenticulostriate small vessels, which results in cerebral and cerebellar abnormalities,

periventricular calcifications, and vasculopathy.[7,45] On CT and MR imaging, brain abnormalities depend on the degree of brain destruction and the timing of the injury, and include lissencephaly, polymicrogyria, white matter volume loss, delayed myelination, small cerebellum, and periventricular calcifications (Fig. 12). Human CMV becomes latent early in life in myeloid precursor cells after asymptomatic infection. Reactivation of the virus can occur in immunocompromised patients. CMV encephalitis is common among immunocompromised patients and usually occurs during systemic CMV infection with myelitis, polyradiculopathy, or retinitis. In patients with AIDS, reactivation occurs at low CD4 counts, usually less than 100 cells/μL. CMV encephalitis often shows a pattern of ependymitis, ventriculitis, polyradiculitis, and necrotizing meningoencephalitis. Sensitivity and specificity of CSF PCR for the detection of CMV DNA are 79% and 95%.[2]

MR imaging can show T2 and FLAIR periventricular white matter hyperintensity with periventricular enhancement, hydrocephalus, and occasionally cortical nodular enhancement, but

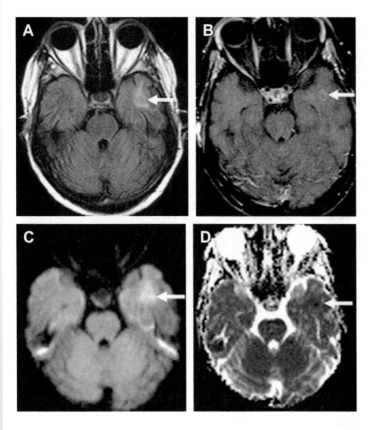

Fig. 8. Human herpesvirus-6 encephalitis. A 28-year-old woman with seizures after allogeneic stem cell transplantation for acute lymphoblastic leukemia. FLAIR image shows a hyperintense lesion (*arrow*) in the left temporal lobe (*A*). Postcontrast T1-weighted image shows mild enhancement in the lesion (*arrow in B*). DWI reveals the lesion as hyperintense (*arrow in C*). ADC map shows decreased ADC of the lesion (*arrow in D*). (*From* Moritani T, Ekholm SE, Westesson PL. Diffusion-weighted MR imaging of the brain. 2nd edition. Berlin, Heidelberg (Germany): Springer-Verlag; 2009. p. 216; with permission.)

imaging is often normal (**Fig. 13**).[2,3] The disease is often fatal within 4 to 6 weeks. CMV replication in arterial endothelial cells may induce atherosclerosis, promoting ischemic stroke.[19] Acyclovir is ineffective. Ganciclovir with or without foscarnet is currently recommended; cidofovir is a possible alternative.[46]

EBV Infection

EBV is a ubiquitous virus and epidemiologically important because it asymptomatically infects more than 90% of the world's population.[3,7] Acute infectious mononucleosis is the commonest manifestation of EBV, and is usually a self-limiting condition. Chronic active EBV infection is rare but often fatal. Following primary infection, it typically remains in a latent state within B lymphocytes regulated by cytotoxic T cells and natural killer (NK) cells.[47] CNS complications of EBV infection range from 0.4% to 7.3% and include meningitis, encephalitis, myelitis, cerebellitis, ADEM, reversible encephalitis, Guillain-Barré syndrome, and neuropsychiatric disturbances.[48,49] EBV

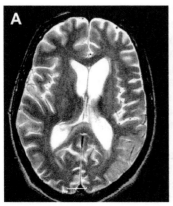
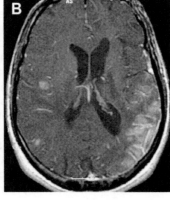

Fig. 9. Human herpesvirus-6 meningoencephalitis. A 44-year-old man with HIV and a progressive memory problem. T2-weighted image show asymmetric hyperintense lesions in the gray and white matter in the temporoparieto-occipital areas bilaterally, left more than right (extrahippocampal involvement) (*A*). Postcontrast T1-weighted image shows extensive leptomeningeal and gyral enhancement (*B*).

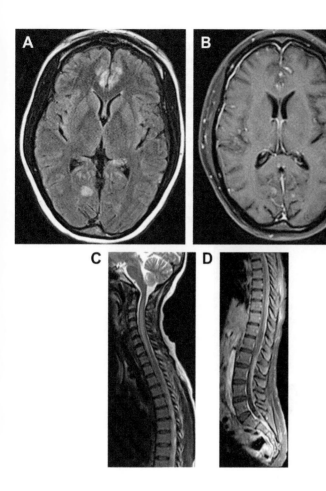

Fig. 10. Disseminated varicella-zoster meningoencephalitis, myelitis and polyradiculitis in a patient with HIV. FLAIR image shows asymmetric patchy hyperintense lesions in bilateral frontal and right occipital lobes (*A*). Postcontrast T1-weighted image shows dural, leptomeningeal, and gyral enhancement consistent with meningoencephalitis (*B*). Sagittal T2-weighted image of cervicothoracic spine reveals longitudinal cord signal abnormality consistent with myelitis (*C*). Sagittal postcontrast T1-weighted image of thoracolumbar spine shows enhancement along the cord and nerve root representing meningitis and radiculomyelitis (*D*).

meningoencephalitis is usually mild with personality changes, depressed level of consciousness, and abnormal movements, and fatal cases secondary to brain encephalitis have been reported. Acyclovir and corticosteroids have been recommended for treatment of EBV encephalitis, but the effectiveness is uncertain. The diagnosis of EBV infection is made with a positive PCR for EBV DNA in CSF and specific EBV immunoglobulin (Ig) M antibodies against viral capsid antigen in serum.[3,48]

Virus-associated hemophagocytic syndrome (VAHS), also called hemophagocytic lymphohistiocytosis (HLH), is a multisystem disorder characterized with aggressive proliferation of macrophages and histiocytes showing hemophagocytosis with an upregulation of the inflammatory cytokines, including macrophage colony–stimulating factor, by T-helper cells.[50,51] HLH can be primary (familial, autosomal recessive) or secondary. EBV is the most common cause of VAHS (secondary HLH). VAHS often follows a brief of viral illness. The diagnostic criteria include fever, hepatosplenomegaly, pancytopenia, hypertriglyceridemia,

hyperferritinemia and/or low fibrin level, and hemophagocytosis in the reticuloendothelial system.[52] In situ hybridization analysis of EBV-encoded small RNAs (EBER) is positive in pathology specimens and diagnostically useful. VAHS affects the CNS in 10% to 73% of patients with variable neurologic symptoms including irritability, seizures, hemiparesis, and coma.[52] The CSF is normal in approximately 50%.[53] Pathology shows initial leptomeningeal and intraparenchymal perivascular lymphocytic infiltration with astrogliosis affecting mainly white matter, followed by areas of necrosis and focal demyelination.

MR imaging findings are parenchymal volume loss with focal necrosis and/or white matter abnormalities (**Fig. 14**).[50–54] Leptomeningeal and perivascular enhancement is frequently seen. Multiple enhancing lesions have also been described. Treatment consists of immunosuppression chemotherapy, including corticosteroids and cyclosporine A, combined with etoposide and, ultimately, bone marrow transplantation. VAHS/HLH may have a relapsing and remitting course, or it may rapidly progress

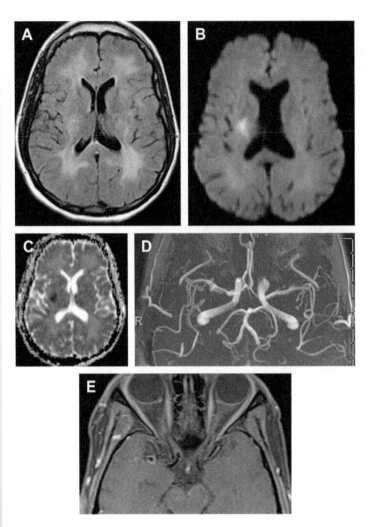

Fig. 11. Varicella-zoster vasculitis. A 26-year-old man with a stroke and a history of HIV infection. FLAIR image shows diffuse white matter hyperintensity consistent with HIV encephalopathy (A). DWI (B) shows hyperintensity in the posterior internal capsule associated with decreased ADC consistent with an acute infarct (C). MR angiography reveals an ectatic M1 portion of the right middle cerebral artery (D). Postcontrast T1-weighted image shows enhancement of the wall of ectatic right middle cerebral artery consistent with arteritis (E).

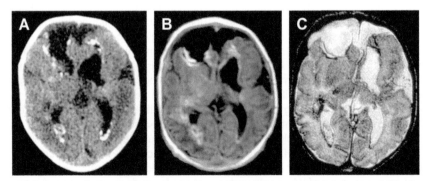

Fig. 12. Congenital cytomegalovirus infection in a 10-day old boy. CT shows periventricular calcifications and ventriculomegaly (A). T1-weighted (B) and T2-weighted (C) images show periventricular calcifications and ventriculomegaly, open-lip schizencephaly in the right frontal lobe, lissencephaly, and polymicrogyria in the bilateral frontoparietal cortices.

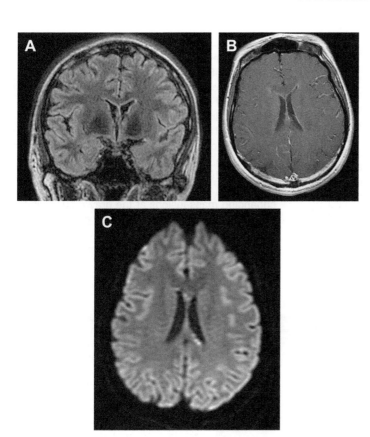

Fig. 13. Cytomegalovirus ependymitis/ventriculitis. A 24-year-old woman with aplastic anemia and cytomegalovirus retinitis. Coronal FLAIR image shows linear high signal intensity along the ventricular wall (*A*). Postcontrast T1-weighted image shows diffuse ventricular wall enhancement consistent with ependymitis/ventriculitis (*B*). DWI reveals multiple diffusion-restricted foci consistent with acute microinfarcts (*C*). (*Courtesy of* Dr Jay Starkey, MD, University of California, San Francisco, CA.)

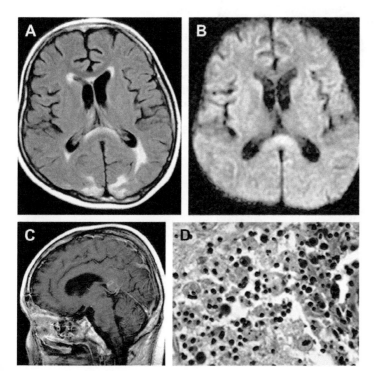

Fig. 14. EBV-associated hemophagocytic syndrome. A 13-year-old boy with mental status change, hepatosplenomegaly, and hypercytokinemia. FLAIR image (*A*) and DWI (*B*) show a splenial lesion as hyperintense. FLAIR-hyperintense lesions in bilateral occipital lobes represent posterior reversible encephalopathy syndrome caused by the treatment of cyclosporine A. Sagittal postcontrast T1-weighted image (*C*) reveals enhancement in the splenial lesion. The patient died with multiorgan failure. Brain at autopsy reveals infiltration of hemophagocytic histiocytes and atypical lymphocytes with edema in the splenial lesion (*D*) ([*D*] hematoxylin-eosin, original magnification ×400). (*Courtesy of* Dr Nobuo Kobayashi, MD, St. Luke's International Hospital, Tokyo, Japan.)

to multiorgan failure and death. Between 30% and 40% of patients with VAHS have poor clinical outcomes.

EBV was the first human tumor virus to be discovered and identified in Burkitt lymphoma (in 1964).[55] When EBV infects B cells in vitro, lymphoblastoid cell lines eventually emerge that are capable of indefinite growth. EBV is associated with several lymphomas and lymphoproliferative disorders that include B-cell, T-cell, and NK-cell neoplasias.[47] These include posttransplant lymphoproliferative disease (PTLD), lymphomatoid granulomatosis (LYG) and AIDS-related CNS lymphoma. EBER in situ hybridization is positive and diagnostically useful for EBV-associated lymphoma and lymphoproliferative disorder.

PTLD

PTLD is defined as a heterogeneous group of lymphoproliferative diseases that occur as a consequence of immunosuppression in the recipient of a solid organ or stem cell allograft. It is EBV infection related in 60% to 70% of cases.[47] PTLD is subdivided into monomorphic, polymorphic, plasmacytic, or Hodgkin lymphoma–like variants. Most of PTLD is B cell in origin but 10% to 15% is of T/K-cell origin.[47] In CNS-PTLD, MR imaging shows multiple necrotic enhancing mass lesions at the gray matter–white matter junction and deep gray matter (Fig. 15).[56,57] Combination immunochemotherapy regimens including rituximab are commonly used, with variable success.

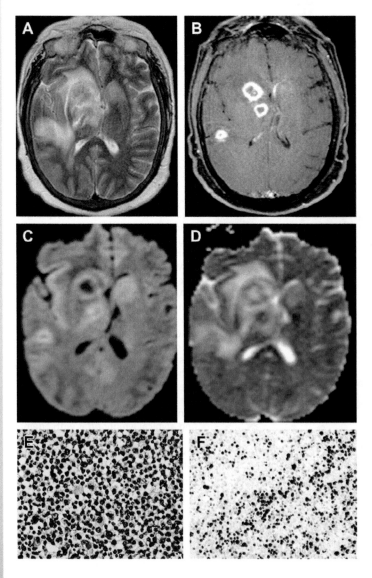

Fig. 15. PTLD. A 54-year-old man after renal transplantation. T2-weighted image shows multiple mildly hyperintense masses with vasogenic edema in the white matter (A). Postcontrast T1-weighted image shows ring or heterogeneous enhancement (B). DWI shows hyperintensity in the ring enhancing solid portion and hypointensity in the central necrosis (C). ADC map shows partially decreased ADC of the solid portion of the mass (D). Brain biopsy reveals a hypercellular atypical lymphoid infiltrate with mitosis and nuclear pleomorphism (E). In situ hybridization analysis of EBER was positive (F) ([E] hematoxylin-eosin, original magnification ×400; [F] original magnification ×400). (From Moritani T, Ekholm SE, Westesson PL. Diffusion-weighted MR imaging of the brain. 2nd edition. Berlin, Heidelberg (Germany): Springer-Verlag; 2009. p. 279; with permission.)

LYG

LYG is a rare lymphoproliferative disorder. Most patients with LYG do not have a history of overt immunodeficiency. There is a predilection for men in a 2:1 ratio to women and it commonly presents between the fourth and sixth decades of life.[47] LYG may arise in the setting of a global deficit in CD8 T cells with selected defects in EBV-specific immunity. On histology, LYG lesions are characterized by angiocentric and angiodestructive lymphoid infiltrate consisting of EBV-positive B cells admixed with a prominent inflammatory background of T cells, plasma cells, and histiocytes. In CNS-LYG, MR imaging typically shows multiple necrotic enhancing mass lesions but a diffuse white matter infiltrative pattern can be seen (**Fig. 16**).[58,59] Treatment with various cytotoxic agents, corticosteroids, and interferon (immunochemotherapy) has been described.

AIDS-related CNS Lymphoma

In patients with HIV/AIDS, most CNS lymphomas are diffuse large B-cell lymphomas and nearly 100% are EBV positive.[47] Detection of EBV in the CSF with a CNS lesion supports the diagnosis of lymphoma. MR imaging shows diffuse or multifocal ring enhancing mass lesions with predominant periventricular location (**Fig. 17**).[60] Treatment consists of combinations of chemotherapy, which include high-dose methotrexate and cytarabine with or without radiotherapy. The addition of rituximab may improve survival rates.

JCV Infection

PML is a noninflammatory demyelinating disease first described in 1958, associated with oligodendrocytes infected with JCV.[61] JCV is a double-stranded circular DNA virus, and a member of Polyomaviridae family first isolated in 1971 and formerly known as papovavirus. JCV is a ubiquitous human pathogen.[62] Primary asymptomatic infection with JCV is presumed to occur during childhood. The reservoir of the virus is thought to be established in the kidneys and B lymphocytes.[63] Reactivation and dissemination may occur under impaired T-cell function. How and when JCV reaches the CNS remains unknown. The symptoms of PML are often psychiatric/behavioral changes or progressive neurologic

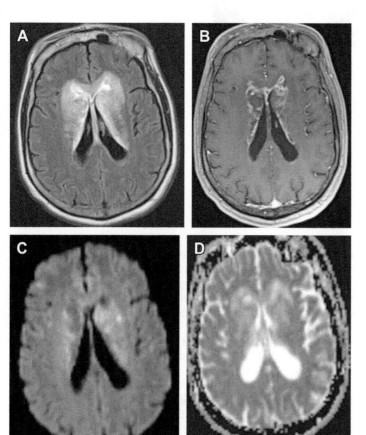

Fig. 16. Lymphomatoid granulomatosis. A 56-year-old man with mental status changes. FLAIR image shows symmetric periventricular hyperintensity (*A*). Postcontrast T1-weighted image reveals heterogeneous enhancement in the lesions (*B*). DWI (*C*) shows mixed hyperintensity and hypointensity associated with heterogeneous ADC values (*D*) representing cellular infiltration and necrosis. In situ hybridization (EBER) was positive for EBV (not shown).

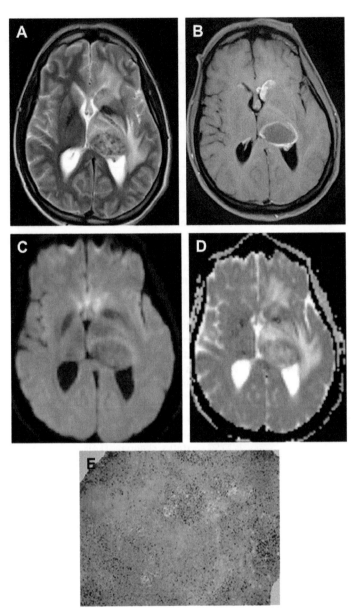

Fig. 17. AIDS-related lymphoma in a 42-year-old man. T2-weighted image shows mildly hyperintense or hypointense masses in the left periventricular region with vasogenic edema in the white matter (A). Postcontrast T1-weighted image shows ring or heterogeneous enhancement (B). DWI reveals hyperintensity in the ring and hypointensity in the center of the mass (C). ADC map shows partially decreased ADC of the solid portion of the mass (D). Brain biopsy reveals lymphoma with necrosis (E). In situ hybridization (EBER) was positive for EBV (not shown) ([E] hematoxylin-eosin, original magnification ×100).

deficits. HIV accounts for approximately 80% of PML cases.[63,64] Other causes of immunodeficiency are organ/stem cell transplant, hematologic malignancy, autoimmune disease or multiple sclerosis treated with immune modulators including monoclonal antibodies (natrizumab, efalizumab, rituximab), and primary immunodeficiency syndrome.[63,65–67]

The pathology of PML typically shows demyelination without evidence of inflammation, swollen oligodendrocytes with densely basophilic nuclear inclusion bodies, and astrocytes with enlarged hyperchromatic nuclei (bizarre astrocytes) resembling neoplastic cells. In advanced cases,

lesions may have cavitary necrosis. PML is, rarely, associated with a marked inflammatory reaction characterized by perivascular mononuclear infiltrates. There are different settings of this type of PML: in patients with HIV with HAART (PML-IRIS), patients with HIV without HAART, or patients without HIV.[68,69] Three other subtypes of JCV-associated disease have been recently recognized: (1) JCV infecting only cerebellar granule cell neurons (JCVGCN), (2) JCV meningoencephalitis, and (3) JCV preferentially infecting cortical pyramidal neurons and astrocytes (JCV encephalopathy [JCE]).[70–72] Before the introduction of HAART, PCR for JCV DNA in the CSF had high sensitivity and specificity (72%–92% and 92%–100%). However, immune restoration with HAART may decrease viral replication, which decreases the sensitivity to 58%.[73] Sensitivity and specificity of brain biopsies are 64% to 96% and 100% retrospectively.

In the HAART era for the treatment of HIV infection, imaging has become more important in the diagnosis of PML.[74,75] MR imaging is the most sensitive imaging tool for PML. Supratentorial white matter lesions are typically asymmetric, multifocal, bilateral, sometimes with confluent lobar involvement, but can be unilateral or there may be a single lesion (Fig. 18). The lesions characteristically extend into the subcortical U fibers. PML can involve deep gray matter such as the thalamus and basal ganglia. Posterior fossa lesions are common and typically affect the middle cerebellar peduncles and adjacent pons and cerebellar hemisphere (Fig. 19) and can extend into the midbrain and medulla. Spinal cord involvement is extremely rare. The degree of enhancement depends on the patient's immunologic status. The peripheral hyperintensity rim on DWI with reduced ADC may represent

JCV-infected, swollen oligodendrocytes in the active margin of the lesions.[76,77] JCVGCN presents with isolated cerebellar atrophy.[70] JCE is initially restricted to hemispheric gray matter with extension to the subcortical white matter.[72] Differential diagnosis includes other opportunistic infection, encephalitis/encephalopathy, lymphoma, or other demyelinating disease. There is no specific treatment of JCV infection. HAART is the best treatment in patients with HIV. HAART increased the 1-year survival rate by 10% to 50%. In HIV-negative patients, reduction of the cause of immunosuppression is indicated as much as is clinically allowable.

WNV Infection

WNV, a single-stranded RNA flavivirus, Japanese encephalitis serocomplex, and arbovirus transmitted by the *Culex* mosquito, was first isolated in 1937 in the West Nile province of Uganda.[78] WNV first emerged in North America in 1999.[79] It is maintained by a bird-mosquito transmission cycle. Humans, horses, and other nonavian vertebrates are incidental hosts. In humans, there are

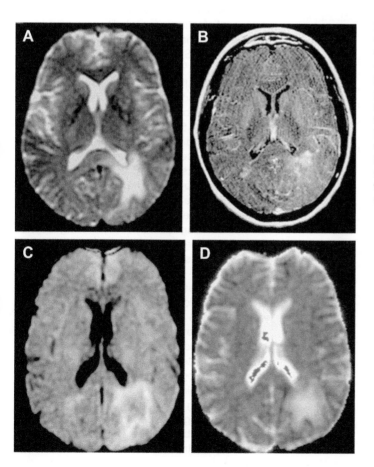

Fig. 18. PML. A 50-year-old woman with right hemianopsia after chemotherapy and bone marrow transplant for chronic lymphocytic leukemia. T2 hyperintense lesions are seen in the posterior part of the corpus callosum and left parieto-occipital white matter extending into the U fibers (A). Postcontrast T1-weighted image reveals multiple patchy enhancement in the white matter lesion (B). DWI (C) reveals a peripheral rim of hyperintensity associated with slightly decreased ADC (D).

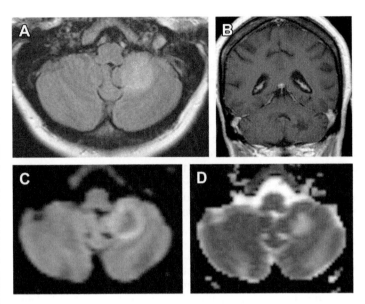

Fig. 19. PML with HIV. A 43-year-old woman presented with ataxia. FLAIR image shows a hyperintense lesion in the left cerebellum (*A*). Postcontrast coronal T1-weighted image reveals no enhancement in the cerebellar lesion (*B*). DWI (*C*) reveals a peripheral rim of hyperintensity associated with slightly decreased ADC (*D*).

4 other patterns of transmission: transfusion, transplanted organ, transplacental, and via breast feeding.[80] Eighty percent of infections are asymptomatic and 20% cause a mild self-limiting illness called WNV fever.[81] Less than 1% of patients infected with WNV develop meningoencephalitis. Common symptoms include fever, headache, weakness, meningismus, myalgia, rash, tremor, and flaccid paralysis with spinal cord involvement.[82] The incubation period is 3 to 14 days. Myositis, hepatitis, and pancreatitis are rare nonneurologic manifestations of WNV infection. Only 35% of patients with neurologic involvement have complete recovery.[83] The mortality is around 10%. Pathology shows microglial nodules composed of lymphocytes and histiocytes, perivascular lymphocytic cuffing, spongiotic changes, and necrosis in the white and gray matter.[81,84] The most efficient diagnostic test is detection of WNV IgM antibody in CSF.[81]

MR imaging shows mildly hyperintense lesions on T2 and FLAIR in the basal ganglia, thalami, mesial temporal lobe, white matter, cerebellum, brain stem (especially the substantia nigra and medulla), and spinal cord (**Fig. 20**).[80–84] MR imaging reveals no abnormalities in 30% of cases. Leptomeningeal enhancement can be seen. DWI can show isolated restricted diffusion in white matter or foci of restricted diffusion within the T2 signal abnormalities. The mainstay of treatment is supportive (intravenous fluid, respiratory support). Ribavirin in high doses and interferon alfa-2b have some activity based on in vitro efficacy against WNV.[81,84]

Measles Virus Infection

Measles is an acute, highly contagious infection caused by a single-stranded RNA virus of the paramyxovirus family. Measles virus causes (1) acute postinfectious encephalitis, (2) acute progressive encephalitis, and (3) the slow measles virus infection SSPE, originally described by Dawson in 1933.[7,85,86] SSPE is a sequela of early measles infection, often before 2 years of age. The virus remains dormant intracellularly and manifests as SSPE between 5 and 15 years of age (mean, 7 years). SSPE is rare in the United States after widespread immunization but can be seen in immigrants, those whose parent refuse immunization, and patients with HIV.[87] SSPE has an insidious onset of behavioral changes followed by mental deterioration, myoclonus, seizures, dementia, and inexorable progression to death. Pathologic findings include predominantly involvement of gray matter with white matter demyelination, perivascular lymphocytic cuffing, neuronophagia, intracellular viral inclusions, and gliosis. Diagnosis is based on clinical findings, electroencephalogram results, and measles antibodies in serum and CSF.

MR imaging reveals no abnormalities in the early stages. Multifocal lesions in the cortex and subcortical white matter may be observed. As the disease progresses, the lesions extend into the periventricular white matter and corpus callosum, resulting in brain atrophy (**Fig. 21**).[87–89] The basal ganglia, thalamus, brain stem, and cerebellum can be involved. Combined oral isoprinosine and intraventricular interferon-alfa can

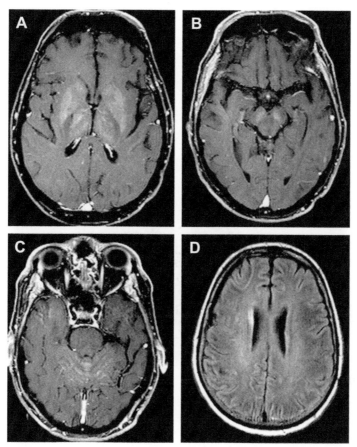

Fig. 20. West Nile encephalitis in a 56-year-old man with fever and tremors with a history of renal transplant. Postcontrast T1-weighted images show symmetric mild enhancement in the basal ganglia, thalami (*A*), and substantia nigra (*B*), and leptomeningeal enhancement in the posterior fossa (*C*). FLAIR image (*D*) and DWI (*E*) show diffuse symmetric hyperintense lesions with decreased ADC (*F*) only in the deep white matter. Brain biopsy shows perivascular lymphocytic cuffing (*G*) and microglial nodules ([*G*] hematoxylin-eosin, original magnification ×400). (*From* Moritani T, Ekholm SE, Westesson PL. Diffusion-weighted MR imaging of the brain. 2nd edition. Berlin, Heidelberg (Germany): Springer-Verlag; 2009. p. 218; with permission.)

result in some improvement. Curative therapy for SSPE is not available.

NONINFECTIOUS VIRUS-ASSOCIATED WHITE MATTER DISEASES

The differential diagnosis of viral meningoencephalitis is diverse and includes other infectious diseases (bacterial, fungal, parasitic), ischemic disease, vasculitis/vasculopathy, neoplastic disease, paraneoplastic syndrome, toxic/metabolic diseases, and other demyelinating and degenerative diseases.[1–3,90,91] This article focuses on noninfectious, virus-associated immune-mediated encephalopathy/encephalitis as differential diagnosis from infectious viral white matter diseases.

These include:

1. ADEM
2. AHLE
3. BBE
4. Acute necrotizing encephalitis (ANE)
5. MERS

ADEM

ADEM is an immune-mediated inflammatory disorder of the CNS, usually triggered by an inflammatory response to viral infections or, rarely, vaccinations.[1,7,92] This condition predominantly affects children and young adults. ADEM presents with abrupt onset of neurologic symptoms 2 to 31 days after a viral illness or vaccination. The neurologic picture of ADEM commonly reflects a multifocal but usually monophasic involvement, whereas multiple sclerosis (MS) is characterized by recurrent episodes disseminated both in time and space. ADEM lesions tend to resolve, partially or completely, and new lesions rarely occur.[92]

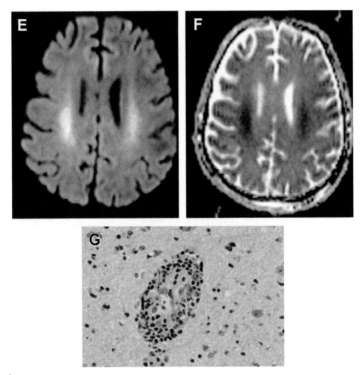

Fig. 20. (*continued*)

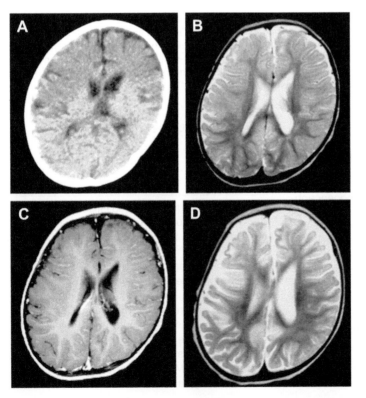

Fig. 21. SSPE. A 6-year-old boy with a remote history of measles infection. CT shows diffuse low density in the bilateral frontal lobes (*A*). T2-weighted image shows diffuse mild hyperintensity with multifocal subcortical white matter lesions in the frontal lobes (*B*). Postcontrast T1-weighted image reveals diffuse leptomeningeal enhancement (*C*). One-year follow-up MR imaging shows progression of atrophy in the bilateral frontoparietal areas (*D*).

A possible mechanism of ADEM is an autoimmune response to myelin basic protein (MBP). The protein by-products from the virus or vaccination have a similar structure to MBP (molecular mimicry), which activates an autoimmune T-cell clone.[1] Pathologic findings include perivenous demyelination, infiltration of lymphocytes and macrophages, hyperemia, edema, endothelial swelling, and hemorrhage.[93] CSF shows lymphocytic pleocytosis with mildly increased protein and may appear similar to viral encephalitis.

MR imaging shows ill-defined T2-hyperintense and FLAIR-hyperintense lesions asymmetrically distributed in the white and gray matter (Fig. 22).[1,7,94] ADEM lesions are observed in the supratentorial and infratentorial white matter, brain stem, spinal cord, and also in the thalami and basal ganglia, especially in children. Involvement of the subcortical white matter is nearly a constant finding. The incidence of gadolinium-enhancing lesions on T1-weighted sequences is variable, depending on the stage of inflammation. DWI usually shows hyperintense lesions with increased ADC in the white matter caused by expanded extracellular space with axonal loss, demyelination, and vasogenic edema.[95] However, in the acute stage, ADEM lesions can show decreased ADC, presumably caused by intramyelinic edema.[96] Mortality in the acute phase is around 20%.[1] Corticosteroid therapy has been the standard of care in ADEM. The average time for recovery has varied between 1 and 6 months.

AHLE

AHLE is an acute, rapidly progressive, and frequently fulminant inflammatory hemorrhagic demyelination, considered a hyperacute form of variant of ADEM.[92] This condition was first described as a pathologic entity by Hurst in 1941(Hurst encephalitis).[97] It is usually triggered by upper respiratory tract infections. CSF analysis shows pleocytosis with predominant polymorphonuclear cells, in contrast with lymphocyte predominance in ADEM.[98,99] Pathology shows demyelination, diffuse neutrophil infiltration, necrotizing vasculitis, and perivascular hemorrhage. MR imaging shows large white matter lesions with surrounding edema and hemorrhage (Fig. 23).[100] Involvement of the basal ganglia,

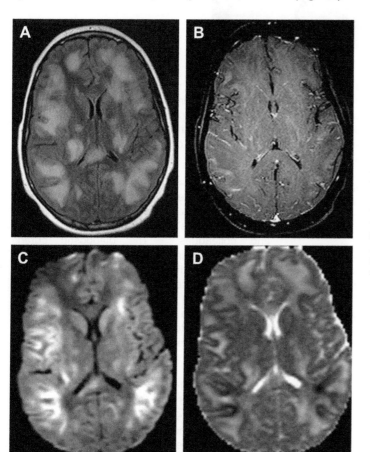

Fig. 22. ADEM. An 11-year-old boy with altered mental status. FLAIR image shows multiple ill-defined, hyperintense lesions in the white matter, corpus callosum and basal ganglia, and thalami (A). Postcontrast T1-weighted image shows mild enhancement in subcortical white matter lesions (B). DWI (C) shows multiple hyperintense lesions with increased ADC and partially decreased ADC in the peripheral area of the lesions (D), which probably represents a combination of cytotoxic and vasogenic edema with demyelination. (*From* Moritani T, Ekholm SE, Westesson PL. Diffusion-weighted MR imaging of the brain. 2nd edition. Berlin, Heidelberg (Germany): Springer-Verlag; 2009. p. 150; with permission.)

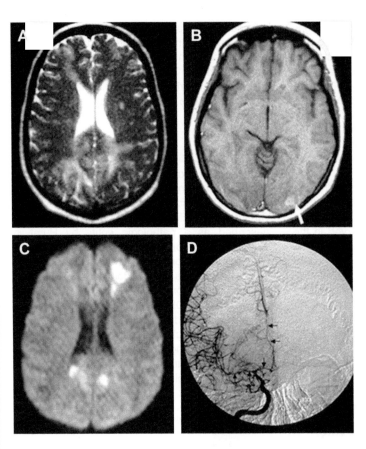

Fig. 23. AHLE. A 48-year-old woman with altered mental status. T2-weighted image shows multiple hyperintense lesions in the anterior and posterior white matter bilaterally (*A*). T1-weighted image reveals a hyperintense area in the left occipital lobe consistent with intracerebral hemorrhage (*arrow*) (*B*). DWI (*C*) shows the lesions as mildly low-intensity or isointense areas with multiple very hyperintense foci consistent with a combination of vasogenic and cytotoxic edema. Digital subtraction angiography shows multiple stenoses in the anterior and middle cerebral arteries (*arrows*) (*D*). This patient died within 1 week. (*From* Moritani T, Ekholm SE, Westesson PL. Diffusion-weighted MR imaging of the brain. 2nd edition. Berlin, Heidelberg (Germany): Springer-Verlag; 2009. p. 151; with permission.)

thalamus, brain stem, cerebellum, and spinal cord may also occur. DWI shows restricted diffusion in the affected areas of the brain, possibly related to acute vasculitis with subsequent vessel occlusion.[92,101] Death from brain edema is common within a week (mortality 70%) and high morbidity ensues in surviving patients.[1] Early and aggressive treatment is necessary using steroids, immunoglobulin, cyclophosphamide, and plasma exchange.

BBE

BBE is a rare life-threatening inflammatory disorder involving the brain stem and cerebellum. It was initially described by Bickerstaff[102] in 1957. The cause is frequently undetermined but is thought to be an immune-mediated process. It often follows a viral infection (HSV, influenza A, enterovirus 71, adenovirus). In some cases, bacteria (*Listeria*, *Mycoplasma*, *Legionella*) and parasites or paraneoplastic syndromes have been implicated. BBE is associated with Miller Fisher and Guillain-Barré syndromes.[1,103,104]

MR imaging shows T2-hyperintense and FLAIR-hyperintense lesions in the brainstem often associated with enhancement.[105] Associated thalamic involvement and white matter changes in the cerebellum and cerebrum can be seen (**Fig. 24**). DWI shows hyperintensity in the lesion with decreased or increased ADC, depending on whether there is cytotoxic or vasogenic edema.

ANE

ANE is an acute encephalopathy with bilateral thalamotegmental involvement in infants and children. It was first described by Mizuguchi and colleagues.[106] The diagnostic criteria include clinical findings of acute encephalopathy following viral disease (most commonly, influenza A, influenza B, HSV, HHV6, mycoplasma) with seizure and deterioration of consciousness. Laboratory data show increased CSF protein without pleocytosis and increase of serum aminotransferase. Although the exact pathogenesis remains unknown, ANE is thought to be associated with a cytokine storm after viral infections. Pathology shows necrosis of neuroglial cells and perivascular hemorrhage with congestion of vessels, acute swelling of oligodendrocytes, and myelin pallor in the thalami. The brainstem tegmentum, periventricular white matter, internal capsule, putamen, and dentate

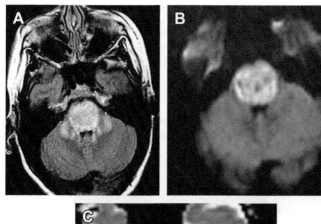

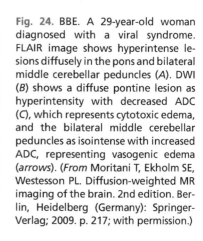

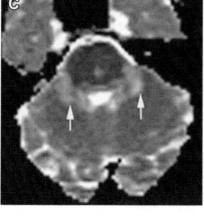

Fig. 24. BBE. A 29-year-old woman diagnosed with a viral syndrome. FLAIR image shows hyperintense lesions diffusely in the pons and bilateral middle cerebellar peduncles (*A*). DWI (*B*) shows a diffuse pontine lesion as hyperintensity with decreased ADC (*C*), which represents cytotoxic edema, and the bilateral middle cerebellar peduncles as isointense with increased ADC, representing vasogenic edema (*arrows*). (*From* Moritani T, Ekholm SE, Westesson PL. Diffusion-weighted MR imaging of the brain. 2nd edition. Berlin, Heidelberg (Germany): Springer-Verlag; 2009. p. 217; with permission.)

nuclei of the cerebellum may be involved. The typical distribution of the lesions and the absence of inflammatory cell infiltration differentiate this entity from ADEM, AHLE, and other immune-mediated disorders.[106,107]

MR imaging shows multiple, bilateral, symmetric, necrotic, hemorrhagic lesions in the thalami, brainstem, putamen, and cerebral white matter (**Fig. 25**).[108] Rim enhancement at the margin of the thalami may occur during the acute phase. DWI shows hyperintensity of the lesions associated with decreased ADC, probably caused by cytotoxic edema of the neuroglial cells.[109] The prognosis is generally poor.

MERS

MERS has been reported not only associated with viral infections (influenza virus, rotavirus, EBV, HHV6, mumps, varicella-zoster, adenovirus, measles) but also with other infections such as *Salmonella*, Legionnaires' disease, and *Escherichia coli* O-157.[10,49,110–116] Although the pathogenesis remains unknown, some type of CNS cytokinopathy is implicated as the cause of

MERS.[10] Reversible splenial lesions have been reported in a wide spectrum of diseases and conditions, including patients with seizures with or without antiepileptic medications, alcoholism and malnutrition, hypoglycemia, osmotic myelinolysis, trauma, medications (5-fluorouracil, metronidazole, intravenous immunoglobulin), systemic lupus erythematosus, and leptomeningeal malignancy.[117–128] The cause of the reversible splenial lesions is presumably related to a combination of a CNS cytokinopathy with excitotoxic mechanisms.[96] Various cytokines activate glial cells (microglia, astrocytes, oligodendrocytes) releasing excitotoxic neurotransmitters such as glutamate that can presumably cause edema of the corpus callosum because the corpus callosum contains a high concentration of glutamate receptors. Complete reversibility of the lesion suggests that the edema represents a purely intramyelinic edema.

Conventional MR imaging shows a nonhemorrhagic, hyperintense lesion on T2-weighted and FLAIR images that is slightly hypointense on T1-weighted images (**Fig. 26**). There is no enhancement after administration of intravenous

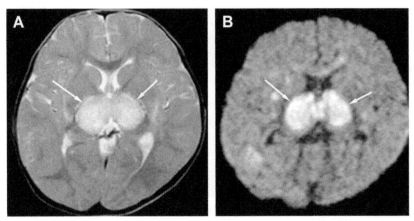

Fig. 25. ANE. A 1-year-old boy with altered mental status and seizures. T2-weighted image shows hyperintensity and swelling in bilateral thalami (*arrows*) (*A*). DWI (*B*) also shows bilateral thalami and right temporo-occipital region (*arrows*) as hyperintensity associated with decreased ADC (not shown). (*From* Moritani T, Ekholm SE, Westesson PL. Diffusion-weighted MR imaging of the brain. 2nd edition. Berlin, Heidelberg (Germany): Springer-Verlag; 2009. p. 320; with permission.)

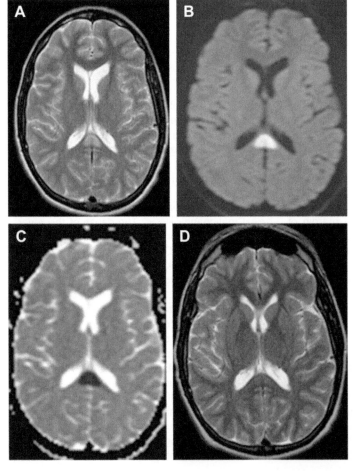

Fig. 26. MERS after upper respiratory infection. A 22-year-old man with fever and headache after upper respiratory infection (no seizures, no special medications). MR imaging shows an oval, splenial, hyperintense lesion on T2-weighted image (*A*) and DWI (*B*) associated with decreased ADC that may represent an intramyelinic edema (*C*). At 2-month follow-up, MR imaging shows complete resolution (*D*).

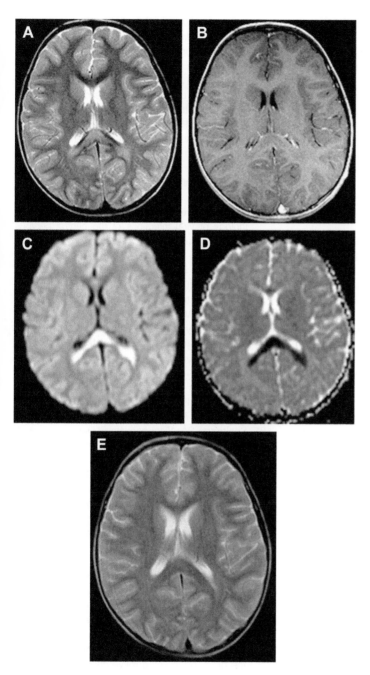

Fig. 27. MERS. A 5-year-old boy with acute encephalopathy after rotavirus gastroenteritis. T2-weighted image shows a hyperintense splenial lesion extending into posterior deep white matter bilaterally and also in the anterior corpus callosum through the callosal body (*A*). Postcontrast T1-weighted image shows no enhancement in the lesion (*B*). DWI (*C*) reveals these lesions as hyperintensity associated with reduced ADC (*D*), which likely represents an intramyelinic edema. These lesions completely resolved at 4-day follow-up MR imaging (*E*).

gadolinium. DWI shows a symmetric round or oval hyperintense lesion associated with decreased ADC in the splenium of the corpus callosum. In general, the diffusion-restricted lesions have been reported to have complete resolution on the follow-up study. It may extend along the callosal fiber laterally or may even extend into the anterior corpus callosum, which can be the spectrum of this type of reversible encephalopathy **(Fig. 27)**.[49,129]

SUMMARY

Imaging findings in virus-related infectious and noninfectious encephalitis/encephalopathy with white matter involvement are described. The differential diagnosis based on the characteristic distribution is discussed. Acute viral encephalitis/encephalopathy is a medical emergency. Prompt introduction of treatment has a significant influence on survival and the extent of permanent brain injury. Differentiation between infectious and noninfectious CNS involvement is paramount because the treatment and outcome are different. Although the confirmation of the diagnosis often requires the detection of specific viral antigens or serologic markers in CSF, neuroimaging (especially MR imaging) provides many clues for the specific diagnosis. Understanding the underlying disorder and pathophysiology is important for the interpretation of the images and therefore the treatment.

REFERENCES

1. Stone MJ, Hawkins CP. A medical overview of encephalitis. Neuropsychol Rehabil 2007;17(4–5): 429–49.

2. Chaudhuri A, Kennedy PG. Diagnosis and treatment of viral encephalitis. Postgrad Med J 2002; 78:575–83.

3. Gupta RK, Soni N, Kumar S, et al. Imaging of central nervous system viral diseases. J Magn Reson Imaging 2012;35:477–91.

4. Solbrig MV, Hasso AN, Jay CA. CNS viruses–diagnostic approach. Neuroimaging Clin N Am 2008; 18(1):1–18.

5. Rumboldt Z. Imaging of topographic viral CNS infections. Neuroimaging Clin N Am 2008;18(1): 85–92.

6. Gupta RK, Jain KK, Kumar S. Imaging of nonspecific (nonherpetic) acute viral infections. Neuroimaging Clin N Am 2008;18(1):41–5.

7. Lo CP, Chen CY. Neuroimaging of viral infections in infants and young children. Neuroimaging Clin N Am 2008;18:119–32.

8. McCarthy M. Newer viral encephalitides. Neurologist 2003;9(4):189–99.

9. Whitley RJ, Gnann JW. Viral encephalitis: familiar infections and emerging pathogens. Lancet 2002; 359(9305):507–13.

10. Tada H, Takanashi J, Barkovich AJ, et al. Clinically mild encephalitis/encephalopathy with a reversible splenial lesion. Neurology 2004;63:1854–8.

11. Steiner I, Budka H, Chaudhuri A, et al. Viral encephalitis: a review of diagnostic methods and guidelines for management. Eur J Neurol 2005; 12(5):331–43.

12. Gottlieb MS, Schroff R, Schanker HM, et al. Pneumocystis carinii pneumonia and mucosal candidiasis in previously healthy homosexual men: evidence of a new acquired cellular immunodeficiency. N Engl J Med 1981;305(24):1425–31.

13. Barré-Sinoussi F, Chermann JC, Rey F, et al. Isolation of a T-lymphotropic retrovirus from a patient at risk for acquired immune deficiency syndrome (AIDS). Science 1983;220(4599):868–71.

14. Yadav A, Collman RG. CNS inflammation and macrophage/microglial biology associated with HIV-1 infection. J Neuroimmune Pharmacol 2009; 4:430–47.

15. Kure K, Llena JF, Lyman WD, et al. Human immunodeficiency virus-1 infection of the nervous system: an autopsy study of 268 adult, pediatric, and fetal brains. Hum Pathol 1991;22(7):700–10.

16. Budka H, Wiley CA, Kleihues P, et al. HIV associated disease of the nervous system: review of nomenclature and proposal for neuropathology-based terminology. Brain Pathol 1991;1(3): 143–52.

17. Shankar SK, Mahadevan A, Kovoor JM. Neuropathology of viral infections of the central nervous system. Neuroimaging Clin N Am 2008;18(1): 19–39.

18. Flowers CH, Mafee MF, Crowell R, et al. Encephalopathy in AIDS patients: evaluation with MR imaging. AJNR Am J Neuroradiol 1990;11:1235–45.

19. Nagel MA, Mahalingam R, Cohrs RJ, et al. Virus vasculopathy and stroke: an under-recognized cause and treatment target. Infect Disord Drug Targets 2010;10:105–11.

20. Connor MD, Lammie GA, Bell JE, et al. Cerebral infarction in adult AIDS patients: observations from the Edinburgh HIV autopsy cohort. Stroke 2000;31:2117–26.

21. Shelburne SA, Visnegarwala F, Darcourt J, et al. Incidence and risk factors for immune reconstitution inflammatory syndrome during highly active antiretroviral therapy. AIDS 2005;19(4): 399–406.

22. Venkataramana A, Pardo CA, McArthur JC, et al. Immune reconstitution inflammatory syndrome in the CNS of HIV-infected patients. Neurology 2006;67(3):383–8.

23. Shelburne SA 3rd, Darcourt J, White AC Jr, et al. The role of immune reconstitution inflammatory syndrome in AIDS-related Cryptococcus neoformans disease in the era of highly active antiretroviral therapy. Clin Infect Dis 2005; 40(7):1049–52.

24. Safriel YI, Haller JO, Lefton DR, et al. Imaging of the brain in the HIV-positive child. Pediatr Radiol 2000;30(11):725–32.

25. Shah SS, Zimmerman RA, Rorke LB, et al. Cerebrovascular complications of HIV in children. AJNR Am J Neuroradiol 1996;17(10):1913–7.

26. Park YD, Belman AL, Kim TS, et al. Stroke in pediatric acquired immunodeficiency syndrome. Ann Neurol 1990;28(3):303–11.

27. Gilden DH, Mahalingam R, Cohrs RJ, et al. Herpesvirus infections of the nervous system. Nat Clin Pract Neurol 2007;3(2):82–94.

28. Goldsmith SM, Whitley RJ. Herpes simplex encephalitis. In: Lambert HP, editor. Infections of the

central nervous system. Philadelphia: BC Decker; 1991. p. 283–99.

29. Whitley RJ. Viral encephalitis. N Engl J Med 1990; 323:242–50.

30. Sämann PG, Schlegel J, Müller G, et al. Serial proton MR spectroscopy and diffusion imaging findings in HIV-related herpes simplex encephalitis. AJNR Am J Neuroradiol 2003;24(10):2015–9.

31. Spuler A, Blaszyk H, Parisi JE, et al. Herpes simplex encephalitis after brain surgery: case report and review of the literature. J Neurol Neurosurg Psychiatry 1999;67(2):239–42.

32. Lakeman FD, Whitley RJ. Diagnosis of herpes simplex encephalitis: application of polymerase chain reaction to cerebrospinal fluid from brain-biopsied patients and correlation with disease. National Institute of Allergy and Infectious Diseases Collaborative Antiviral Study Group. J Infect Dis 1995; 171(4):857–63.

33. Leonard JR, Moran CJ, Cross DT 3rd, et al. MR imaging of herpes simplex type 1 encephalitis in infants and young children: a separate pattern of findings. AJR Am J Roentgenol 2000;174(6): 1651–5.

34. Dhawan A, Kecskes Z, Jyoti R, et al. Early diffusion-weighted magnetic resonance imaging findings in neonatal herpes encephalitis. J Paediatr Child Health 2006;42(12):824–6.

35. Obeid M, Franklin J, Shrestha S, et al. Diffusion-weighted imaging findings on MRI as the sole radiographic findings in a child with proven herpes simplex encephalitis. Pediatr Radiol 2007;37: 1159–62.

36. Küker W, Nägele T, Schmidt F, et al. Diffusion-weighted MRI in herpes simplex encephalitis: a report of three cases. Neuroradiology 2004;46(2): 122–5.

37. Heiner L, Demaerel P. Diffusion-weighted MR imaging findings in a patient with herpes simplex encephalitis. Eur J Radiol 2003;45(3):195–8.

38. McCabe K, Tyler K, Tanabe J. Diffusion-weighted MRI abnormalities as a clue to the diagnosis of herpes simplex encephalitis. Neurology 2003;61(7): 1015–6.

39. Provenzale JM, vanLandingham KE, Lewis DV, et al. Extrahippocampal involvement in human herpesvirus 6 encephalitis depicted at MR imaging. Radiology 2008;249:955–63.

40. Noguchi T, Mihara F, Yoshiura T, et al. MR imaging of human herpesvirus-6 encephalopathy after hematopoietic stem cell transplantation in adults. AJNR Am J Neuroradiol 2006;27:2191–5.

41. Gorniak RJ, Young GS, Wiese DE, et al. MR imaging of human herpesvirus-6-associated encephalitis in 4 patients with anterograde amnesia after allogeneic hematopoietic stem-cell transplantation. AJNR Am J Neuroradiol 2006;27:887–91.

42. Yao K, Honarmand S, Espinosa A, et al. Detection of human herpesvirus-6 in cerebrospinal fluid of patients with encephalitis. Ann Neurol 2009;65(3): 257–67.

43. Gilden D, Cohrs RJ, Mahalingam R, et al. Varicella zoster virus vasculopathies: diverse clinical manifestations, laboratory features, pathogenesis, and treatment. Lancet Neurol 2009;8(8):731–40.

44. Silver B, Nagel MA, Mahalingam R, et al. Varicella zoster virus vasculopathy: a treatable form of rapidly progressive multi-infarct dementia after 2 years' duration. J Neurol Sci 2012;323(1–2):245–7.

45. Barkovich AJ, Lindan CE. Congenital cytomegalovirus infection of the brain: imaging analysis and embryologic considerations. AJNR Am J Neuroradiol 1994;15(4):703–15.

46. Enting R, de Gans J, Reiss P, et al. Ganciclovir/foscarnet for cytomegalovirus meningoencephalitis in AIDS. Lancet 1992;340(8818):559–60.

47. Dunleavy K, Roschewski M, Wilson WH. Lymphomatoid granulomatosis and other Epstein-Barr virus associated lymphoproliferative processes. Curr Hematol Malig Rep 2012;7(3):208–15.

48. Ono J, Shimizu K, Harada K, et al. Characteristic MR features of encephalitis caused by Epstein-Barr virus: a case report. Pediatr Radiol 1998; 28(8):569–70.

49. Hagemann G, Mentzel HJ, Weisser H, et al. Multiple reversible MR signal changes caused by Epstein-Barr virus encephalitis. AJNR Am J Neuroradiol 2006;27(7):1447–9.

50. Forbes KP, Collie DA, Parker A. CNS involvement of virus-associated hemophagocytic syndrome: MR imaging appearance. AJNR Am J Neuroradiol 2000;21:1248–50.

51. Shinoda J, Murase S, Takenaka K, et al. Isolated central nervous system hemophagocytic lymphohistiocytosis: case report. Neurosurgery 2005; 56(1):E187–90.

52. Ozgen B, Karli-Oguz K, Sarikaya B, et al. Diffusion-weighted cranial MR imaging findings in a patient with hemophagocytic syndrome. AJNR Am J Neuroradiol 2006;27(6):1312–4.

53. Chung TW. CNS involvement in hemophagocytic lymphohistiocytosis: CT and MR findings. Korean J Radiol 2007;8(1):78–81.

54. Ishikura R, Ando K, Hirota S, et al. Callosal and diffuse white matter lesions with restricted water diffusion in hemophagocytic syndrome. Magn Reson Med Sci 2010;9(2):91–4.

55. Epstein MA, Barr YM. Cultivation in vitro of human lymphoblasts from Burkitt's malignant lymphoma. Lancet 1964;1(7327):252–3.

56. Castellano-Sanchez AA, Li S, Qian J, et al. Primary central nervous system posttransplant lymphoproliferative disorders. Am J Clin Pathol 2004;121:246–53.

57. Brennan KC, Lowe LH, Yeaney GA. Pediatric central nervous system posttransplant lymphoproliferative disorder. AJNR Am J Neuroradiol 2005; 26(7):1695–7.

58. Tateishi U, Terae S, Ogata A, et al. MR imaging of the brain in lymphomatoid granulomatosis. AJNR Am J Neuroradiol 2001;22:1283–90.

59. Lucantoni C, De Bonis P, Doglietto F, et al. Primary cerebral lymphomatoid granulomatosis: report of four cases and literature review. J Neurooncol 2009;94:235–42.

60. Chang L, Ernst T. MR spectroscopy and diffusion-weighted MR imaging in focal brain lesions in AIDS. Neuroimaging Clin N Am 1997;7: 409–26.

61. Aström KE, Mancall EL, Richardson EP Jr. Progressive multifocal leukoencephalopathy; a hitherto unrecognized complication of chronic lymphatic leukaemia and Hodgkin's disease. Brain 1958; 81(1):93–111.

62. Padget BL, Walker DL, Zu Rhein GM, et al. Cultivation of papova-like virus from human brain with progressive multifocal leucoencephalopathy. Lancet 1971;29:1257–60.

63. Bag AK, Curé JK, Chapman PR, et al. JC virus infection of the brain. AJNR Am J Neuroradiol 2010;31(9):1564–76.

64. Whiteman ML, Post MJ, Berger JR, et al. Progressive multifocal leukoencephalopathy in 47 HIV-seropositive patients: neuroimaging with clinical and pathologic correlation. Radiology 1993; 187(1):233–40.

65. Kharfan-Dabaja MA, Ayala E, Greene J, et al. Two cases of progressive multifocal leukoencephalopathy after allogeneic hematopoietic cell transplantation and a review of the literature. Bone Marrow Transplant 2007;39(2):101–7.

66. Van Assche G, Van Ranst M, Sciot R, et al. Progressive multifocal leukoencephalopathy after natalizumab therapy for Crohn's disease. N Engl J Med 2005;353(4):362–8.

67. Kleinschmidt-DeMasters BK, Tyler KL. Progressive multifocal leukoencephalopathy complicating treatment with natalizumab and interferon beta-1α for multiple sclerosis. N Engl J Med 2005;353(4): 369–74.

68. Tan K, Roda R, Ostrow L, et al. PML-IRIS in patients with HIV infection: clinical manifestations and treatment with steroids. Neurology 2009; 72(17):1458–64.

69. Huang D, Cossoy M, Li M, et al. Inflammatory progressive multifocal leukoencephalopathy in human immunodeficiency virus-negative patients. Ann Neurol 2007;62(1):34–9.

70. Dang X, Koralnik IJ. A granule cell neuron-associated JC virus variant has a unique deletion in the VP1 gene. J Gen Virol 2006;87(Pt 9):2533–7.

71. Blake K, Pillay D, Knowles W, et al. JC virus associated meningoencephalitis in an immunocompetent girl. Arch Dis Child 1992;67(7):956–7.

72. Wüthrich C, Dang X, Westmoreland S, et al. Fulminant JC virus encephalopathy with productive infection of cortical pyramidal neurons. Ann Neurol 2009;65(6):742–8.

73. Marzocchetti A, Di Giambenedetto S, Cingolani A, et al. Reduced rate of diagnostic positive detection of JC virus DNA in cerebrospinal fluid in cases of suspected progressive multifocal leukoencephalopathy in the era of potent antiretroviral therapy. J Clin Microbiol 2005;43(8):4175–7.

74. Thurnher MM, Post MJ, Rieger A, et al. Initial and follow-up MR imaging findings in AIDS-related progressive multifocal leukoencephalopathy treated with highly active antiretroviral therapy. AJNR Am J Neuroradiol 2001;22(5):977–84.

75. Post MJ, Yiannoutsos C, Simpson D, et al. Progressive multifocal leukoencephalopathy in AIDS: are there any MR findings useful to patient management and predictive of patient survival? AIDS Clinical Trials Group, 243 Team. AJNR Am J Neuroradiol 1999; 20(10):1896–906.

76. Buckle C, Castillo M. Use of diffusion-weighted imaging to evaluate the initial response of progressive multifocal leukoencephalopathy to highly active antiretroviral therapy: early experience. AJNR Am J Neuroradiol 2010;31(6):1031–5.

77. Bergui M, Bradac GB, Oguz KK, et al. Progressive multifocal leukoencephalopathy: diffusion-weighted imaging and pathological correlations. Neuroradiology 2004;46(1):22–5.

78. Smithburn KC, Hughes TP, Burke AW, et al. A neurotropic virus isolated from the blood of a native of Uganda. Am J Trop Med Hyg 1940;20:471–92.

79. Nash D, Mostashari F, Fine A, et al. The outbreak of West Nile virus infection in New York City area in 1999. N Engl J Med 2001;344:1807–14.

80. Petropoulou KA, Gordon SM, Prayson RA, et al. West Nile virus meningoencephalitis: MR imaging findings. AJNR Am J Neuroradiol 2005;26:1986–95.

81. Zak IT, Altinok D, Merline JR, et al. West Nile virus infection. AJR Am J Roentgenol 2005;184:957–61.

82. Kraushaar G, Patel R, Stoneham GW. West Nile virus: a case report with flaccid paralysis and cervical spinal cord: MR imaging findings. AJNR Am J Neuroradiol 2005;26:26–9.

83. Ali M, Safriel Y, Sohi J, et al. West Nile virus infection: MR imaging findings in the nervous system. AJNR Am J Neuroradiol 2005;26:289–97.

84. Rosas H, Wippold FJ 2nd. West Nile virus: case report with MR imaging findings. AJNR Am J Neuroradiol 2003;24:1376–8.

85. Lee KY, Cho WH, Kim SH, et al. Acute encephalitis associated with measles: MRI features. Neuroradiology 2003;5(2):100–6.

86. Dawson JR. Cellular inclusions in cerebral lesions of lethargic encephalitis. Am J Pathol 1933;9(1): 7–16.3.

87. Brismar J, Gascon GG, von Steyern KV, et al. Subacute sclerosing panencephalitis: evaluation with CT and MR. AJNR Am J Neuroradiol 1996;17: 761–72.

88. Aydin K, Okur O, Tatli B, et al. Reduced gray matter volume in the frontotemporal cortex of patients with early subacute sclerosing panencephalitis. AJNR Am J Neuroradiol 2009;30(2):271–5.

89. Sener RN. Subacute sclerosing panencephalitis findings at MR imaging, diffusion MR imaging, and proton MR spectroscopy. AJNR Am J Neuroradiol 2004;25(5):892–4.

90. Maschke M, Kastrup O, Forsting M, et al. Update on neuroimaging in infectious central nervous system disease. Curr Opin Neurol 2004;17(4): 475–80.

91. Rumboldt Z, Thurnher MM, Gupta RK. Central nervous system infections. Semin Roentgenol 2007; 42(2):62–91.

92. Tenembaum S, Chitnis T, Ness J, et al, International Pediatric MS Study Group. Acute disseminated encephalomyelitis. Neurology 2007;68:S23–36.

93. Garg RK. Acute disseminated encephalomyelitis. Postgrad Med J 2003;79(927):11–7.

94. Caldemeyer KS, Smith RR, Harris TM, et al. MRI in acute disseminated encephalomyelitis. Neuroradiology 1994;36(3):216–20.

95. Bernarding J, Braun J, Koennecke HC. Diffusion and perfusion-weighted MR imaging in a patient with acute demyelinating encephalomyelitis (ADEM). J Magn Reson Imaging 2002;15:96–100.

96. Moritani T, Smoker WR, Sato Y, et al. Diffusion-weighted imaging of acute excitotoxic brain injury. AJNR Am J Neuroradiol 2005;26:216–28.

97. Hurst EW. Acute hemorrhagic leukoencephalitis previous undefined entity. Med J Aust 1941;2:16.

98. Lee HY, Chang KH, Kim JH, et al. Serial MR imaging findings of acute hemorrhagic leukoencephalitis: a case report. AJNR Am J Neuroradiol 2005; 26(8):1996–9.

99. Kuperan S, Ostrow P, Landi MK, et al. Acute hemorrhagic leukoencephalitis vs ADEM: FLAIR MRI and neuropathology findings. Neurology 2003; 60(4):721–2.

100. Gibbs WN, Kreidie MA, Kim RC, et al. Acute hemorrhagic leukoencephalitis: neuroimaging features and neuropathologic diagnosis. J Comput Assist Tomogr 2005;29(5):689–93.

101. Mader I, Wolff M, Niemann G, et al. Acute haemorrhagic encephalomyelitis (AHEM): MRI findings. Neuropediatrics 2004;35:143–6.

102. Bickerstaff ER. Brain-stem encephalitis; further observations on a grave syndrome with benign prognosis. Br Med J 1957;1(5032):1384–7.

103. Al-Din AN, Anderson M, Bickerstaff ER, et al. Brainstem encephalitis and the syndrome of Miller Fisher: a clinical study. Brain 1982;105(Pt 3):481–95.

104. Odaka M, Yuki N, Yamada M, et al. Bickerstaff's brainstem encephalitis: clinical features of 62 cases and a subgroup associated with Guillain-Barré syndrome. Brain 2003;126(Pt 10):2279–90.

105. Wasenko JJ, Park BJ, Jubelt B, et al. Magnetic resonance imaging of mesenrhombencephalitis. Clin Imaging 2002;26:237–42.

106. Mizuguchi M, Tomonaga M, Fukusato T, et al. Acute necrotizing encephalopathy with widespread edematous lesions of symmetrical distribution. Acta Neuropathol 1989;78:108–11.

107. Mizuguchi M, Hayashi M, Nakano I, et al. Concentric structure of thalamic lesions in acute necrotizing encephalopathy. Neuroradiology 2002;44(6):489–93.

108. Wong AM, Simon EM, Zimmerman RA, et al. Acute necrotizing encephalopathy of childhood: correlation of MR findings and clinical outcome. AJNR Am J Neuroradiol 2006;27(9):1919–23.

109. Albayram S, Bilgi Z, Selcuk H, et al. Diffusion-weighted MR imaging findings of acute necrotizing encephalopathy. AJNR Am J Neuroradiol 2004; 25(5):792–7.

110. Takanashi J, Barkovich AJ, Yamaguchi K, et al. Influenza-associated encephalitis/encephalopathy with a reversible lesion in the splenium of the corpus callosum: a case report and literature review. AJNR Am J Neuroradiol 2004;25(5):798–802.

111. Bulakbasi N, Kocaoglu M, Tayfun C, et al. Transient splenial lesion of the corpus callosum in clinically mild influenza-associated encephalitis/encephalopathy. AJNR Am J Neuroradiol 2006;27:1983–6.

112. Fuchigami T, Goto K, Hasegawa M, et al. 4-year-old girl with clinically mild encephalopathy with a reversible splenial lesion associated with rotavirus infection. J Infect Chemother 2013;19:149–53.

113. Kobata R, Tsukahara H, Nakai A, et al. Transient MR signal changes in the splenium of the corpus callosum in rotavirus encephalopathy: value of diffusion-weighted imaging. J Comput Assist Tomogr 2002;26(5):825–8.

114. Natsume J, Naiki M, Yokotsuka T, et al. Transient splenial lesions in children with "benign convulsions with gastroenteritis". Brain Dev 2007;29(8):519–21.

115. Fukuda S, Kishi K, Yasuda K, et al. Rotavirus-associated encephalopathy with a reversible splenial lesion. Pediatr Neurol 2009;40(2):131–3.

116. Ogura H, Takaoka M, Kishi M, et al. Reversible MR findings of hemolytic uremic syndrome with mild encephalopathy. AJNR Am J Neuroradiol 1998; 19:1114–345.

117. Cohen-Gadol AA, Britton JW, Jack CR Jr, et al. Transient postictal magnetic resonance imaging abnormality of the corpus callosum in a patient

with epilepsy. Case report and review of the litera-ture. J Neurosurg 2002;97:714–7.

118. Kim SS, Chang KH, Kim ST, et al. Focal lesion in the splenium of the corpus callosum in epileptic pa-tients: antiepileptic drug toxicity? AJNR Am J Neu-roradiol 1999;20:125–9.

119. Maeda M, Shiroyama T, Tsukahara H, et al. Transient splenial lesion of the corpus callosum associated with antiepileptic drugs: evaluation by diffusion-weighted MR imaging. Eur Radiol 2003;13(8):1902–6.

120. Cecil KM, Halsted MJ, Schapiro M, et al. Revers-ible MR imaging and MR spectroscopy abnormal-ities in association with metronidazole therapy. J Comput Assist Tomogr 2002;26:948–51.

121. Appenzeller S, Faria A, Marini R, et al. Focal tran-sient lesions of the corpus callosum in systemic lupus erythematosus. Clin Rheumatol 2006;25: 568–71.

122. Polster T, Hoppe M, Ebner A. Transient lesion in the splenium of the corpus callosum: three further cases in epileptic patients and a pathophysiolog-ical hypothesis. J Neurol Neurosurg Psychiatry 2001;70:459–63.

123. Maeda M, Tsukahara H, Terada H, et al. Reversible splenial lesion with restricted diffusion in a wide spectrum of diseases and conditions. J Neuroradiol 2006;33:229–36.

124. Takanashi J, Barkovich AJ, Shiihara T, et al. Widening spectrum of a reversible splenial lesion with transiently reduced diffusion. AJNR Am J Neu-roradiol 2006;27:836–8.

125. da Rocha AJ, Reis F, Gama HP, et al. Focal tran-sient lesion in the splenium of the corpus callosum in three non-epileptic patients. Neuroradiology 2006;48:731–5.

126. Kim JH, Choi JY, Koh SB, et al. Reversible splenial abnormality in hypoglycemic encephalopathy. Neuroradiology 2007;49:217–22.

127. Doherty MJ, Jayadev S, Watson NF, et al. Clinical implications of splenium magnetic resonance im-aging signal changes. Arch Neurol 2005;62:433–7.

128. Conti M, Salis A, Urigo C, et al. Transient focal lesion in the splenium of the corpus callosum: MR imaging with an attempt to clinical-physiopathological expla-nation and review of the literature. Radiol Med 2007; 112:921–35.

129. Sreedharan SE, Chellenton J, Kate MP, et al. Reversible pancallosal signal changes in febrile encephalopathy: report of 2 cases. AJNR Am J Neuroradiol 2011;32(9):E172–4.

Neuroimaging of Vascular Dementia

Sangam Kanekar, MD[a,b,]*, Jeffrey D. Poot, DO[a]

KEYWORDS

- Vascular dementia • MR imaging • Subcortical vascular dementia • CADASIL
- Cerebral amyloid angiopathy (CAA)

KEY POINTS

- Vascular dementia (VaD) is the third leading cause of progressive and irreversible dementia after Alzheimer disease (60%–70%) and dementia with Lewy bodies (10%–25%).
- Because of the high variability of cerebrovascular pathologic conditions and its causative factors, there are no accepted neuropathologic criteria for diagnosing VaD.
- Brain pathology may show diffuse confluent age-related white matter changes, multi-lacunar state (état lacunaire), multiple (territorial) infarcts, strategic cortical-subcortical or watershed lesions, cortical laminar necrosis (granular cortical atrophy), and delayed postischemic demyelination and hippocampal sclerosis.
- Subcortical VaD is the most common subtype of small-vessel VaD and constitutes approximately 50% of VaD cases.

INTRODUCTION

Cerebrovascular disease (CVD) is the second most prominent cause of dementia either alone or in combination with Alzheimer disease (AD).[1] In the past, the term *vascular dementia* (VaD) was used to define the cognitive impairment resulting from CVD and ischemic or hemorrhagic brain injury.[2] The definition and diagnostic criteria of VaD remains unclear and generates much confusion in clinical practice. In addition, it was not able to classify patients who develop a cognitive impairment that does not fulfill the traditional criteria for dementia but that nonetheless has a significant impact on the patients' quality of life and ability to carry out activities of daily living. The term *vascular cognitive impairment* (VCI) was introduced to encompass all of the effects of vascular diseases or lesions on cognition and incorporate the complex interactions between vascular causes, risk factors, and cellular changes within the brain and cognition.[3] VCI refers to "a syndrome with evidence of clinical stroke or subclinical vascular brain injury and cognitive impairment affecting at least one cognitive domain." VCI also includes both pure (CVD alone) and mixed (CVD with other pathologic conditions, such as that of AD). It is important to understand that VCI is not a disease like AD but is rather a syndrome or phenotype that results from CVD, subsequently leading to vascular brain injury that disrupts the brain network for memory and thinking. VaD is a subset of the broader designation VCI.

PREVALENCE

Dementia from all causes has a prevalence of about 8% in individuals aged more than 65 years.[1,3] In the Western literature, VaD is the third leading cause of progressive and irreversible

[a] Department of Radiology, Penn State Milton S. Hershey Medical Center and College of Medicine, The Pennsylvania State University, 500 University Drive, Hershey, PA 17033, USA; [b] Department of Neurology, Penn State Milton S. Hershey Medical Center and College of Medicine, The Pennsylvania State University, 500 University Drive, Hershey, PA 17033, USA

* Corresponding author. Department of Radiology and Neurology, Penn State Milton S. Hershey Medical Center and College of Medicine, The Pennsylvania State University, 500 University Drive, Hershey, PA 17033.

E-mail address: skanekar@hmc.psu.edu

Radiol Clin N Am 52 (2014) 383–401
http://dx.doi.org/10.1016/j.rcl.2013.11.004
0033-8389/14/$ – see front matter © 2014 Elsevier Inc. All rights reserved.

dementia after AD (60%–70%) and dementia with Lewy bodies (10%–25%).[4] The incidence of VaD shows a wide variation in the patient population (age, sex), geographic location, and use of clinical methods. Of all causes of dementia, 13% to 19% are from pure vascular causes, whereas mixed dementia whereby vascular causes are part of the disease is seen in 11% to 43%.[3,4] The proportion of cases caused by VaD decreases with increasing age, but the prevalence of all dementia increases so rapidly with age that the prevalence of VaD also increases, from 0% to 2% in the 60- to 69-year-old age group and up to 16% (3%–6% for men) in individuals aged 80 to 89 years.[5] Globally, VaD seems to be more common in men, especially before 75 years of age. The incidence in women and men aged 85 years and older is around 9.3% and 15.9%, respectively. Epidemiologic studies suggest that the incidence of VaD in Europe accounts for about 15% to 20% of the cases, whereas in Japan it accounts for around 50% of the cases.[1,6] VaD is also more prevalent in populations affected by cerebral small-vessel disease (SVD), such as Asians, African Americans, and Hispanics.

The introduction of the new term *VCI* encompasses all of the effects of vascular disease on cognition leading to a change in the epidemiology. In patients younger than 74 years, VCI may be the single most common cause of cognitive impairment. In those individuals aged 75 to 84 years, cases of pure VCI, VaD, and those with a vascular component in the context of mixed disease outnumber those with pure AD.[7] In a Canadian study, the prevalence of VCI has been estimated at 5% in people older than 65 years.[1,5] The cognitive outcome of patients with VaD may be as severe as in AD, but their morbidity and mortality are usually worse.

DIAGNOSTIC CRITERIA

The concept of CVD leading to cognitive decline and dementia has been recognized since the seventeenth century. In the latter half of the nineteenth century, Kraepelin and colleagues coined the term *atherosclerotic dementia*.[8] In 1974, Vladimir Hachinski and colleagues[9] introduced the term *multi-infarct dementia* (MID). Since then, because of the advances in imaging techniques, our understanding of the disease process has significantly evolved. Unfortunately, because of the high variability of cerebrovascular pathologic conditions and its causative factors, there are no accepted neuropathologic criteria for diagnosing VaD or VCI, as agreed for AD or dementia with Lewy bodies. Unlike AD, vascular lesions are classified based on the morphologic characteristics rather than by their pathogenesis. The criteria from the *Diagnostic and Statistical Manual of Mental Disorders*, (Fourth Edition) (*DSM-IV*) for VaD were proposed by the American Psychiatric Association from a general definition of dementia (**Box 1**).[10] The major limitations for these criteria are the following: They are purely clinical. No neuroimaging findings are incorporated. No criteria are mentioned to establish a causal relationship between dementia and vascular disease. The cross-sectional neuroimaging modalities computed tomography (CT) and magnetic resonance (MR) imaging have significantly improved our understanding of SVD, MID, and VaD. In 1993, the National Institute of Neurologic Disorders and Stroke (NINDS)–Association Internationale pour la Recherche et l'Enseignement en Neurosciences (AIREN) formulated criteria that incorporated the structural neuroimaging as a crucial element for the diagnosis of VaD (**Box 2**).[11] To enhance their clinical implementation, operational definitions for the radiological part of the NINDS-AIREN's criteria were subsequently modified in 2003.[12] To diagnose VaD, the current criteria require the presence of the syndrome of dementia and a pathophysiologic mechanism.

Box 1
DSM-IV criteria for VaD

a. There are multiple cognitive deficits manifested by both memory impairment and one or more of the following cognitive disturbances: aphasia, apraxia, agnosia, or disturbance in executive functioning.

b. The cognitive deficits cause significant impairment in social or occupational activities and represent a significant decline from a previous level of functioning.

c. There are focal neurologic signs and symptoms (eg, exaggeration of deep tendon reflexes, extensor plantar response, pseudobulbar palsy, gait abnormalities, weakness of an extremity) or laboratory evidence indicating CVD (eg, multiple infarcts involving the cortex and the underlying white matter) that are judged to be etiologically related to the disturbance.

d. The deficits do not exclusively occur during the course of a delirium.

From American Psychiatric Association. Diagnostic and Statistical Manual of Mental Disorders. 4th edition. Washington, DC: American Psychiatric Association; 1994. p. 9–36; with permission.

Box 2
Operational definitions for the radiological part of the NINDS-AIREN's criteria (2003)

Topography

Large-vessel stroke

- Large-vessel stroke is an infarction defined as a parenchymal defect in an arterial territory involving the cortical gray matter.
  - ○ ACA: Only bilateral ACA infarcts are sufficient to meet the NINDS-AIREN's criteria.
  - ○ PCA: Infarcts in the PCA territory can be included only when they involve the following regions:
    - ■ Paramedian thalamic infarct
    - ■ Inferior medial temporal lobe lesions
- Association areas: MCA infarcts need to involve the following regions:
  - ○ Parietotemporal lobe (eg, angular gyrus)
  - ○ Temporo-occipital cortex
- Watershed carotid territories (between the MCA and PCA or the MCA and ACA)

SVD

- Multiple basal ganglia and frontal white matter lacunes
- Extensive periventricular white matter lesions (leukoaraiosis)
- Bilateral thalamic lesions

Severity

- Large-vessel disease of the dominant hemisphere
- Bilateral large-vessel hemispheric strokes
- Leukoencephalopathy involving at least 25% of the total white matter

Fulfillment of radiological criteria for probable VaD

- Large-vessel disease: Both the topography and severity criteria should be met (a lesion must be scored in at least 1 subsection of both topography and severity).
- SVD: For white matter lesions, both the topography and severity criteria should be met.

Abbreviations: ACA, anterior cerebral artery; MCA, middle cerebral artery; PCA, posterior cerebral artery.
  Modified from Roman GC, Tatemichi TK, Erkinjuntti T, et al. Vascular dementia: diagnostic criteria for research studies. Report of the NINDS-AIREN International Workshop. Neurology 1993;43:250–60; with permission.

PATHOPHYSIOLOGY

The risk factors for VCI are the same as that for CVD, stroke, and white matter lesions (WMLs), which include arterial hypertension, atrial fibrillation, myocardial infarction, coronary artery disease, diabetes, generalized atherosclerosis, lipid abnormalities, smoking, family history, and specific genetic features.[13] The pathophysiology of VCI and VaD is thought to be multifactorial and is attributed to causes like CVD, infarcts, diffuse WMLS, atrophy, and host factors. These lesions are either diffuse or in the strategic location and cause interruptions of the various white matter

tracts and cortical and subcortical neuronal circuits leading to various cognitive declines and dementia. The neuropathologic changes associated with VaD include multifocal and/or diffuse disease or as a single focal lesion in the strategic location. Brain pathology may show diffuse confluent age-related white matter changes, multi-lacunar state (état lacunaire), multiple (territorial) infarcts, strategic cortical-subcortical or watershed lesions, cortical laminar necrosis (granular cortical atrophy), and delayed postischemic demyelination and hippocampal sclerosis.[14] It is the combinations of these findings seen that often cause the cognitive decline. Histopathology specimens show cellular processes, such as demyelination, axonal damage, diaschisis or retrograde degeneration, and atrophy.

At the neurotransmitter level, cholinergic dysfunction has been well documented in the experimental animal models of ischemic VaD.[15] Deficits in cholinergic markers and cholinergic receptors have also been documented in human cases of VaD. These changes are most pronounced in the basal forebrain nuclei, which are supplied by penetrating arterioles from the middle cerebral artery (MCA), anterior communicating artery, and anterior cerebral artery (ACA). In addition, vascular insults affecting the white matter and basal ganglia can also interrupt the cholinergic projections from the basal forebrain.

NEUROIMAGING

The imaging appearance of VaD can be broadly divided into (1) large-vessel VaD, (2) small-vessel VaD, and (3) microhemorrhage and dementia (Box 3).

LARGE-VESSEL VAD
MID (Poststroke Dementia)

Large-vessel VaD may be either caused by multiple or single cortical or subcortical infarcts or

---

Box 3
Neuroimaging classification of VaD

LARGE-VESSEL VaD

1. Multi-infarct dementia (multiple large complete infarcts involving cortical and subcortical areas)
2. Watershed infarction
3. Strategic single-infarct dementia
4. Hypoperfusion and ischemic encephalopathy

SMALL-VESSEL VaD

1. Subcortical VaD
2. Lacunes
3. Perivascular spaces
4. Silent cerebral infarcts

MICROHEMORRHAGE AND DEMENTIA

CAA, cerebral amyloid angiopathy; CADASIL, cerebral autosomal dominant arteriopathy with subcortical infarcts and leukoencephalopathy; CARASIL, cerebral autosomal recessive arteriopathy with subcortical infarcts and leukoencephalopathy; HERNS, hereditary endotheliopathy retinopathy nephropathy and stroke.

---

caused by a cerebrovascular lesion involving the strategic regions like the hippocampus, paramedian thalamus, and thalamocortical networks.[11] The source of these infarcts may be due to atherosclerosis, vasculitis, or embolic phenomenon. Occlusion of the extracranial arteries, the internal carotid artery, the main intracranial arteries including the MCA, medium-sized arteries in the leptomeninges, and proximal perforating arteries can lead to VaD. The damage can be worse depending on the presence of hypertension and related CVD. The NINDS-AIREN's criteria define probable VaD as a cognitive decline from a previously higher level of functioning in memory and 2 or more cognitive domains, with the decline being severe enough to interfere with activities of daily living.[11] For the diagnosis of the VaD, both clinical criteria and neuroimaging evidence of CVD are required. The clinical criteria may have 2 of the following: (1) onset of dementia within 3 months after a recognized stroke, (2) abrupt deterioration in cognition (days to weeks), and/or (3) stepwise deterioration.[16] Imaging plays a supportive role by identifying the type (hemorrhagic vs nonhemorrhagic) and localizing the anatomic site of the abnormality.

VaD largely depends on the site of the blocked vessel and the affected brain parenchyma. Up to one-third of stroke survivors exhibit dementia within 3 months after their stroke, whereby memory loss may not be the primary symptom. In classic poststroke patients, cortical cognitive deficits, such as agnosia, apraxia, alexia, aphasia, and visuospatial or constructional difficulty, are seen, often without motor deficit.

Cross-sectional imaging with CT and MR along with CT angiography or MR angiography have become the imaging modalities to evaluate patients with VaD.[17] These modalities are very sensitive in confirming the size and location of the symptomatic as well as asymptomatic (silent) strokes. MR is also very helpful in the diagnosis of microbleeds, anoxic/hypoxic brain injury, and identifying the changes of gliosis and encephalomalacia. The parenchymal perfusion status may also be obtained using CT or MR perfusion. Diffusion-weighted imaging (DWI)–apparent diffusion coefficient (ADC) has an established role in the diagnosis of hyperacute infarction. An infarcted area, which has a decrease in Brownian motion, is seen on the DWI sequence as restricted diffusion with low ADC. In the subacute-chronic stage of infarction, imaging is characterized by local brain atrophy, gliosis, cavity formation, and ex vacuo dilatation of the ipsilateral ventricle. Encephalomalacia and gliosis are seen on T2 and fluid-attenuated inversion recovery (FLAIR) images as a loss of parenchymal tissue with hyperintensity in the infarcted and subjacent tissue with prominence of cerebrospinal fluid (CSF) space (**Fig. 1**). Calcification and deposition of blood products (hemosiderin) may be seen on T2 and gradient echo (GRE) sequences. Corticospinal tract degeneration (ie, Wallerian degeneration) is also seen with hemispheric infarction. There is a loss of brain tissue and its corresponding function. Strokes involving the left hemisphere were shown to have a higher incidence of dementia as compared with the right. Also, a strong correlation is seen between dementia and infarctions in the left posterior cerebral artery (PCA) and the ACA and parietal areas (**Fig. 2**).[18] Cortical laminar necrosis, neuronal ischemia accompanied by gliosis, and layered deposition of fat-laden macrophages may be seen in the infarcted region. Gray matter is more vulnerable to hypoxia than white matter. On MR,

laminar necrosis is seen as hyperintensity in the cortex on T1-weighted and FLAIR images (**Fig. 3**). These changes are visible 2 weeks after infarction and are most prominent at 1 to 3 months.

Watershed Infarctions

Watershed infarctions are seen at the junction of the distal fields of the 2 nonanatomizing major cerebral arteries. They are classified into cortical and internal watershed infarcts.[19] Cortical watershed infarcts may occur symmetrically or unilaterally in circular border zones between the deep and superficial branches of ACA, MCA, and PCA. The pathogenesis of watershed infarction remains debatable and is thought to be multifactorial.[19,20] A hemodynamic mechanism, which includes internal carotid stenosis or occlusion, systemic

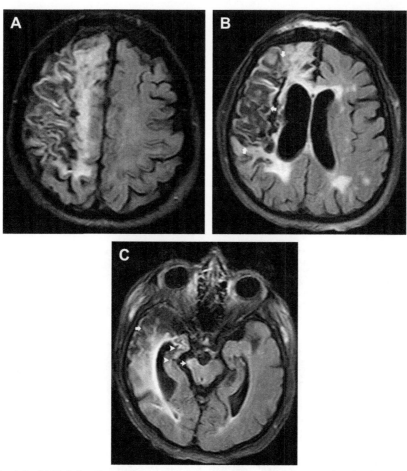

Fig. 1. Chronic right MCA infarction with severe cognitive decline. Axial FLAIR (*A–C*) MR images show large chronic right MCA infarct with encephalomalacia and surrounding hyperintensity caused by gliosis (*fat arrows*). There is ex vacuo dilatation of the ipsilateral lateral ventricle. There is atrophy of the right side of the brainstem with hyperintensity in the cerebral peduncles caused by Wallerian degeneration (*small arrow* in *C*). Also seen is severe atrophy of the head and body of the right hippocampus (*arrowheads* in *C*).

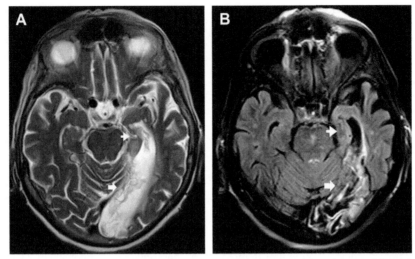

Fig. 2. PCA infarct in a 69-year-old male patient with dementia. Axial T2 (*A*) and FLAIR (*B*) MR images show a large left temporo-occipital chronic infarct with mild ex vacuo dilatation of the temporal horn (*thin arrow*). There is mild volume loss of the head of left hippocampus (*fat arrow*).

hypotension, and embolic events, is a major cause of watershed infarction. They are caused by hypotension with misery perfusion (ie, diminished flow in distal vessels or showers of microemboli).[21] Watershed infarction may affect eloquent areas of the brain and may be associated with a strategic infarct dementia. The superior frontal area, between the distal supply of the ACA and MCA, and the posterior parieto-occipital junction, among ACA, MCA, and PCA, are frequently involved with watershed infarction. Associated hypoxia may also cause alterations in the hippocampal subareas CA-1 and CA-4, the outer half

of the caudate nucleus and putamen, and the anterior and dorsomedial nucleus of the thalamus. Damage to these areas is often associated with the development of cognitive decline and dementia.

MR is very sensitive and specific in the diagnosis of watershed infarction. In acute events, DWI is very sensitive for the diagnosis of both cortical watershed infarct and internal watershed infarct. Classically, cortical watershed infarcts appear as fan- or wedge-shaped hyperintensities extending from the lateral margins of the lateral ventricle toward the cortex, whereas internal watershed

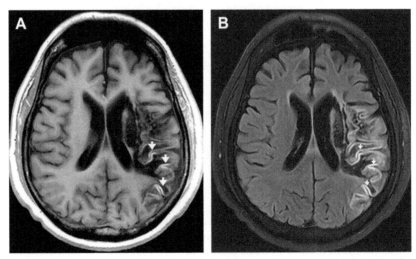

Fig. 3. Laminar necrosis. Axial T1 (*A*) and FLAIR (*B*) MR images reveal large chronic left MCA infarction with encephalomalacia and gliosis. Hyperintensity seen along the gyri on T1 and FLAIR images within the infarcted area is suggestive of cortical laminar necrosis (*arrows*).

infarcts are seen as hyperintensities running parallel to the lateral ventricles, either confluent or focal, and may be unilateral or bilateral (**Fig. 4**).[22]

Strategic Single-Infarct Dementia

Strategic infarct dementia is characterized by focal, ischemic lesions in areas that control or participate in cognition and behavior or higher cortical functions. The strategic *cortical* sites include the hippocampal formation, angular gyrus, and cingulate gyrus, whereas the *subcortical* sites leading to impairment are the thalamus, fornix, basal forebrain, caudate, globus pallidus, and the genu or anterior limb of the internal capsule.[23] The mechanism by which the strategic single infarct leads to dementia is not completely understood, but it is thought to be caused by the interruption of frontal-subcortical circuits.[11,24] The general organization of these circuits includes the frontal lobes, striatum, globus pallidus/substantia nigra, and the thalamus.

Cognitive decline and the clinical symptoms largely depend on the strategic area involved. *Caudate nucleus infarctions* can lead to abulia, restlessness and hyperactivity, language deficits, and poor memory. The cognitive domains mostly affected in caudate infarcts are decreased problem-solving ability, impaired recent and remote memory with preservation of recognition memory, and decreased attention. Ischemic stroke or a subarachnoid hemorrhage from ruptured aneurysms involving the *mesial temporal lobe* and thalamus may cause memory and other

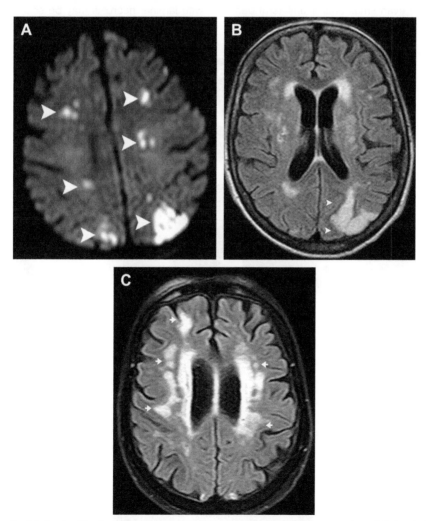

Fig. 4. Watershed infarct with dementia. Axial DWI (*A*) and FLAIR (*B*) MR images show bilateral deep cortical watershed infarctions bilaterally (*arrowheads*). Sixteen months following the event, the patient presented with gradual cognitive decline. Axial FLAIR (*C*) MR image shows mild global atrophy with diffuse white matter changes (*arrows*) suggestive of chronic microangiopathic changes.

cognitive deficits because of the interruption of the cholinergic projections to the cholinergic nuclei in the basal forebrain (Fig. 5). These patients may present with severe anterograde amnesia for verbal or visuospatial material, along with severe apathy, lack of initiative and spontaneity, and executive dysfunction. These patients are also unable to encode and consolidate new verbal material, such as facts, events, short stories, names, and concepts. This inability may be difficult clinically to differentiate from AD. A *thalamic stroke* produces a peculiar form of thalamic VaD (Fig. 6). These patients show a depressed level of consciousness impairments in attention, motivation, initiative, executive functions, and memory, as well as dramatic verbal and motor slowness and apathy. Thalamic lesions may cause thalamic amnesia because of the damage to the mammillothalamic tract; even small and/or unilateral damage to this structure may affect memory,

executive functioning, and attention. *PCA infarcts* may cause damage to the hippocampus, isthmus, entorhinal and perirhinal cortex, and parahippocampal gyrus (see Fig. 2). Therefore, patients may present with amnesia.

Hypoperfusion and Ischemic Encephalopathy

Diseases of the large arteries and the heart can lead to cerebral hypoperfusion and have been associated with the development of dementia after stroke. Hypoperfusion may affect both gray and white matter. Hypoperfusion affecting white matter may lead to leukoaraiosis and incomplete infarction, which comprises zones of partial neuronal or axonal loss with demyelination, increased perivascular spaces, reactive astrocytosis, and gliosis.[25] Damage to the cerebral cortex with laminar necrosis may be seen at the arterial border zones following hypoxia. These zones are

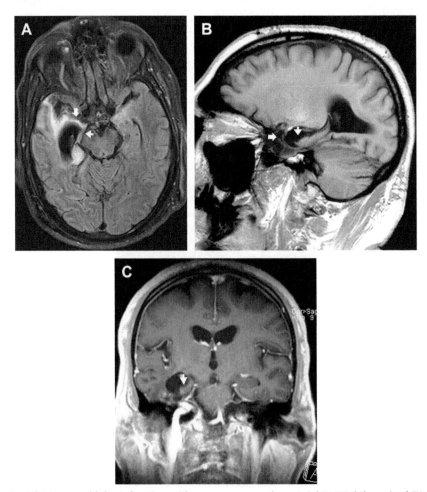

Fig. 5. Chronic right temporal lobe infarction with severe memory loss. Axial FLAIR (*A*), sagittal T1 (*B*), and coronal T1 (*C*) MR images show chronic infarction of the anterior temporal lobe with ex vacuo dilatation of the right temporal horn. There is striking atrophy of the right amygdala (*fat arrow*) and hippocampus (*thin arrow*).

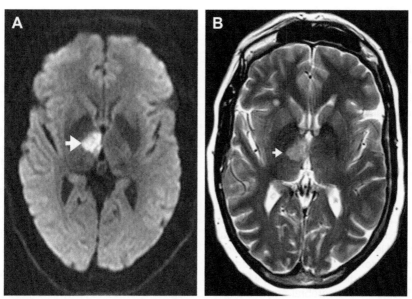

Fig. 6. 61-year-old man with acute-onset amnesia. Axial DWI (*A*) and T2 (*B*) MR images show hyperintensity in the anteromedial aspect of the right thalamus (*arrows*) caused by acute thalamic stroke.

often associated with diffuse white matter damage and cerebellar atrophy. Hypoperfusion can also produce hippocampal neuronal loss or severe white matter changes leading to hippocampal sclerosis. There is severe gliosis and neuronal loss in the CA-1 region of the hippocampus and in the subiculum, which present as cognitive decline often with marked memory impairment.[26] It predominantly co-occurs with AD but is also seen associated with frontotemporal lobar degeneration and tauopathies. Dedicated coronal T2 and FLAIR images show decreased size of the hippocampus with increased signal intensity (Fig. 7). There may be bilateral atrophy of the temporal lobes with associated T2 hyperintensity changes in the white matter. It is often accompanied by multiple small infarcts in other brain regions, leukoencephalopathy, or both.

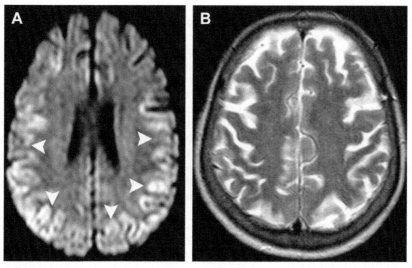

Fig. 7. Dementia caused by global hypoxia in a 54-year-old man. Axial DWI (*A*) MR image shows restricted diffusion in the cerebral cortex bilaterally (*arrowheads*), suggestive of diffuse hypoxic injury from hypotension. Follow-up scan performed 2 years later for early signs of dementia shows advanced cortical atrophy for the age of the patient on T2 MR image (*B*).

SMALL-VESSEL VAD (WMLS AND DEMENTIA)

With the advent of MR imaging, diffuse or focal WMLs are detected with higher sensitivity. These lesions are also related to various cognitive decline and VaD. In neuropathology literature, these lesions are described under various synonyms, such as subcortical arteriosclerotic encephalopathy or Binswanger disease, diffuse white matter disease, WMLs, leukoaraiosis, periventricular arteriosclerotic (leuko) encephalopathy or leukomalacia, subcortical vascular encephalopathy, and periventricular lucency.

Subcortical VaD

As per the NINDS–AIREN's diagnostic criteria, small-vessel VaD is classified into 2 types: *subcortical and cortical* forms.[11,12,27] The subcortical form is a classic subcortical VaD (SCVD), whereas the cortical SVD is mostly cerebral amyloid angiopathy (CAA). SCVD is the most common subtype of small-vessel VaD and constitutes approximately 50% of VaD cases.[27,28] SCVD is attributed to SVD and is characterized by focal and diffuse ischemic WMLs, lacunar infarcts, and incomplete ischemic injury. All of these disease conditions may coexist.

The risk factors for the SCVD are similar to stroke (smoking, hypertension, diabetes, cholesterol). Cerebral arterial small vessels arise superficially from the subarachnoid circulation as terminations of medium-sized arteries and deeply as arterial perforators from larger vessels at the base of the brain. These vessels supply deep white matter structures. Like the rest of the organs of the body, these cerebral blood vessels also undergo progressive age-related changes. These changes include perivascular collagen deposits, also referred to as *microvascular fibrosis* and *basement membrane thickening*, which are mainly seen in the end-arteries and arterioles. The primary target is the small vessels of the white matter; however, the gray matter vessels are affected. Small-vessel changes of fibrohyalinosis in the white matter and angionecrosis and lipohyalinosis in the gray matter, including the basal ganglia and the thalamus. These vessel changes lead to small-vessel cortical microinfarcts, infarcts of the perforating deep small vessels, état criblé (multiple enlarged deep gray matter Virchow–Robin spaces [VRS]), microbleeds, and diffuse WMLs (incomplete infarctions).[27,28] Histopathology shows focal areas of white matter demyelination, loss of axons, gliosis, widening of perivascular spaces, and loss of blood-brain–barrier integrity.[27] These changes are found mainly in the frontal, parietal, and occipital white matter and in the periventricular areas. Various parenchymal changes lead to a loss of neural integrity and retrograde neuronal dysfunction in the basal ganglia and the cerebral cortices, thereby resulting in vascular parkinsonism and dementia.

Because SVD is a slowly progressive disease, it usually lacks the classic stepwise decline more typical of large-vessel VaD. They commonly present with *subcortical cognitive syndrome,* which includes executive dysfunction, mental slowness, decision-making problems, poor organizational ability, adaptability difficulties, attention deficit, and apathy. It is attributed to preferential damage to the prefrontal subcortical circuits.[27] Because the primary anatomic target of SCVD and AD are different, their clinical cognitive and mental profiles are different. Memory loss is relatively mild in SCVD, but the loss of executive control function is prevalent.

Neuroimaging plays an important role in the diagnosis of SCVD, especially because it is a very slow progressive disease. MR can show changes before the symptoms are evident clinically. The most commonly seen abnormality on MR is a *diffuse hyperintensity* on T2-weighted imaging (T2WI) primarily in the centrum semiovale and around the ventricles.[27,29] Confluent areas of hyperintensities (leukoaraiosis) may also be commonly seen in occipital, periventricular, and sometimes frontal white matter (**Fig. 8**). On T1WI, corresponding areas may or may not show hypointensity. If these areas are isointense on T1WI, then they represent areas of incomplete infarctions; if they show hypointensity, then they are caused by complete infarction and represent tissue destruction. Ex vacuo dilatation of the ventricles may be seen because of softening of the periventricular white matter. Newer imaging techniques, such as CT or MR perfusion, may show a diffuse decrease in the cerebral blood flow and volume in the cerebral white matter. For the diagnosis of Binswanger disease, it is important to have associated clinical cognitive decline from a previously higher level of functioning in memory and 2 or more cognitive domains, in addition to the white matter changes on neuroimaging (**Fig. 9**).[30,31] The decline must at least be severe enough to interfere with activities of daily living. Without clinical findings, such findings on imaging are to be termed *leukoaraiosis.*

The second most common imaging finding seen with SVD is focal WMLs. WMLs have been found in 22% of patients younger than 40 years and in 27% to 60% of those patients older than 65 years, whereas in patients with AD and VaD, they are detected by MR in almost 100% of patients.[32] The WMLs can be categorized into *periventricular WMLs* (PVWMLs), which are attached to the

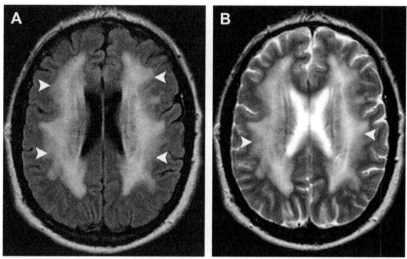

Fig. 8. Diffuse SVD with subcortical dementia. Axial FLAIR (*A*) and T2 (*B*) MR images reveal diffuse confluent hyperintensity in the white matter (*arrowheads*) in a 71-year-old man with hypertension, hyperlipidemia, and long-standing diabetes.

ventricular system, and *deep WMLs* (DWMLs), which are located in subcortical white matter. On T2/FLAIR images, PVWMLs may be further differentiated into smooth, well-defined hyperintensities versus irregular PVWMLs.[32,33] DWMLs and irregular PVWMLs are more likely to be caused by microcystic ischemic lesions. Irregular PVWMLs are more frequently seen with atherosclerosis and thought to be more hemodynamically determined, whereas DWML might be more attributed to SVD, which is seen more commonly with hypertension. Studies have shown that the risk of dementia and the severity of cognitive impairment is preferentially associated with PVWML (**Fig. 10**), whereas mood disorders were more likely seen with DWML (**Fig. 11**).[32,33]

Lacunes

Lacunes are defined as focal complete infarcts of deep small vessels that are less than 2 cm in size.[22] They are the second most common imaging finding seen in patients with subcortical dementia. Lacunae result from SVD with lumen occlusion secondary to arteriolosclerosis caused by microatheroma and lipohyalinosis or embolism, usually in patients with arterial hypertension.[34] These changes are mostly seen in the deep perforators, such as lenticulostriate, thalamoperforating, and long medullary arterioles. Therefore, lacunae are mostly seen in the basal ganglia, the upper two-thirds of the putamen, the internal capsule, the thalamus, the paramedian and lateral regions of the brain stem, the corona radiata, and the centrum semiovale. These regions play an important role in

several aspects of cognition. On histopathology, lacunes are often scattered within the areas of pallor in the white matter. They show cavitary and noncavitary infarctions or areas of vacuolation, with a loss or pallor of myelin, loss of axons and oligodendroglia, and areas of reactive astrocytosis, with or without macrophage reaction.

MR imaging is more sensitive than CT for the diagnosis of acute and chronic lacunar infarctions. Signal intensity of a lacunar infarct largely depends on the stage of the infarct. Acute lacunes show a small area of restricted diffusion with corresponding low ADC signal changes. In the chronic stages, these lesions are seen as round, oval, or slitlike, small cavitated infarcts ranging from a few millimeters to 1.5 cm. These lesions are hyperintense on T2 and FLAIR images and remain hypointense on T1WI (**Fig. 12**). In very late stages, lacunes may be hypointense on FLAIR with an irregular rim of hyperintensity around. A common differential diagnosis includes VRS, which follow CSF signal on all MR imaging sequences. In practice, the 2 forms of subcortical ischemic VaD, lacunae and deep WMLs, are often seen together, presumably because of their common origin.

Perivascular Spaces

Perivascular spaces (PVS) or VRS represent subpial interstitial spaces surrounding the penetrating arteries and arterioles.[35] They are seen most commonly along the path of lenticulostriate arteries entering the basal ganglia or along the perforating medullary arteries entering the cortical gray matter. Prominent VRS may occur in all age

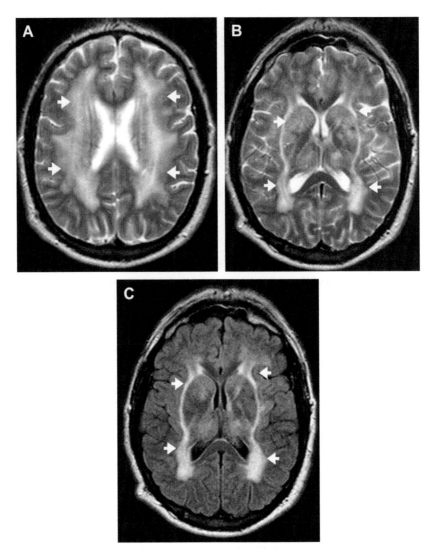

Fig. 9. Binswanger disease in a 67-year-old male patient with cognitive decline. Axial T2 (*A, B*) and FLAIR (*C*) MR images show extensive symmetric hyperintensity in the white matter sparing the U fibers (*arrows*). Increased signal intensity is also noted in the deep gray matter nuclei bilaterally.

groups and are regarded as incidental findings without much clinical significance. However, when they are prominent in elderly patients, they indicate the shrinkage of the surrounding white matter. On histopathology, there is no evidence of necrosis, macrophages, or tissue debris in the VRS. Dilated PVS may contain an insignificant and dispersed population of lipid-rich or iron pigment-laden macrophages. Dilatation of the VRS is common in disorders associated with microvascular diseases, and they are as important as periventricular hyperintensity in the scoring of cognitive deficiency. Multiple enlarged VRS in the basal ganglia is called *état criblé* and may present clinically, either with movement disorders or cognitive decline (**Fig. 13**).[36]

On MR, the PVS appears oval, with a well-defined, smooth margin that is isointense to CSF on all pulse sequences and demonstrates no enhancement after contrast administration. They are usually bilateral but may be unilateral and are localized at the level of anterior commissure, basal ganglia, cerebral convexity, midbrain, or inferior putamen. The most common differential diagnosis is lacunar infarcts, which are hyperintense on FLAIR and proton-density images.

Silent Cerebral Infarcts

Infarcts are defined as silent if they lack strokelike symptoms. Although they are termed *silent strokes*, they do present as subtle deficits in

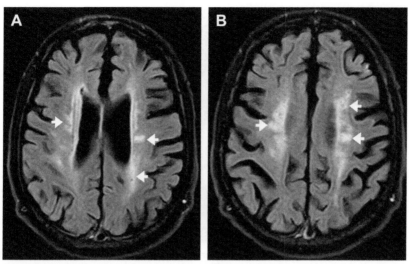

Fig. 10. Periventricular white matter lesions in a female patient with mild cognitive decline. Axial FLAIR (*A, B*) MR images show multiple focal hyperintensities in the periventricular white matter (*arrows*). Most of these lesions are seen abutting the lateral margin of the lateral ventricle.

physical and cognitive function that commonly go unnoticed. Moreover, the presence of silent infarcts more than doubles the risk of subsequent stroke and dementia. The relationship between silent brain infarcts and the risk of dementia and cognitive decline in the general population has been well established following the Rotterdam Scan study.[37] The study showed that the presence of silent brain infarcts more than doubles the risk of dementia, including AD. Silent brain infarcts were also shown to be the risk factor for mild cognitive impairment in the Cardiovascular Health Study. Silent brain infarcts are common among the general population. They are far more common than strokes, both with respect to prevalence and incidence. The overall prevalence of silent infarct ranges from 8% to 28% and increases with age.[38] Their risk factors are similar to infarction, with hypertension being, by far, the strongest modifiable risk factor.

The cumulative effect of this silent infarct can give rise to deficits in cognitive function. The symptoms totally depend on the area and the white matter connections disrupted, with memory performance being most affected by silent thalamic lesions. WMLs and cortical microinfarcts

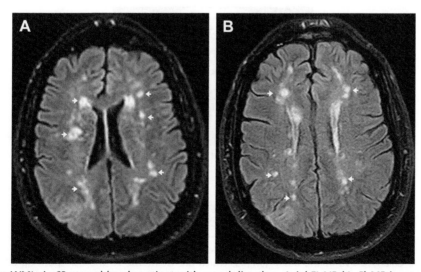

Fig. 11. Deep WMLs in 63-year-old male patient with mood disorders. Axial FLAIR (*A, B*) MR images show multifocal, rounded hyperintensities in the deep white matter bilaterally (*arrows*).

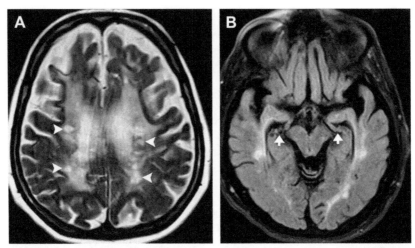

Fig. 12. SVD with lacunes. Axial T2 (*A*) and FLAIR (*B*) MR images show diffuse confluent hyperintensity in the white matter with multiple tiny lacunes (*arrowheads* in *A*). There is atrophy of the hippocampus bilaterally (*arrows* in *B*).

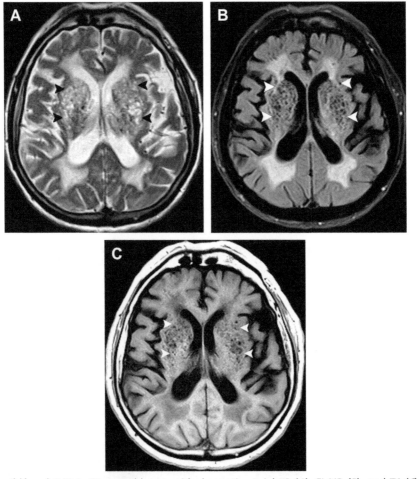

Fig. 13. État criblé and SVD in 71-year-old man with dementia. Axial T2 (*A*), FLAIR (*B*), and T1 (*C*) MR images reveal multiple enlarged PVS in the basal ganglia, which are isointense to the CSF space on all 3 sequences (*arrowheads*). There is generalized prominence of convexity sulci, ventricular system, and diffuse periventricular white matter hyperintensity caused by ischemic SVD.

from the silent infarctions results in disruption and degradation of white matter pathways connecting the cortical (particularly frontal) and subcortical structures.[39] It is also presumed that the vascular lesions somehow also increase the development of plaques and tangles.

MICROHEMORRHAGE AND DEMENTIA

Primary, large, intracerebral hemorrhage is a rare cause of dementia. A primary bleed can cause cognitive decline only if they are in a strategic location, such as basal ganglia and thalamus. With the advent of susceptibility-weighted imaging techniques, MR is capable of detecting millimeter-sized paramagnetic blood products including hemosiderin stored in macrophages from the leakage of small blood vessels in the basal ganglia or subcortical white matter. Microbleeds are defined as small, rounded, hypointense foci on T2* or susceptibility-weighted images not attributable to vessels, calcification, or other pathologic conditions like cavernomas. Microbleeds caused by sporadic SVD are often central in distribution involving the basal ganglia, whereas their distribution is mostly cortical-subcortical (lobar) in specific disorders, such as CAA.[40]

CAA

CAA has been defined as an amyloid deposition in the cerebral vessels sufficient to cause vascular dysfunction, mainly microhemorrhages.[41,42] CAA may be either hereditary or sporadic. Sporadic CAA is a common cerebrovascular pathology of the elderly and is caused by the deposition of β-amyloid in the media and adventitia of small- to medium-sized cerebral arteries.[41,42] Age is the strongest risk factor for sporadic occurrence of CAA. The prevalence of CAA on autopsy is around 2% at 50 years of age and increases to 74% to 100% in patients older than 90 years.[43] In sporadic CAA, the apolipoprotein E e2 and e4 alleles are risk factors: the latter leads to a higher propensity for β-amyloid 40 to be deposited in vessel walls.[41,42,44] Histopathologically, degenerative vascular changes are mainly seen affecting the capillaries, arterioles, and small- and medium-sized arteries of the cerebral cortex, overlying leptomeninges, and cerebellum. White and deep gray matter vessels are relatively spared. Changes in the vessel include amyloid deposition, fibrous thickening of the vessel wall, fibrinoid necrosis, and leakage of blood through the degenerated vessel wall.

There are also hereditary forms of amyloidosis, the most widely studied is the APP gene on chromosome 21 having specific point mutations.[45] The age of onset of hereditary CAA is almost 3 decades earlier (30–60 years) to the sporadic aging-related CAA (60–80 years).[45,46] In all of these APP-related CAAs, meningocortical arteries are affected by β-amyloid deposits, leading to aneurysmal dilatation or thinning of the vessel wall and to fibrinoid necrosis. Vessels in the deep hemispheric structures and brainstem are relatively spared.

In both types of CAA, patients may present with focal neurologic signs, including spasticity, ataxia, facial paralysis, occasional seizures, and cognitive impairment often leading to dementia. It is mostly the subcortical type of dementia. Stroke, a common feature of sporadic CAA, is slightly less common in the hereditary type of CAA. Rapid decline of cognitive functions is thought to be caused by diffuse white matter changes. Neuroimaging, especially MR with susceptibility-weighted images, plays a vital role in the diagnosis of the CAA. On T2WI, white matter shows diffuse hyperintensities with lacunes caused by ischemia. One of the main findings is the presence of multiple microhemorrhages at the corticomedullary junctions on GRE or susceptibility weighted imaging (SWI) images (Fig. 14). There may be superficial siderosis caused by cortical bleeds. Patients may also show large acute or subacute lobar bleeds on CT or MR.

Cerebral Autosomal Dominant Arteriopathy With Subcortical Infarcts and Leukoencephalopathy

Cerebral autosomal dominant arteriopathy with subcortical infarcts and leukoencephalopathy (CADASIL) is an autosomal dominant arteriopathy with complete penetrance.[43] The estimated prevalence in Western countries is around 5 cases in 100,000.[47] Clinical symptoms may be seen as early as 10 years of age. Migraines, usually with auras, are the most common symptom. Other clinical features include transient ischemic attacks, recurrent strokes, depression, ataxia, cognitive decline, and dementia. CADASIL is caused by single missense mutations or exon deletions in the Notch3 gene on chromosome 19.[48] The gene encodes a type 1 transmembrane protein (Notch3), which is essential during development and for regulating cellular differentiation. A definitive diagnosis requires skin biopsy and genetic testing. Pathologically, the vessels show severe arteriopathy caused by deposition of the granular osmophilic material in the media of small vessels (diameter 100–400 μm).[49] A loss of vascular smooth muscle cells in the brain leads to wall thickening and fibrosis in small- and

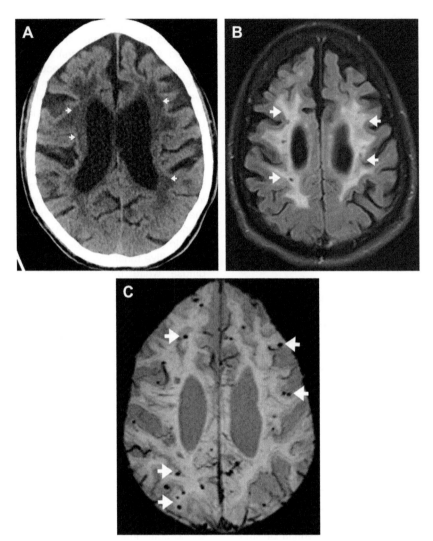

Fig. 14. Cerebral amyloid angiopathy. Axial CT (*A*) image shows generalized prominence of convexity sulci, dilatation of ventricular system, and diffuse hypodensity in the white matter (*arrows*). Axial FLAIR (*B*) MR image shows global cerebral atrophy with diffuse white matter hyperintensity (*arrows*) caused by ischemic SVD. Axial SWI (*C*) MR image shows multiple hypointensities in the cortical and subcortical region (*arrows*), suggestive of microhemorrhages.

medium-sized penetrating arteries. The wall thickening and fibrosis leads to a reduction in both cerebral blood flow and blood volume in the affected white matter with effects on the hemodynamic reserve by decreasing the vasodilatory response. The affected vessels progress to obliteration and/or thrombosis, leading to multiple subcortical infarcts predominantly involving the fronto-temporal white matter and lacunar infarcts, mainly in the basal ganglia.

An MR may show 2 main abnormalities in CADASIL: first, 0.5- to 2.0-cm linear or punctate sharply defined, lacunar infarcts in the periventricular deep white matter, subcortical white matter, external capsule, brainstem, basal ganglia, and

thalamus and, second, large, confluent white matter changes predominately in the subcortical regions of the anterior temporal and frontal lobes with involvement of the subcortical U fibers. These changes are often symmetric (**Fig. 15**). Ribbonlike hyperintensities may also be seen in the external capsule, which are characteristic for CADASIL. Temporal white matter and paramedian superior frontal white matter regions and arcuate fiber involvement is the major finding differentiating CADASIL from Binswanger disease. An MR may also show areas of low signal intensity within the deep gray matter nuclei on T2 and GRE images thought to be caused by increased iron deposition, possibly resulting from disturbed axonal iron transport.

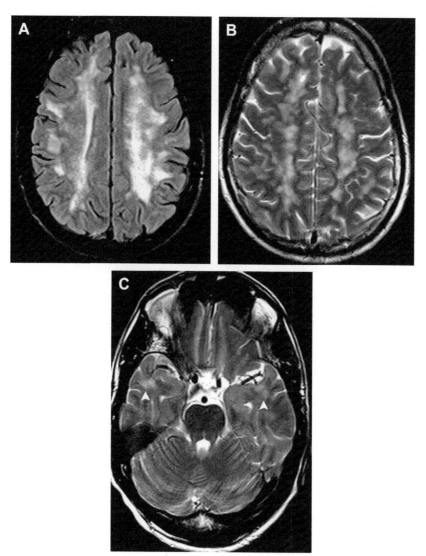

Fig. 15. CADASIL. A 43-year-old male patient with mild cognitive decline. Axial FLAIR (*A*), T2 (*B, C*) MR images reveal extensive white matter abnormalities with characteristic symmetric involvement of the anterior aspect of the temporal lobes (*arrowheads*).

SUMMARY

As people live longer, there is a corresponding increase in neurodegenerative disorders and dementia. More than 24.3 million people are currently estimated to have dementia, and 4.6 million new cases are diagnosed each year. It is predicted that worldwide, a new case of dementia is diagnosed every 7 seconds. When atrophy is seen on imaging in adult patients, it does not necessarily represent AD. Many cases of dementia or cognitive decline could be caused by reversible or preventable disease, such as VaD. This article familiarizes the physician with various types of vascular lesions leading to dementia and cognitive decline and their imaging appearances. Neuroimaging plays an important role in identifying vascular lesions of the brain very early, even before the clinical manifestation of the cognitive decline symptoms and, thus, can help to prevent or delay the symptoms related to the various vascular pathologic conditions.

REFERENCES

1. Rockwood K, Wenzel C, Hachinski V, et al. Prevalence and outcomes of vascular cognitive impairment. Neurology 2000;54:447–51.
2. Erkinjuntti T, Rockwood K. Vascular dementia. Semin Clin Neuropsychiatry 2003;8:37–45.

3. O'Brien JT, Erkinjuntti T, Reisberg B, et al. Vascular cognitive impairment. Lancet Neurology 2003;2:89–98.

4. Ganguli M. Epidemiology of dementia. In: Abou-Saleh MT, Katona C, Kumar A, editors. Principles and practice of geriatric psychiatry. 3rd edition. Hoboken (NJ): Wiley; 2011. Chapter 38.

5. Bowler JV. Vascular cognitive impairment. J Neurol Neurosurg Psychiatry 2005;76(Suppl V):v35–44.

6. Lobo A, Launer LJ, Fratiglioni L, et al. Prevalence of dementia and major subtypes in Europe: a collaborative study of population-based cohorts. Neurologic Diseases in the Elderly Research Group. Neurology 2000;54:S4–9.

7. Hebert R, Brayne C. Epidemiology of vascular dementia. Neuroepidemiology 1995;14:240–57.

8. Kraepelin E. Das senile und präsenile Irresein. In: Psychiatrie: Ein Lehrbuch für Studierende und Ärzte. Leipzig (Germany): Johann Ambrosius Barth; 1910. p. 533–632.

9. Hachinski VC, Lassen NA, Marshall J. Multi infarct dementia. A cause of mental deterioration in the elderly. Lancet 1974;2:207–10.

10. DSM-IV criteria American Psychiatric Association. Diagnostic and statistical manual of mental disorders. 4th edition. Washington, DC: American Psychiatric Association; 1994.

11. Roman GC, Tatemichi TK, Erkinjuntti T, et al. Vascular dementia: diagnostic criteria for research studies. Report of the NINDS-AIREN International Workshop. Neurology 1993;43:250–60.

12. van Straaten EC, Scheltens P, Knol DL, et al. Operational definitions for the NINDS-AIREN criteria for vascular dementia: an interobserver study. Stroke 2003;34:1907–12.

13. Gorelick PB, Brody J, Cohen D, et al. Risk factors for dementia associated with multiple cerebral infarcts. A case-control analysis in predominantly African-American hospital-based patients. Arch Neurol 1993;50:714–20.

14. Pasquier F, Henon H, Leys D. Risk factors and mechanisms of post-stroke dementia. Rev Neurol (Paris) 1999;155:749–53.

15. Swartz RH, Sahlas DJ, Black SE. Strategic involvement of cholinergic pathways and executive dysfunction: does location of white matter signal hyperintensities matter? J Stroke Cerebrovasc Dis 2003;12:29–36.

16. Erkinjuntti T. Diagnosis and management of vascular cognitive impairment and dementia. J Neural Transm Suppl 2002;(63):91–109.

17. Guermazi A, Miaux Y, Rovira-Cañellas A, et al. Neuroradiological findings in vascular dementia. Neuroradiology 2007;49:1–22.

18. Pohjasvaara T, Mantyla R, Salonen O, et al. How complex interactions of ischemic brain infarcts, white matter lesions, and atrophy relate to post-stroke dementia. Arch Neurol 2000;57:1295–300.

19. Momjian-Mayor I, Baron JC. The pathophysiology of watershed infarction in internal carotid artery: review of cerebral perfusion studies. Stroke 2005; 36:567–77.

20. Bladin CF, Chambers BR. Frequency and pathogenesis of hemodynamic stroke. Stroke 1994;25: 2179–82.

21. Baron JC, Bousser MG, Rey A, et al. Reversal of focal "misery perfusion syndrome" by extra-intracranial arterial bypass in hemodynamic cerebral ischemia: a case study with 150 positron emission tomography. Stroke 1981;12:454–9.

22. Marks MP. Cerebral ischemia and infarction. In: Atlas SW, editor. Magnetic resonance imaging of the brain and spine, vol. 1, 4th edition. Philadelphia: Williams & Wilkins; 2009. p. 772–825.

23. Ferro JM. Hyperacute cognitive stroke syndromes. J Neurol 2001;248:841–9.

24. Desmond DW. Vascular dementia: a construct in evolution. Cerebrovasc Brain Metab Res 1996;8: 296–325.

25. Jellinger KA. The enigma of vascular cognitive disorder and vascular dementia. Acta Neuropathol 2007; 113:349–88.

26. Attems J, Jellinger KA. Hippocampal sclerosis in Alzheimer disease and other dementias. Neurology 2006;66:775.

27. Tomimoto H. Subcortical vascular dementia. Neuroscience Research 2011;71:193–9.

28. Yoshitake T, Kiyohara Y, Kato I, et al. Incidence and risk factors of vascular dementia and Alzheimer's disease in a defined elderly Japanese population: the Hisayama Study. Neurology 1995;45:1161–8.

29. Salonen O, Autti T, Raininko R, et al. MRI of the brain in neurologically healthy middle-aged and elderly individuals. Neuroradiology 1997;39:537–45.

30. Bennett DA, Gilley DW, Wilson RS, et al. Clinical diagnosis of Binswanger's disease. J Neurol Neurosurg Psychiatry 1990;53:961–5.

31. Roman GC. New insight into Binswanger disease. Arch Neurol 1999;56:1061–2.

32. Vernooij MW, Smits M. Structural neuroimaging in aging and Alzheimer's disease. Neuroimaging Clin N Am 2012;22(1):33–55.

33. Galluzzi S, Lanni C, Pantoni L, et al. White matter lesions in the elderly: pathophysiological hypothesis on the effect on brain plasticity and reserve. J Neurol Sci 2008;273(1–2):3–9.

34. Ay H, Oliveira-Filho J, Buonanno F, et al. Diffusion-weighted imaging identifies a subset of lacunar infarction associated with embolic source. Stroke 1999;30:2644–50.

35. Vital C, Julien J. Expanding lacunae causing triventricular hydrocephalus. J Neurosurg 2000;93:155–6.

36. Adachi M, Hosoya T, Haku T, et al. Dilated Virchow-Robin spaces: MRI pathological study. Neuroradiology 1998;40:27–31.

37. Vermeer SE, Prins ND, Den Heijer T, et al. Silent brain infarcts and the risk of dementia and cognitive decline. N Engl J Med 2003;348(13):1215–22.

38. Boon A, Lodder J, Heuts-van Raak L, et al. Silent brain infarcts in 755 consecutive patients with a first-ever supratentorial ischemic stroke. Relationship with index-stroke subtype, vascular risk factors, and mortality. Stroke 1994;25:2384–90.

39. Fein G, Di Sclafani V, Tanabe J, et al. Hippocampal and cortical atrophy predict dementia in subcortical ischemic vascular disease. Neurology 2000;55: 1626–35.

40. Revesz T, Ghiso J, Lashley T, et al. Cerebral amyloid angiopathies: a pathologic, biochemical, and genetic view. J Neuropathol Exp Neurol 2003;62:885–98.

41. Weller RO, Preston SD. The spectrum of vascular disease in dementia. From ischaemia to amyloid angiopathy. Adv Exp Med Biol 2001;487:111–22.

42. Good CD, Ng VW, Clifton A, et al. Amyloid angiopathy causing widespread miliary haemorrhages within the brain evident on MRI. Neuroradiology 1998;40:308–11.

43. Dichgans M, Mayer M, Uttner DP, et al. The phenotypic spectrum of CADASIL: clinical findings in 102 cases. Ann Neurol 1998;44:731–9.

44. Attems J. Sporadic cerebral amyloid angiopathy: pathology, clinical implications, and possible pathomechanisms. Acta Neuropathol (Berl) 2005;110: 345–59.

45. Wattendorff AR, Frangione B, Luyendijk W, et al. Hereditary cerebral haemorrhage with amyloidosis, Dutch type (HCHWA-D): clinicopathological studies. J Neurol Neurosurg Psychiatry 1995;58:699–705.

46. Zhang-Nunes SX, Maat-Schieman ML, van Duinen SG, et al. The cerebral beta-amyloid angiopathies: hereditary and sporadic. Brain Pathol 2006;16:30–9.

47. Kalimo H, Ruchoux MM, Viitanen M, et al. CADASIL: a common form of hereditary arteriopathy causing brain infarcts and dementia. Brain Pathol 2002;12: 350–9.

48. Joutel A, Favrole P, Labauge P, et al. Skin biopsy immunostaining with a NOTCH3 monoclonal antibody for CADASIL diagnosis. Lancet 2001;358: 2049–51.

49. Mayer M, Straube A, Bruening R, et al. Muscle and skin biopsies are a sensitive diagnostic tool in the diagnosis of CADASIL. J Neurol 1999;246: 526–32.

Metabolic White Matter Diseases and the Utility of MR Spectroscopy

Macey D. Bray, DO[a],*, Mark E. Mullins, MD, PhD[b]

KEYWORDS

- Brain tumor • Demyelination • Inborn errors of metabolism • Leukodystrophy
- Mitochondrial disorders • MR Spectroscopy (MRS) • Radiation therapy • Voxel

KEY POINTS

- Magnetic resonance spectroscopy (MRS) can be useful as an adjuvant diagnostic tool to traditional MR imaging of the brain.
- MRS can provide both quantitative and qualitative information about white matter pathologic abnormality.
- It is important to interpret MRS in conjunction with other clinical factors including but not limited to additional diagnostic neuroimaging, history and physical examination findings, and genetics.

INTRODUCTION

The diagnosis of white matter disease poses a special challenge to the radiologist for many reasons. First, outside of specialized referral centers, many of these diseases affect the pediatric population, are rare, and may only be encountered a handful of times in clinical practice. Second, there is much overlap in distribution of disease and imaging characteristics, many of which are nonspecific. Pattern recognition may be less useful if involvement is diffuse. Third, the spectrum of etiologies is broad, ranging from tumors and demyelinating disease to toxic/ischemic injury and inborn errors of metabolism. Finally, morphologic changes in the brain may either be nonspecific or not be seen. In addition to other advanced imaging techniques that focus more on anatomy and physiology, magnetic resonance spectroscopy (MRS) can provide complementary information based on physiologic and chemical properties of abnormal white matter. To date, there is a wide range of clinical applications for MRS. Some examples include demyelinating disease, epilepsy, infections, metabolic disorders, neurodegenerative diseases, stroke, and tumors.[1–7] This article focuses on the utility of MRS as a complementary technique to traditional and other advanced MR imaging techniques to further characterize disease processes that predominantly or entirely affect the white matter.

In a patient with an abnormal appearance of the white matter on conventional T2-weighted and fluid attenuated inversion recovery (FLAIR) sequences, MRS can provide information that differs from other advanced imaging techniques. Both MR and computed tomographic perfusion have been used to evaluate hemodynamic parameters in the brain including cerebral blood flow, cerebral blood volume, and mean transit time. Dynamic contrast-enhanced MR perfusion is performed with a gadolinium-based contrast agent that is currently an "off-label" use in accordance with the US Food and Drug Administration. Positron emission tomography–computed tomography has been

Financial Disclosures: None.

[a] Department of Radiology, University of New Mexico, MSC10 5530, 1 University of New Mexico, Albuquerque, NM 87131, USA; [b] Department of Radiology and Imaging Sciences, Emory University, 1364 Clifton Road Northeast, Room D125A, Atlanta, GA 30345, USA

* Corresponding author.

E-mail address: mbray@atsu.edu

Radiol Clin N Am 52 (2014) 403–411
http://dx.doi.org/10.1016/j.rcl.2013.11.012
0033-8389/14/$ – see front matter © 2014 Elsevier Inc. All rights reserved.

used to show areas of FDG uptake in the brain based on glucose metabolism.[8] Diffusion tensor imaging is a method that can assess damage to the microstructure of the brain and may be useful to assess for axonal injury.[9] MRS differs from the above techniques by looking at brain metabolites that may be elevated, decreased, or absent in some diseases. Possible indications for MRS for use as an adjunct to traditional MR imaging in the setting of white matter disease include but are not limited to distinguishing recurrent predominant high-grade brain tumor from predominant radiation necrosis,[9] differentiating low-grade from high-grade brain tumors,[10] and evaluation of rare inherited inborn errors of metabolism affecting the central nervous system.[3,11] White matter diseases can have either a specific or a nonspecific appearance on standard T2-weighted sequences. These patterns can be focal or diffuse, confluent or discontinuous, and unifocal or multifocal. MRS can be a helpful tool to analyze the biochemical components of the areas of signal change.

Metabolic white matter diseases fall into broad categories presenting a particular challenge to the referring clinician and radiologist alike due to the wide range of MR imaging appearances as well as overlapping clinical and imaging findings of many of these processes. Several factors can be used to help distinguish many of these diseases, including the age of the patient, laboratory and genetic analysis, and especially imaging. Traditionally, diagnostic imaging has been a form of qualitative analysis based on conventional MR imaging sequences. With advanced MR imaging techniques, quantitative analysis can be obtained with the unique properties of MRS.

Gamut of Magnetic Resonance

Before the development of what is now considered advanced MR imaging techniques, there were "standard" sequences to evaluate the brain, including T1, T2, FLAIR, and gradient recalled echo to name a few. With improvements in technology came more sophisticated methods to evaluate different brain pathologic abnormalities, especially in the setting of white matter disease. Examples of specialized MR imaging sequences and scans include diffusion weighted imaging, diffusion tensor imaging and tractography, magnetization transfer, MR perfusion, susceptibility weighted imaging, functional MR imaging, and the subject matter of this article, MRS.

MRS Fundamentals/Methodology

MRS is used to measure brain chemistry by identifying metabolites in body tissues. Due to

the relatively high concentration in the human body compared with other nuclei, the ^{1}H (proton) is most commonly used (known as proton spectroscopy) and provides much higher signal-to-noise than either sodium or phosphorus.[12] By the excitation of different isotopes within a particular molecular arrangement, the proton spectrum spreads out the different metabolites, referred to as chemical shift, and is expressed in terms of metabolite frequency in parts per million (ppm) on the x-axis. Signal intensity on the y-axis is a measure of peak amplitude. The spectrum "reads" from right to left (**Fig. 1**).

A region of interest in the brain, which can be either gray or white matter, can be obtained as a single voxel or multivoxel, and is selected using specific software on the MR imaging scanner. Representing the 3D version of a pixel, the voxel or volume element corresponds to a region or volume of tissue. Whether using the single-voxel or multivoxel method, the decision to apply a short or long echo time can change the composition of the spectrum. In general, the single-voxel method applies a short TE of 30 ms and is used to make the initial diagnosis due to higher signal-to-noise and more accurate quantitation of metabolites.[13] At longer TEs, the signal decreases due to T2 relaxation and signal from most of the metabolites is lost. The multivoxel method frequently uses a longer TE of 135 or 270 ms and therefore metabolites with a long TE are shown, producing a spectrum comprising primarily choline (Cho), creatine (Cr), and N-acetylaspartate (NAA). The multivoxel method allows for advantages including a large area of brain to be evaluated at the same time but suffers from decreased signal-to-noise and voxel bleed compared with the single-voxel method. By analyzing more than one voxel,

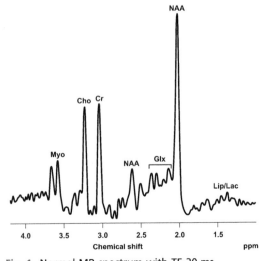

Fig. 1. Normal MR spectrum with TE 30 ms.

this method also allows for more accurate interpretation of the signal peak along the "y"-axis without the necessity of an external reference. It also can confirm that the spectroscopy worked in an instance of complete absence of signal from a particular voxel or voxels, which may be in a region of necrosis.

Metabolites

The commonly observable proton metabolites of the brain in order of increasing ppm are listed in **Table 1**.[13] Each of these presumably reflects a particular cellular process. NAA has the highest peak in normal brain tissue and is found exclusively in the nervous system, both central and peripheral.[13] NAA is a marker of axonal viability and, when decreased, indicates presumed neuronal loss or destruction.[14] Cr is a marker of cellular energy metabolism and its concentration is relatively stable, making it a good internal reference in calculating metabolite ratios.[15] Cho is a marker of cellular membrane turnover and thus likely reflects cellular proliferation.[16] Additional metabolites that are commonly helpful if found include lactate, lipids, and myo-inositol (Myo). Lactate is typically undetectable in the normal adult brain and its concentration increases with anaerobic metabolism, such as ischemia, hypoxia, seizures, and metabolic disorders. Lipids are components of cell membranes and their peaks are absent or minimally detectable in the normal brain. An abnormal lipid peak occurs with cellular membrane breakdown or necrosis. Myo is a simple sugar and considered a glial marker because it is primarily synthesized in astrocytes.[17] Myo is elevated with proliferation of glial cells or increase in glial cell size. Glutamine and glutamate (Glx) and glycine are better seen at shorter TEs and increased ppm, the neurotransmitter glutamate, as well as the amino acids glutamine and glycine, can be found, which can also have clinical implications.[7,13]

ANALYSIS

MRS can provide both qualitative and quantitative information from a region of brain tissue represented by the voxel. The qualitative analysis is viewed in the form of graphs or spectra based on the chemical shift of the metabolite. Quantitatively, each metabolite in a particular spectrum has a peak height, which represents the relative concentration of the metabolite. The area under the curve is proportional to the total concentration. Using the multivoxel method, comparing the peak heights across many voxels can be achieved. It should be stated that absolute peak assessment is achieved with spin counting methods, which are beyond the scope of this article. Normal brain tissue has reproducible concentrations of the 3 most commonly analyzed metabolites: NAA, Cr, and Cho. By drawing a line through the peak heights of these particular metabolites, Hunter's angle is formed and in normal tissue has a slope of approximately 45° (**Fig. 2**). In abnormal brain tissue, the concentration of one or all of these metabolites may be abnormally high or low and Hunter's angle is not preserved. An additional way to analyze spectra is by looking at metabolite ratios, specifically NAA/Cr, NAA/Cho, and Cho/Cr. For example, in highly malignant brain tumors, NAA and Cr decrease and Cho, lipids, and lactate increase, resulting in decreased NAA/Cr and NAA/Cho ratios and a lipid/lactate peak at short TEs. At intermediate TEs, the lactate peak

Metabolites	ppm	Properties
Lipids	0.9–1.4	Biproduct of brain destruction
Lactate	1.3	Biproduct of anaerobic glycolysis
NAA	2.0	Neuronal marker
Glutamine/ GABA	2.2–2.4	Neurotransmitters
Creatine	3.0	Energy metabolism
Choline	3.2	Cell membrane marker
Myo-inositol	3.5	Glial cell marker, osmolyte hormone receptor mechanisms

Table 1
Observable proton metabolites of the brain in order of increasing ppm

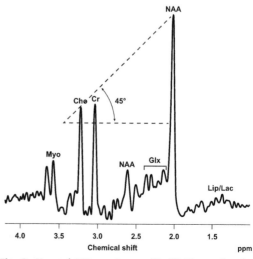

Fig. 2. Normal MR spectrum with TE 30 ms showing Hunter's angle.

inverts and can be found below the baseline, thus distinguishing it from lipids.

Imaging Technique

Depending on where the signal changes are in the brain, an area of interest can be chosen to construct a particular metabolic protocol that may include the deep gray nuclei, white matter, or peripheral gray matter in the cortex. Either a single-voxel or a multivoxel technique may be used for a specific purpose. The single-voxel technique, for reasons already discussed, usually results in a high-quality spectrum, a shorter scan time, and good field homogeneity.[13] The multivoxel method uses a grid placed over a larger spatial distribution and can be adjusted after acquisition. Traditionally MR spectra are obtained on either a 1.5- or 3-T magnet preceded by a triplanar FLAIR sequence, which usually shows the white matter abnormality to best advantage. Typical single- and multivoxel techniques would include a voxel size of 10 × 10 × 10 mm, specifically placed to include the area of interest and also to avoid fat (eg, in bone marrow and scalp), air (eg, in the paranasal sinuses and mastoid air cells), and calcium (eg, in bone). Water suppression pulse sequences, either PRESS or STEAM, are necessary to eliminate the large signal peak from water molecules.[18,19] Shimming is a technique used to minimize the inherent magnetic field inhomogeneities, thereby reducing "noise" in the baseline and resulting in more reliable metabolite quantification. As explained above, the single-voxel technique often uses a short spin-echo TE 30 ms and the multivoxel technique uses a long spin-echo TE of 135 or 270 ms. The TR of 1500 ms is the same with both. A total of 512 data points are collected over a spectral bandwidth of 1000 Hz. A Fourier transform is then applied to the data to separate the signal into individual frequencies.[12,13]

Clinical Applications

Metabolic disorders

There are many thousands of endogenous or common metabolites in the human body. The concentration of many of these molecules can be abnormally high or low in many processes, some of which include inborn errors of metabolism, mitochondrial disorders, and the leukodystrophies. Although the proton spectrum changes may only reflect general pathologic abnormality such as demyelination or ischemia, the combination with other clinical, genetic, and biochemical information may help to establish the diagnosis. Sometimes the identification of a specific biomarker with either increased or decreased concentration may aid in the diagnosis. As well, the spectrum may demonstrate a pathologic metabolite that might serve as a diagnostic clue. Therefore, MRS can, it is thought, be useful in the workup of a pediatric patient with a suspected disorder that affects the white matter.

Caution should be used in the evaluation of MRS in the pediatric population, especially in the newborn. In the immature brain in infants less than 2 years of age, the concentration of brain metabolites can differ considerably from the normal spectrum in an adult. For instance, Myo and Cho are elevated in the brain spectra of newborns and NAA is decreased, correlating with the lack of myelination for age.[20,21] This same spectrum would be considered abnormal in the adult patient. A small amount of lactate may be seen in the newborn brain normally.[22] In certain circumstances, it may be necessary to consult a pediatric neuroradiologist or spectroscopy expert. In elderly adults, the literature is inconsistent in regards to MRS, with some studies showing a reduction in NAA and higher Cho and Cr with increasing age.[23] Other studies have shown relatively stable concentrations in NAA in older patients but increased Cho and/or Cr.[24] Another study found "a 17%–30% reduction in the amount of white matter NAA/Cho in 85 year old subjects relative to younger adults."[25]

Inborn Errors of Metabolism, Mitochondrial Disorders, and Leukodystrophy

MRS is somewhat limited in the imaging evaluation of metabolic disorders, especially to differentiate them as distinct disorders, and is apparently related to decreased sensitivity from concentration thresholds of metabolites and decreased specificity related to overlap of many of their imaging features.[26] However, in some patients MRS may be extremely useful for diagnosis. The prototypical example is Canavan disease, which is one of the leukodystrophies with an autosomal-recessive inheritance resulting in a deficiency in the enzyme aspartoacylase. This deficiency results in abnormal accumulation of the metabolite NAA in the central nervous system, which impairs normal myelination and results in spongiform degeneration.[11] The spectrum of the abnormal white matter shows a markedly elevated NAA peak on proton MRS (Fig. 3). Another example of a rare inborn error of metabolism showing a specific proton spectrum is nonketotic hyperglycinemia. This autosomal-recessive disorder is the second most common disorder of amino acid metabolism (following phenylketonuria), due to

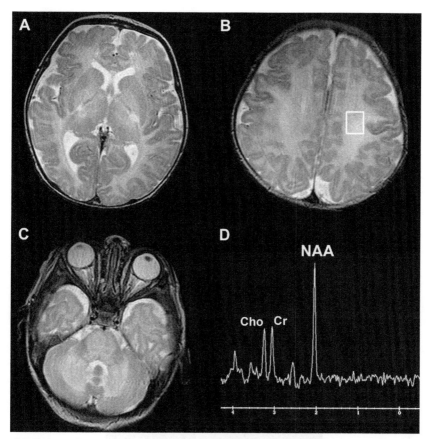

Fig. 3. Images (*A–C*) show abnormal T2 prolongation throughout the visualized supratentorial and infratentorial white matter on these T2-weighted sequences. The MR spectrum (*D*) obtained from the voxel on image (*B*) shows the characteristic markedly elevated NAA peak at 2 ppm. The spectrum also shows an abnormally decreased Cho peak relative to the NAA peak for this 5-week-old neonate with hypertonia and horizontal nystagmus since birth diagnosed with Canavan disease. (*Courtesy of* Tina Young Poussaint, MD, Children's Hospital Boston and Harvard Medical School, Boston, MA.)

defects in the glycine cleavage system.[27] This defect results in an abnormal accumulation of glycine in the brain, which can be found on proton MRS with a longer TE such as 288 ms at 3.55 ppm (**Fig. 4**). A longer TE is necessary to separate the Glycine peak from the myo-inositol peak.[26]

Mitochondrial diseases represent a set of disorders that differ from other abnormalities of white matter due to disruption of the respiratory chain. Clinically, tissues in the brain and muscle are usually the most affected because of the high oxidative demands. MRS has been shown to aid in this diagnosis based on the assumption that lactic acidosis is a primary feature.[26] However, it should be noted that elevated lactate is neither sensitive nor specific for mitochondrial disorders in the absence of conventional imaging and clinical factors. The first of 2 examples discussed in this article include MELAS (Mitochondrial Encephalomyopathy, Lactic Acidosis, and Stroke-like episodes), which clinically combines symptoms of

generalized mitochondrial disease and strokelike events (**Fig. 5**). Using routine T2-weighted MR imaging sequences of the brain, patients with this type of disease can typically be found to have abnormal signal changes with superimposed defined areas of infarction, many of differing ages. MRS in the areas of abnormal signal characteristically shows an elevated lactate peak in the acute and subacute stages.[13,28] Another complex mitochondrial disorder (or group of disorders) resulting in defective oxidative metabolism from several genetic and biochemical processes is known in the literature as Leigh syndrome. Several enzymes in this metabolic pathway, when impaired, can result in Leigh syndrome. Examples of culprit deficient enzymes include complex I, cytochrome oxidase, and pyruvate dehydrogenase, with the common feature being impaired energy production and elevated lactate. Consequently, this disorder also typically shows an elevated lactate peak on proton MRS.[29] MR imaging features in

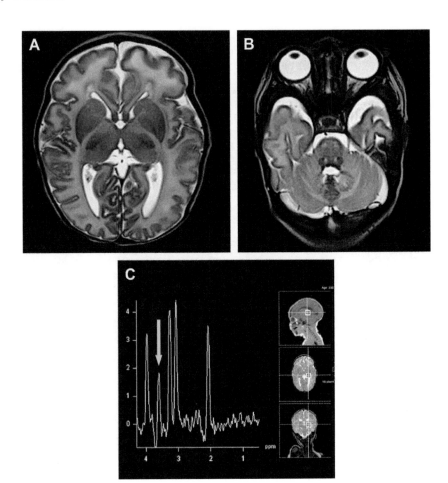

Fig. 4. T2-weighted images (*A, B*) obtained at the level of the basal ganglia and cerebellum show abnormal T2 prolongation throughout the white matter in this 23-day-old female patient. The MR spectrum (*C*) shows an elevated glycine peak at 3.5 ppm (*arrow*), obtained from a voxel in the region of the posterior limb of the internal capsule and corticospinal tracts. A diagnosis of nonketotic hyperglycinemia was suggested and was later confirmed by plasma glycine, cerebrospinal fluid /plasma glycine ratio, and genetic analysis. (*Courtesy of* Seena Dehkharghani, MD, Emory University, Atlanta, GA.)

patients with this disease often show bilateral and symmetric T2 hyperintensity in the putamina as one potential manifestation of this complex disorder (Fig. 6).

ADDITIONAL CLINICAL APPLICATIONS
Differentiating Predominant Tumor Progression from Predominant Radiation Necrosis

A common diagnostic dilemma for both the referring clinician and the radiologist alike is differentiating predominant tumor progression from predominant radiation necrosis on brain MR imaging wherein a patient has a brain tumor and has received surgery, chemotherapy, and radiation therapy. Both of these primary differential diagnostic entities tend to occur within or near the original tumor site, enhance on postcontrast images,

and may have similar mass effect and edema. Although biopsy is presumably the most definitive means to establish a diagnosis, it is by definition invasive. In theory, the spectral patterns for each of these processes are distinct and may be able to differentiate the two. The hallmark of malignant gliomas arising in the white matter is an elevation in Cho signifying increased membrane turnover in rapidly dividing cells. There is also a decrease in NAA and little or minor change in Cr. Therefore, one would expect predominant recurrent tumor to have significantly increased Cho/NAA and Cr/NAA ratios compared with predominant radiation necrosis. Spectroscopic changes that occur in predominant radiation necrosis have been reported and include slight depression of NAA and variable changes in Cho and Cr.[9] MRS has also been shown in the literature to be useful in differentiating high-grade primary,

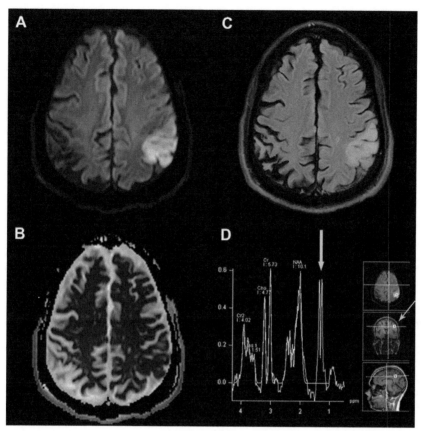

Fig. 5. Axial diffusion weighted imaging and apparent diffusion coefficient images (*A, B*) Area of reduced diffusion involving cortex and subcortical white matter in the posterolateral left frontal lobe with corresponding FLAIR signal hyperintensity (*C*) compatible with infarction. The MR spectrum (*D*) obtained from the voxel (*small arrow*) placed in the left frontal lobe shows a lactate doublet (*large arrow*) at approximately 1.3 ppm in this patient diagnosed with MELAS syndrome. (*Courtesy of* Otto Rapalino, MD, Massachusetts General Hospital and Harvard Medical School, MA.)

low-grade primary, and metastatic brain tumors.[30] Unfortunately, there can be much overlap in the MR spectra of these neurologic processes.

Pearls, Pitfalls, and Variants

- It is the authors' opinion that MRS should be interpreted in conjunction with conventional MR imaging of the brain and clinical history to avoid misinterpretation. Specifically, structural information from standard T1- and T2-weighted sequences, postcontrast imaging, and physiologic information (including diffusion and perfusion imaging) when available can possibly help avoid this potential pitfall.[31] For example, MRS performed on a tumefactive multiple sclerosis plaque may appear identical to a high-grade primary brain tumor.[32]
- There are several inherent disadvantages of MRS based on the nature of the technique. One disadvantage is the presence of voxel

bleed[33] whereby the spectrum may be "contaminated" by signals originating from adjacent voxels due to the limited matrix size. In other words, the selected voxel is contaminated by surrounding tissues and substances.[22,34] A similar concept applies when there is admixture of different tissue components within a particular sample. For example, in patients with primary high-grade neoplasms who have received radiation therapy, MRS may not be able to differentiate predominant tumor progression from predominant radiation necrosis.[35] As well, with inborn errors of metabolism, only small metabolites with sufficiently high concentrations can be observed by MRS.[34]
- Probably the greatest disadvantage of MRS is the lack of specificity in "general" white matter processes that result in neuronal loss or destruction; many of these disorders show decreased NAA and are indistinguishable on MRS alone.

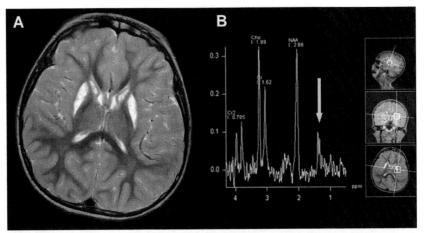

Fig. 6. An axial T2-weighted image at the level of the basal ganglia (*A*) shows bilateral and symmetric T2 prolongation in the caudate head nuclei, putamina, and dorsal thalami in this patient with Leigh syndrome. The MR spectrum (*B*) obtained from a voxel centered in the left putamen shows a decreased NAA/Cr ratio and a lactate doublet at 1.3 ppm (*arrow*). (*Courtesy of* Otto Rapalino, MD, Massachusetts General Hospital and Harvard Medical School, MA.)

What the Referring Physician Needs to Know

- As stated previously in this article, the importance of providing pertinent clinical history to the radiologist remains paramount in the setting of neuroimaging, especially regarding MRS. The referring physician should be aware of the inherent limitations of MRS including lack of specificity, but that also it can be useful in certain diseases.
- Finally, at the time of this writing and to the best of the authors' knowledge, MRS is not paid for by many third-party payers, and may be, therefore, discretionary. It is recommended that you determine whether or not MRS is reimbursable in your own system.

SUMMARY

As a complementary technique to traditional MR imaging of the brain, MRS can provide unique information based on the analysis of brain metabolites, which can be especially helpful in the setting of white matter disease. The specific diagnosis of white matter disease remains a diagnostic challenge due to the decreased specificity of imaging features and considerable overlap in many of the disorders, which is especially true in the pediatric population. MRS can be the key imaging study in individual cases as described in the substance of this article. Despite some inherent limitations of MRS, with continued advances in technology and imaging it is the authors' hope that MRS will become more mainstream as an additional diagnostic tool in the application of white matter diseases.

REFERENCES

1. Majos C, Aguilera C, Alonso J, et al. Proton MR spectroscopy improves discrimination between tumor and pseudotumoral lesion in solid brain masses. AJNR Am J Neuroradiol 2009;30(3):544–51. http://dx.doi.org/10.3174/ajnr.A1392. PubMed PMID: 19095788.
2. Hollingworth W, Medina LS, Lenkinski RE. A systematic literature review of magnetic resonance spectroscopy for the characterization of brain tumors. AJNR Am J Neuroradiol 2006;27:1404–11.
3. Cheon JE, Kim IO, Hwang YS, et al. Leukodystrophy in children: a pictorial review of MR imaging features. Radiographics 2002;22(3):461–76. PubMed PMID: 12006681.
4. Thompson JE, Castillo M, Kwock L, et al. Usefulness of proton MR spectroscopy in the evaluation of temporal lobe epilepsy. AJR Am J Roentgenol 1998;170(3):771–6. http://dx.doi.org/10.2214/ajr.170.3.9490972. PubMed PMID: 9490972.
5. Huisman TA. Tumor-like lesions of the brain. Cancer Imaging 2009;9(Spec No A):S10–3. http://dx.doi.org/10.1102/1470-7330.2009.9003. PubMed PMID: 19965288; PubMed Central PMCID: PMC2797474.
6. Bitsch A, Bruhn H, Vougioukas V, et al. Inflammatory CNS demyelination: histopathologic correlation with in vivo quantitative proton MR spectroscopy. AJNR Am J Neuroradiol 1999;20(9):1619–27. Epub 1999/10/30. PubMed PMID: 10543631.
7. Agarwal N, Renshaw PF. Proton MR spectroscopy-detectable major neurotransmitters of the brain: biology and possible clinical applications. AJNR Am J Neuroradiol 2012;33(4):595–602. http://dx.doi.org/10.3174/ajnr.A2587. PubMed PMID: 22207303.
8. Hasuuinger D. Introduction to protein structure bioinformatics 2004 NMR spectroscopy 2004.

9. Mullins ME, Barest GD, Schaefer PW, et al. Radiation necrosis versus glioma recurrence: conventional MR imaging clues to diagnosis. AJNR Am J Neuroradiol 2005;26(8):1967–72. PubMed PMID: 16155144.

10. Porto L, Kieslich M, Franz K, et al. MR spectroscopy differentiation between high and low grade astrocytomas: a comparison between paediatric and adult tumours. Europ J Paediatr Neurol 2011;15(3):214–21. http://dx.doi.org/10.1016/j.ejpn.2010.11.003. PubMed PMID: 21145271.

11. Gripp KW, Zimmerman RA, Wang ZJ, et al. Imaging studies in a unique familial dysmyelinating disorder. AJNR Am J Neuroradiol 1998;19(7):1368–72.

12. Hesselink J. Fundamentals of MR Spectroscopy.

13. Castillo M, Kwock L, Mukherji SK. Clinical applications of proton MR spectroscopy. AJNR Am J Neuroradiol 1996;17:1–15.

14. Pirko I, Fricke ST, Johnson AJ, et al. Magnetic resonance imaging, microscopy, and spectroscopy of the central nervous system in experimental animals. NeuroRx 2005;2(2):250–64. http://dx.doi.org/10.1602/neurorx.2.2.250. PubMed PMID: 15897949; PubMed Central PMCID: PMC1064990.

15. Butteriss DJ, Ismail A, Ellison DW, et al. Use of serial proton magnetic resonance spectroscopy to differentiate low grade glioma from tumefactive plaque in a patient with multiple sclerosis. Br J Radiol 2003;76(909):662–5. http://dx.doi.org/10.1259/bjr/85069069.

16. Croteau D, Scarpace L, Hearshen D, et al. Correlation between magnetic resonance spectroscopy imaging and image-guided biopsies: semiquantitative and qualitative histopathological analyses of patients with untreated glioma. Neurosurgery 2001;49(4): 823–9.

17. Castillo M, Smith JK, Kwock L. Correlation of myo-inositol levels and grading of cerebral astrocytomas. AJNR Am J Neuroradiol 2000;21(9):1645–9. PubMed PMID: 11039343.

18. Constantinidis I. MRS methodology. Adv Neurol 2000;83:235–46. PubMed PMID: 10999205.

19. Gillies RJ, Morse DL. In vivo magnetic resonance spectroscopy in cancer. Annu Rev Biomed Eng 2005;7:287–326. http://dx.doi.org/10.1146/annurev.bioeng.7.060804.100411. PubMed PMID: 16004573.

20. Fayed N, Olmos S, Morales H, et al. Physical basis of magnetic resonance spectroscopy and its application to central nervous system diseases. Am J Appl Sci 2006;3(5):1836–45.

21. Dezortova M, Hajek M. 1H MR spectroscopy in pediatrics. Clin Imaging 2009;33(1):78.

22. Mullins ME. MR spectroscopy: truly molecular imaging; past, present and future. Neuroimaging Clin N Am 2006;16(4):605–18. http://dx.doi.org/10.1016/j.nic.2006.06.008 viii. PubMed PMID: 17148022.

23. Soares DP, Law M. Magnetic resonance spectroscopy of the brain: review of metabolites and clinical applications. Clin Radiol 2009;64(1):12–21. http://dx.doi.org/10.1016/j.crad.2008.07.002. PubMed PMID: 19070693.

24. Soher BJ, van Zijl PC, Duyn JH, et al. Quantitative proton MR spectroscopic imaging of the human brain. Magn Reson Med 1996;35(3):356–63.

25. Kadota T, Horinouchi T, Kuroda C. Development and aging of the cerebrum: assessment with proton MR spectroscopy. AJNR Am J Neuroradiol 2001;22(1): 128–35.

26. Cecil KM. MR spectroscopy of metabolic disorders. Neuroimaging Clin N Am 2006;16(1):87–116. http://dx.doi.org/10.1016/j.nic.2005.10.004 viii. PubMed PMID: 16543087.

27. Heindel W, Kugel H, Roth B. Noninvasive detection of increased glycine content by proton MR spectroscopy in the brains of two infants with nonketotic hyperglycinemia. AJNR Am J Neuroradiol 1993; 14(3):629–35. PubMed PMID: 8517351.

28. Bianchi MC, Tosetti M, Battini R, et al. Proton MR spectroscopy of mitochondrial diseases: analysis of brain metabolic abnormalities and their possible diagnostic relevance. AJNR Am J Neuroradiol 2003; 24(10):1958–66. PubMed PMID: 14625217.

29. Saneto RP, Friedman SD, Shaw DW. Neuroimaging of mitochondrial disease. Mitochondrion 2008;8(5–6): 396–413. http://dx.doi.org/10.1016/j.mito.2008.05.003. PubMed PMID: 18590986; PubMed Central PMCID: PMC2600593.

30. Bulakbasi N, Kocaoglu M, Ors F, et al. Combination of single-voxel proton MR spectroscopy and apparent diffusion coefficient calculation in the evaluation of common brain tumors. AJNR Am J Neuroradiol 2003;24(2):225–33. PubMed PMID: 12591638.

31. Atlas SW. Magnetic resonance imaging of the brain and spine. 2009.

32. Barkovich AJ, Raybaud C. Normal development of the neonatal and infant brain, skull and spine. In: Barkovich AJ, Raybaud C, editors. Pediatric neuroimaging. 5th edition. Philadelphia: Lippincott Williams & Wilkins; 2012. p. 20–80.

33. Goelman G, Liu S, Gonen O. Reducing voxel bleed in Hadamard-encoded MRI and MRS. Magn Reson Med 2006;55(6):1460–5. http://dx.doi.org/10.1002/mrm.20903. PubMed PMID: 16685718.

34. van der Graaf M. In vivo magnetic resonance spectroscopy: basic methodology and clinical applications. Eur Biophys J 2010;39(4):527–40. http://dx.doi.org/10.1007/s00249-009-0517-y. PubMed PMID: 19680645; PubMed Central PMCID: PMC2841275.

35. Sundgren PC. MR spectroscopy in radiation injury. AJNR Am J Neuroradiol 2009;30(8):1469–76. http://dx.doi.org/10.3174/ajnr.A1580. PubMed PMID: 19369613.

Diffusion Tensor Imaging of Cerebral White Matter
Technique, Anatomy, and Pathologic Patterns

Asim F. Choudhri, MD[a,b,c,d,*], Eric M. Chin, BS[a],
Ari M. Blitz, MD[e], Dheeraj Gandhi, MD[f,g,h]

KEYWORDS

- Diffusion tensor imaging • White matter • Physiologic imaging • Magnetic resonance imaging
- Anatomy • Brain

KEY POINTS

- Diffusion tensor imaging is a magnetic resonance (MR) imaging technique that allows visualization of location, orientation, and integrity of white matter pathways.
- Mathematical constructs underlying diffusion tensor imaging are complex, but a basic understanding can guide interpretation.
- Interpretation of diffusion tensor parameter maps in conjunction with conventional MR imaging techniques can aid in diagnosis of white matter development and disorders.
- Processing diffusion tensor imaging data via diffusion tensor fiber tracking tractography allows mapping of individual tracts, which can be useful in surgical planning.

INTRODUCTION

The use of diffusion-weighted imaging (DWI) is well established in the rapid diagnosis and evaluation of cerebral infarction,[1] as well as for identifying lesions such as epidermoids and, more recently, characterizing the cellularity of tumors.[2] Diffusion tensor imaging (DTI), an advanced form of DWI, is an important tool in evaluating white matter anatomy and in pathology.[3,4] Although originally a research tool and only used in academic centers,

DTI has become a valuable part of the clinical evaluation of brain development, and in surgical planning for brain tumors.[5–8] The use of DTI has recently been investigated in the spinal cord.[9–11]

This article reviews the techniques of DTI and provides a practical approach for clinical implementation and interpretation. The anatomy of the white matter tracts, previously largely unseen by the radiologist, is increasing in importance (Table 1). This article reviews the fundamental

Disclosures: None.
[a] Department of Radiology, University of Tennessee Health Science Center, 848 Adams Avenue, G216, Memphis, TN 38103, USA; [b] Department of Neurosurgery, University of Tennessee Health Science Center, 848 Adams Avenue, G216, Memphis, TN 38103, USA; [c] Department of Ophthalmology, University of Tennessee Health Science Center, 848 Adams Avenue, G216, Memphis, TN 38103, USA; [d] Le Bonheur Neuroscience Institute, Le Bonheur Children's Hospital, 848 Adams Avenue, G216, Memphis, TN 38103, USA; [e] Division of Neuroradiology, Department of Radiology and Radiological Science, Johns Hopkins University, 600 N Wolfe Street, B100, Baltimore, MD 21287, USA; [f] Division of Neuroradiology, Department of Radiology, University of Maryland, 22 S Greene Street, Baltimore, MD 21201, USA; [g] Department of Neurology, University of Maryland, 22 S Greene Street, Baltimore, MD 21201, USA; [h] Department of Neurosurgery, University of Maryland, 22 S Greene Street, Baltimore, MD 21201, USA
* Corresponding author. Department of Radiology, Le Bonheur Children's Hospital, 848 Adams Avenue, G216, Memphis, TN 38103.
E-mail address: achoudhri@uthsc.edu

Radiol Clin N Am 52 (2014) 413–425
http://dx.doi.org/10.1016/j.rcl.2013.11.005
0033-8389/14/$ – see front matter © 2014 Elsevier Inc. All rights reserved.

Table 1
Major white matter tracts

Tract	Origin	Destination	Course	Function
Corticospinal tract	Precentral gyrus	Anterior horn cells of spinal cord	Traverses PLIC, cerebral peduncle, pyramidal decussation, lateral columns of spinal cord	Motor control for body
Corticobulbar tract	Precentral gyrus (inferiorly)	Pons	Traverses PLIC, cerebral peduncle, pyramidal decussation	Motor control for cranial nerves
Spinothalamic tract	Posterior horn cells of spinal cord	Rostral ventromedial thalamus	Lateral and anterior tracts in cord, anterior white commissure decussation, posterolateral pons, and midbrain	Sensory information from body to the thalamus
Geniculocalcarine tract	Lateral geniculate nucleus	Juxtacalcarine occipital cortex	Lateral margin of atrium and occipital horn of lateral ventricles	Visual fibers
Forceps major	Occipital cortex	Contralateral occipital cortex (homotopic)	Splenium of corpus callosum	Visual association
Forceps minor	Frontal pole cortex	Contralateral occipital cortex (homotopic)	Genu of corpus callosum	Frontal association
Central Tegmental Tract				
Ascending fibers	Solitary tract nucleus	Ventral posteromedial nucleus of thalamus	Midbrain and pons	Ascending taste fibers

Descending fibers (rubro-olivary tract)	Red nucleus (parvocellular)	Inferior olivary nucleus	—	Connection to contralateral cerebellar hemisphere
Transverse pontocerebellar fibers	Cerebellum	Contralateral cerebellum	Basilar pons and middle cerebellar peduncle	Not fully understood; impairment likely involved in MSA-C[32]
Arcuate fasciculus	Wernicke area (typically in region of planum temporale)	Broca area (typically in region of pars opercularis and pars triangularis)	Frontoparietotemporal opercular	Conveys information about the sound within words (not the meaning)
Superior longitudinal fasciculus	Multidirectional fiber bundles connecting frontal, parietal, occipital, and posterior temporal lobes	Multidirectional fiber bundles connecting frontal, parietal, occipital, and posterior temporal lobes	Frontal, temporal, and parietal lobes, lateral to corona radiata	Intrahemispheric association bundles
Inferior longitudinal fasciculus	Bidirectional between temporal and occipital lobes	Bidirectional between temporal and occipital lobes	Temporal and occipital lobes, lateral to lateral ventricle	Intrahemispheric association bundles
Uncinate fasciculus	Limbic system (including amygdala and hippocampus)	Orbitofrontal cortex	Temporal uncus and stem, inferior frontal lobes	Likely extension of limbic system

Abbreviations: MSA-C, multisystem atrophy with predominant cerebellar signs; PLIC, posterior limb of the internal capsule.

anatomic structures visible on DTI that are important to the understanding of white matter pathways and associated pathologic conditions (**Table 2**).

IMAGING TECHNIQUE
Techniques of DTI

Although the physics of DTI can seem daunting, a conceptual understanding is facilitated by understanding the terminology. Perhaps the most important term to understand is anisotropy, a word that is less complex than it might seem. "Iso" is the prefix meaning same and "tropic" is a suffix meaning turning toward or changing, and thus isotropic means moving the same in all directions. In the absence of barriers to movement, a molecule of water randomly moves in all directions in a process known as brownian motion, giving the system isotropic diffusion characteristics. The prefix "an" means not, and therefore anisotropic means movement that is not the same in all directions. Anatomic structures, such as white matter tracts, in which diffusion is highly constrained in some directions (eg, perpendicular to the direction of the contained axons) but remains unrestricted in other directions (eg, parallel to the direction of the

axons) thus demonstrate highly anisotropic diffusion characteristics.

DTI: Theory and Techniques

DTI is a magnetic resonance (MR) imaging technique that allows quantification in tissue of water diffusion characteristics such as anisotropy and the direction of greatest diffusivity. In white matter imaging, these parameters can be used to infer the paths and integrity of individual white matter tracts.[1,3,12]

In white matter, the high degree of anisotropy observed[13] is thought to be caused by bundled parallel axons. Perpendicular to the long axis of the axons (ie, radial movement), diffusion is impeded by the axonal cell membrane and myelin sheath. In contrast, along the long axis of the axons (ie, axial movement), diffusion is less constrained. Thus, if axonal microstructure or myelination is compromised by a disease process, a corresponding decrease in anisotropy can be measured.

In DWI, a pulsed field gradient is used (in contrast with the normal homogeneous magnetic field used for T1-weighted and T2-weighted

---

Table 2
Major white matter anatomic structures

White Matter Structure	Fiber Tracts Contained Within	Function
Corpus callosum		Interhemispheric Association
Genu/rostrum	Forceps minor	• Frontal
Body	—	• Frontal/perirolandic
Isthmus	—	• Perirolandic/precuneus
Splenium	Forceps major	• Occipital
Internal capsule		
ALIC	Various	Various
PLIC	Corticospinal tract	Motor for body
	Corticobulbar tract	Motor for head/face
	Optic tract	Visual information
Optic nerve and tract	Optic pathway	Visual information
Cerebral peduncles	Corticospinal tract	Motor to body
	Corticobulbar tract	Motor to head/face
	Spinothalamic tracts	Sensory fibers
Cerebellar peduncles		
Superior	Ventral spinocerebellar tract, dentatothalamic tract, trigeminocerebellar fibers	Proprioception, various
Middle	Pontocerebellar fibers	Various
Inferior	Dorsal spinocerebellar tract, olivocerebellar tract	Various
Anterior commissure	—	Commissural fibers connecting temporal lobes and amygdalae

images); this causes water molecules to gyrate throughout the tissue. In addition, all diffusion sequences apply a spin echo by producing another gradient pulse in the opposite direction to refocus the water molecules (ie, bringing them back into phase). Because diffusion has a defocusing effect, increased diffusivity nonlinearly attenuates the signal received. However, because diffusion-weighted sequences rely on a field gradient, they are sensitive to diffusion only in a single direction. Sequences used in DTI are an extension of those used in DWI. By repeating the sequence 6 or more times while varying the gradient direction, what is known as the diffusion tensor can be reconstructed: a mathematical entity describing the diffusion characteristics at each voxel imaged, roughly corresponding with the summation of all vectors of water molecule diffusion in the voxel. This tensor is used to calculate the various metrics described later (eg, fractional anisotropy [FA]; axial, radial, and mean diffusivity). In general, current clinical use of DTI can be classified as (1) direct semiquantitative interpretation of maps of these metrics to assess axonal health and myelin status, (2) use of these metrics as an adjunct with other modalities (such as conventional T1-weighted and T2-weighted sequences) to better characterize tissue abnormalities, and (3) use of tractography (described later) to identify the paths of key white matter tracts in surgical planning.

A minimum of 6 directions of encoding are required to obtain directional information and FA calculation, but a larger number of encoding directions improves white matter characterization. High-resolution clinical studies, such as for tumor surgical planning, often use 15 to 30 directions of encoding, and research studies at times use more than 100 directions of encoding.

FA

FA is a dimensionless value that describes the extent of unidirectional water movement, and is scaled from 0 to 1. An FA of 0 indicates no anisotropy in water movement, which is the case for true isotropic movement such as is expected in a glass of water, or within a collection of cerebrospinal fluid such as the ventricular system. An FA of 1 indicates purely unidirectional movement of water, something that does not typically exist in organisms. However, parallel white matter fibers without significant interstitial space, such as in the myelinated corpus callosum, can have an FA of 0.85 or higher (Fig. 1A). FA increases as the brain myelinates.[14,15] Lower FA values do not necessarily indicate decreased white matter integrity, but only less unidirectional water motion. As an example, crossing white matter fibers in the deep white matter may be fully myelinated and intact; however, because of the multidirectional orientation, FA is less than if the same fibers were parallel. FA is also decreased if a greater percentage of a voxel is interstitial space, where there is more isotropic movement and a corresponding lower FA.

Evaluating FA on a quantitative basis can be done comparing homotopic structures between the two hemispheres. FA values are typically symmetric, and any asymmetry should raise suspicion for an abnormality, typically with the abnormal side showing a lower FA value.

FA can be computed on a structure-by-structure basis, such as for the posterior limb of the internal capsule (PLIC) and compared with age-related normative values. A histogram analysis can be performed of FA on either a whole-brain or a regional basis. Although the region is typically an anatomically defined area (voxel-based analysis), such as the PLIC, histogram analysis can also be performed on a white matter bundle that does not have defined anatomic boundaries (eg, the arcuate fasciculus) in a process known as tract-based spatial statistics (TBSS). Identifying the tract for TBSS is typically performed by diffusion tensor fiber tracking (DT-FT), which is discussed further later. More complex (but automated) FA analyses are being investigated to quantify progression of myelination.[16]

Display of FA maps can take place in 3 ways. First is a map on which the grayscale value represents the FA value (see Fig. 1A); to facilitate windowing and leveling on picture archiving and communications systems (PACS), FA maps are typically scaled from 0 to 1000, or 0 to 10,000. Thus, a value in the corpus callosum of 8200 likely indicates an FA of 0.82; confirmation of this should be made for MR and PACS vendor combinations before clinically using these values. Color encoding can be performed based on a lookup table (LUT), in which different ranges of FA values are given different colors (see Fig. 1B), and that can be created from any grayscale FA DICOM dataset; however, typically these are not used clinically. Possibly the most important visual display mechanism of FA data is a directionally encoded (DE) FA map (DE-FA; see Fig. 1C), commonly referred to as color-coded FA maps but described here as DE-FA to distinguish them from the LUT-based color FA maps. DE-FA maps cannot be created solely from a grayscale FA map without additional information (derived from the source diffusion images) about the predominant direction of water movement in a voxel. In DE-FA, the FA value of a voxel is represented by brightness, so voxels

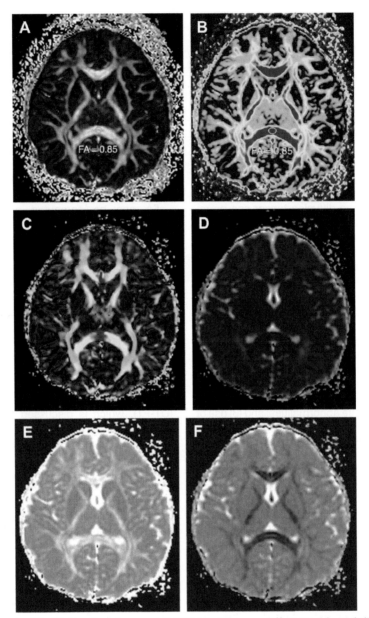

Fig. 1. (A) FA, (B) color FA, (C) directionally encoded (DE) FA, (D) mean diffusivity, (E) axial diffusivity, (F) radial diffusivity.

with high FA appear brighter. The color used for each voxel is based on the direction of the primary axis of water diffusion, with the convention stating that red represents movement along the transverse axis, green along the anterior-posterior axis, and blue along the craniocaudal axis. The features on a scan that most clearly show the directional color scheme are the red commissural fibers of the corpus callosum, the green fibers of the optic radiations (or geniculocalcarine tract), and the blue appearance of the descending fibers of the corticospinal tract within the PLIC.

In DWI, the rate of signal decay is calculated between 2 different time values, typically 0 and 1000 milliseconds (ie, B-0 and B-1000). A similar value exists for DTI, which takes the mean value for the diffusion coefficient among the various encoding directions, a value known as mean diffusivity (MD; see Fig. 1D). MD can be helpful in clinical evaluations in which DTI is performed instead of DWI, and it is required to determine whether bright signal on B-1000 images is related to reduced water diffusion (low apparent diffusion coefficient [ADC] and MD values) or to increased water content (T2 shine-through, which has high ADC and MD values). However, DTI offers additional information: diffusion coefficients can be calculated for the rate of water movement along the primary axis of water movement, known as axial diffusivity (AxD; see **Fig. 1E**). The rate of diffusion in a plane perpendicular to the long axis can be calculated, representing a value known as radial diffusivity (RD; see **Fig. 1F**). Note that the corpus callosum has free diffusion of water along the long axis

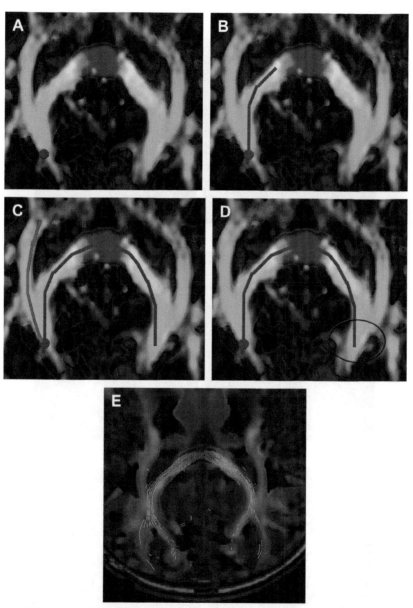

Fig. 2. (A) DE-FA of bilateral occipital cortex with a seed location placed in the right occipital deep white matter. (B) Deterministic DT-FT of the forceps major (red line) beginning from the seed location and progressing toward the splenium of the corpus callosum. (C) Deterministic DT-FT of the forceps major (red line) extending to a homotopic location in the left occipital lobe, as well as the geniculocalcarine tract (pink line) extending toward the lateral geniculate nucleus. (D) Deterministic DT-FT, similar to parts A to C, but with a target region of interest (ROI) placed in the left occipital lobe (blue circle). The forceps major (red line) is unchanged from parts A to C, but the geniculocalcarine tract is no longer present. (E) Axial T1-weighted (T1W) image with DE-FA overlay, as well as overlay of DT-FT mapping the forceps major. The DT-FT is calculated by deterministic tractographic analysis with the ROI placed in the right occipital white matter showing connection to the contralateral occipital lobe through the splenium of the corpus callosum.

and reduced water movement perpendicular to the long axis. The significant difference between these two values is related to the same properties that result in a high FA. If AxD and RD are equal, then FA = 0. Gray matter has intermediate but similar AxD and RD, and a corresponding low FA. AxD and RD are important concepts, but are not routinely used in clinical practice.

Although DTI parameters such as DE-FA are related to the direction and integrity of white matter tracts, perhaps the most intriguing uses of DTI are related to DT-FT. DT-FT, a technique

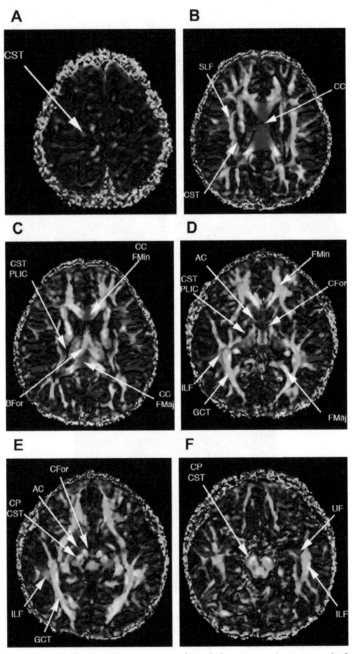

Fig. 3. Axial DE-FA maps at multiple levels (superior to inferior) showing various tracts, including the corticospinal tract (CST; A–I), corpus callosum (CC; B, C); forceps major (FMaj; C, D), forceps minor (FMin; C, D), PLIC (C, D), cerebral peduncles (CP; E, F), superior cerebellar peduncle (SCP; G), decussation of the superior cerebellar peduncle (SCP-D; G), middle cerebellar peduncle (MCP; H, I), inferior cerebellar peduncle (ICP; I), transverse pontocerebellar fibers (TPF; H, I), central tegmental tract (CTT; H, I), geniculocalcarine tract (GCT; D, E), uncinate fasciculus (UF; F, G), superior longitudinal fasciculus (SLF; B), and inferior longitudinal fasciculus (ILF; D–F).

commonly referred to as tractography, is a process whereby the integrity and directions of white matter in adjacent voxels can be processed to postulate the location of white matter fiber pathways. To do this, a starting point is chosen (Fig. 2A), known as a DT-FT seed. Knowing that the voxel anterior to this has a predominantly anterior-posterior motion (indicated by green), a line can be drawn suggesting a possible white matter tract taking this course (see Fig. 2B); in this case the fibers of the forceps major. A similar set of connections can be made for the geniculo-calcarine tract (ie, optic radiations; pink line in Fig. 2C). By selecting a target region of interest (ROI) in the left occipital lobe, only fibers between the seed and target are included (see Fig. 2D). DT-FT often shows multiple fibers (see Fig. 2E). Once tracts are identified, they can be overlaid on structural imaging for purposes such as surgical planning, or can be used to define an ROI for quantitative analysis of FA data in TBSS.

To know which voxels to connect and which to not connect, 2 parameters must be determined. First is an FA threshold. Whichever threshold is chosen, if a voxel has an FA value less than this it is assumed that the proposed tract does not continue through that voxel. The second parameter is the angle threshold. White matter tracts do not necessarily travel in a straight line, but they do not typically make sharp turns either. A determination can be made for an angle threshold less than which it is assumed that the fiber tract is continuous, and more than which it is assumed that a white matter tract does not continue. This method of DT-FT is known as deterministic DT-FT, and is the most commonly used in clinical settings. Research protocols may use probability theory to determine the most likely course of white matter tracts; a method known as probabilistic tracking, which is intended to have improved performance in following crossing fibers.

Common FA thresholds for deterministic tracking are approximately 0.2 to 0.3, and common angle thresholds are approximately 20° to 40°. Changing these parameters can change the outcome of DT-FT significantly, which, coupled with variability in seed and target locations and DTI acquisition parameters, can potentially change results and clinical outcomes.

ANATOMY

When evaluating conventional MR, white matter is often evaluated based on structural features, such

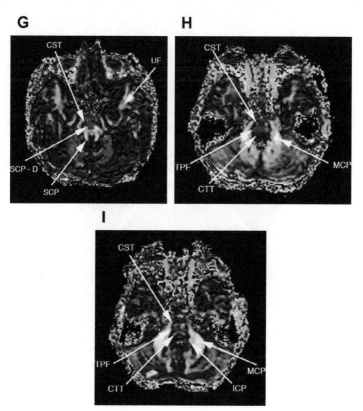

Fig. 3. (continued)

as the corpus callosum and the internal capsule. DTI and DT-FT allow further evaluation of specific tracts within these structures that may perform different functions. For instance, the PLIC carries motor innervation to the cranial nerves through the corticobulbar tract; motor innervation to the body through the corticospinal tract; and, in the posterior-most portion, carries visual fibers within the geniculocalcarine tract.

Innumerable white matter pathways exist within the cerebral hemispheres; however, they can largely be placed into 3 categories. There are commissural fibers, which traverse the midline to the contralateral hemisphere; association fibers, which communicate within a hemisphere; and projection fibers, which leave the cerebral hemispheres and communicate with the brainstem, cerebellum, and spinal cord.

Corona radiata and centrum semiovale are terms that are commonly misused. The corona radiata represents the white matter that extends from the internal capsule superiorly into the cerebral hemispheres. Centrum semiovale represents all the white matter in a cerebral hemisphere. Therefore corona radiata is a subset of centrum semiovale, and the centrum semiovale also contains commissural and intrahemispheric association fibers. The distinction between these two entities is unrelated to their relationship to the lateral ventricles, contrary to commonly misstated definitions.

Further confusion about white matter anatomy comes from the sometimes alternating use of descriptions based on its structure, function, and specific tracts. For instance, the optic radiations are structures that perform the function of the visual pathway, and the specific tract is known as the geniculocalcarine tract because the fibers connect the lateral geniculate nucleus to the juxtacalcarine occipital cortex. Major white matter structures and tracts can be identified on DE-FA maps (Fig. 3).

A comprehensive review of white matter anatomy is beyond the scope of this article, but detailed anatomic references are available.[17–20]

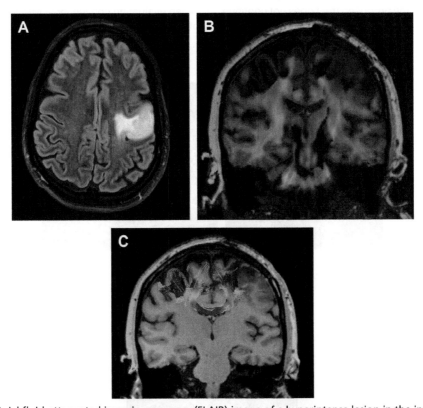

Fig. 4. (A) Axial fluid-attenuated inversion recovery (FLAIR) image of a hyperintense lesion in the inferior aspect of the left precentral gyrus. (B) Coronal T1W image with DE-FA overlay showing diminished FA within infiltrated white matter, without signs of displacement of white matter tracts, suggesting an infiltrative tumor. (C) Coronal T1W image with DT-FT overlay showing diminished extension of commissural fibers to the involved parenchyma, identified by seed-ROI placement in the midbody of the corpus callosum.

IMAGING FINDINGS/PATHOLOGIC CONDITIONS

A common use of DTI and DT-FT is for presurgical planning in patients with brain lesions presumed to be tumors.[7] Some tumors have circumscribed margins and some have indistinct infiltrating margins. DTI may be able to determine whether a tumor that distorts structural anatomy infiltrates white matter tracts or only displaces them (Fig. 4). The concept is that, if there is infiltration of a white matter tract, resection will disrupt whichever function is performed by the infiltrated tract(s), whereas the function of displaced tracts will likely be spared. The identification of tracts potentially infiltrated by neoplasm allows the neurosurgeon to have an informed discussion with the patient regarding whether or not they will be resected, allowing some degree of prediction of the associated potential postoperative neurologic deficits. At times, the surgeon and patient may elect to perform a full resection, with understanding of the possible rehabilitation required because of the disrupted pathway. At other times, surgeons may selectively spare portions of the tumor, anticipating treating those portions with adjunctive measures such as chemotherapy and/or radiation, or possibly just close observation.

DT-FT can be combined with other physiologic imaging techniques such as blood oxygen level–dependent (BOLD) functional MR (fMR) imaging.

fMR imaging may identify an area of cortex that controls a motor or language task (Fig. 5).

Although DT-FT is most commonly used to localize white matter fibers or confirm their integrity, it can also be used to confirm disconnection, such as after a corpus callosotomy (Fig. 6).[21–23]

Vasogenic edema decreases FA by increasing the water content in the interstitial space. There is facilitated diffusion in all directions, in contrast with cytotoxic edema, which has reduced water diffusion in all directions. Decreased FA can also be seen in the setting of wallerian degeneration.[24]

FA changes as the pediatric brain matures, increasing as the brain myelinates.[13,14] An altered FA maturation pattern has been shown in multiple white matter pathways in patients with autism spectrum disorder (ASD),[6] with accelerated maturation and FA greater than controls at 6 months of age followed by an early plateau with FA lower than controls by 24 months of age. Although these trends have been shown on a population basis, threshold values have not yet been validated for this to be used as a tool for early diagnosis of ASD.

In patients with tuberous sclerosis complex (TSC), there is decreased FA in the white matter of cortical tubers and their associated white matter migration lines.[5,25] Studies have shown that treatment with mammalian target of rapamycin (mTOR) inhibitors such as everolimus can partially reverse these FA abnormalities.[26] White matter

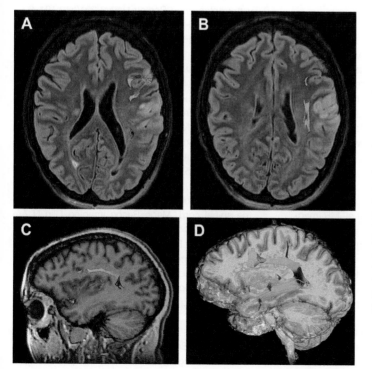

Fig. 5. (A) Axial FLAIR image with BOLD-fMR imaging overlay of areas of cortical activation corresponding with expressive language (Broca area, in pink) in the left pars opercularis and pars triangularis. DT-FT performed using the language centers as seed locations identifies the arcuate fasciculus. (B) Axial FLAIR image showing DT-FT of the arcuate fasciculus coursing beneath a left inferior perirolandic mass. (C) Sagittal T1W image showing DT-FT of the arcuate fasciculus coursing posteriorly to the region of the planum temporale. (D) Lateral projection of a three-dimensional rendering of the brain with cutout of the lateral aspect of the left hemisphere, with DT-FT of the arcuate fasciculus, showing a thicker bundle of fibers than is typically seen on any two-dimensional planar view.

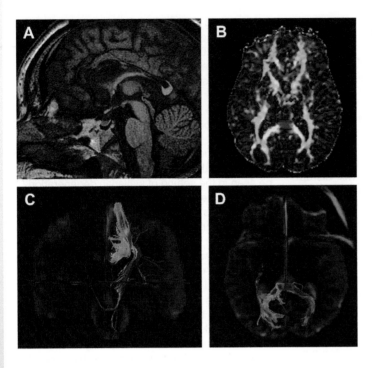

Fig. 6. (A) Sagittal T1W image in a patient after a splenium-sparing corpus callosotomy shows non-visualization of nearly all of the corpus callosum, and a normal appearance of the splenium. (B) Axial DE-FA map shows an absence of transversely oriented red diffusion within the genu of the corpus callosum, but preservation of the splenium. (C) Posterior projection DT-FT with ROI placed in the right frontoparietal deep white matter shows no commissural fibers traversing the midline through the genu, body, or isthmus of the corpus callosum. (D) Superior projection DT-FT performed with ROI in the right occipital deep white matter shows preservation of fibers of the forceps major traversing the midline within the splenium of the corpus callosum.

abnormalities such as this may be related to altered functional connectivity and increased incidence of ASD in patients with TSC.[5,27,28]

Atrophic changes in the transverse pontocerebellar fibers are related to the hot-cross-buns sign seen in multiple system atrophy, which can be shown on DTI.[29-31]

SUMMARY

DTI is a powerful tool for evaluating white matter anatomy and associated abnormalities. DTI was previously a research tool, but is entering clinical practice. Understanding the terminology and basic concepts of this technique can aid in the clinical implementation and interpretation of this blend of structural and physiologic white matter evaluation.

REFERENCES

1. Le Bihan D, Breton E, Lallemand D, et al. MR imaging of intravoxel incoherent motions: application to diffusion and perfusion in neurologic disorders. Radiology 1986;161:401–7.
2. Rumboldt Z, Camacho DL, Lake D, et al. Apparent diffusion coefficients for differentiation of cerebellar tumors in children. AJNR Am J Neuroradiol 2006; 27(6):1362–9.
3. Pierpaoli C, Jezzard P, Basser PJ, et al. Diffusion tensor MR imaging of the human brain. Radiology 1996;201:637–48.
4. Lee SK, Kim DI, Kim J, et al. Diffusion-tensor MR imaging and fiber tractography: a new method of describing aberrant fiber connections in developmental CNS anomalies. Radiographics 2005;25: 53–65 [discussion: 66–8].
5. Krishnan ML, Commowick O, Jeste SS, et al. Diffusion features of white matter in tuberous sclerosis with tractography. Pediatr Neurol 2010;42:101–6.
6. Wolff JJ, Gu H, Gerig G, et al. Differences in white matter fiber tract development present from 6 to 24 months in infants with autism. Am J Psychiatry 2012;169(6):589–600.
7. Pillai JJ, Zaca D, Choudhri A. Clinical impact of integrated physiologic brain tumor imaging. Technol Cancer Res Treat 2010;9:359–80.
8. Choudhri AF, Narayana S, Rezaie R, et al. Same day tri-modality functional brain mapping prior to resection of lesion involving eloquent cortex. Neuroradiol J 2013;26(5):548–54.
9. Thurnher MM, Law M. Diffusion-weighted imaging, diffusion-tensor imaging, and fiber tractography of the spinal cord. Magn Reson Imaging Clin N Am 2009;17:225–44.
10. Thurnher MM, Bammer R. Diffusion-weighted magnetic resonance imaging of the spine and spinal cord. Semin Roentgenol 2006;41:294–311.
11. Ducreux D, Lepeintre JF, Fillard P, et al. MR diffusion tensor imaging and fiber tracking in 5 spinal cord astrocytomas. AJNR Am J Neuroradiol 2006;27: 214–6.
12. Mukherjee P, Berman JI, Chung SW, et al. Diffusion tensor MR imaging and fiber tractography: theoretic

underpinnings. AJNR Am J Neuroradiol 2008;29: 632–41.

13. Moseley ME, Cohen Y, Kucharczyk J, et al. Diffusion-weighted MR imaging of anisotropic water diffusion in cat central nervous system. Radiology 1990;176: 439–45.

14. Provenzale JM, Isaacson J, Chen S, et al. Correlation of apparent diffusion coefficient and fractional anisotropy values in the developing infant brain. Am J Roentgenol 2010;195:W456–62.

15. Provenzale JM, Liang L, Delong D, et al. Diffusion tensor imaging assessment of brain white matter maturation during the first postnatal year. Am J Roentgenol 2007;189:476–86.

16. Chin EM, Choudhri AF. Myelination age: establishing normal ranges for myelination status during development using a histogram-based fractional anisotropy metric. In: Proceedings of the 51st Annual Meeting of the American Society of Neuroradiology, n.d. 2013. p. 280–81.

17. Naidich TP, Duvernoy HM, Delman BN, et al. Duvernoy's atlas of the human brain stem and cerebellum. New York: Springer; 2009.

18. Nieuwenhuys R, Voogd J, Christiaan VH. The human central nervous system: a synopsis and atlas. New York: Springer; 2007.

19. Mori S, van Zijl PC, Oishi K, et al. MRI atlas of human white matter. Waltham (MA): Academic Press; 2010.

20. Schmahmann J, Pandya D. Fiber pathways of the brain. New York: Oxford University Press; 2009.

21. Moreno-Jiménez S, San-Juan D, Lárraga-Gutiérrez JM, et al. Diffusion tensor imaging in radiosurgical callosotomy. Seizure 2012;21:473–7.

22. Pizzini FB, Polonara G, Mascioli G, et al. Diffusion tensor tracking of callosal fibers several years after callosotomy. Brain Res 2010;1312:10–7.

23. Choudhri AF, Whitehead MT, McGregor AE, et al. Diffusion tensor imaging to evaluate commissural disconnection after corpus callosotomy. Neuroradiology 2013;55(11):1397–403.

24. Beaulieu C, Does MD, Snyder RE, et al. Changes in water diffusion due to wallerian degeneration in peripheral nerve. Magn Reson Med 1996;36:627–31.

25. Makki MI, Chugani DC, Janisse J, et al. Characteristics of abnormal diffusivity in normal-appearing white matter investigated with diffusion tensor MR imaging in tuberous sclerosis complex. AJNR Am J Neuroradiol 2007;28:1662–7.

26. Tillema JM, Leach JL, Krueger DA, et al. Everolimus alters white matter diffusion in tuberous sclerosis complex. Neurology 2012;78:526–31.

27. Rezaie R, Zouridakis G, Choudhri AF. Functional connectivity in tuberous sclerosis complex with autistic spectrum disorder preliminary findings. Journal of Pediatric Neurology 2013;11(2):79–82.

28. Simao G, Raybaud C, Chuang S, et al. Diffusion tensor imaging of commissural and projection white matter in tuberous sclerosis complex and correlation with tuber load. AJNR Am J Neuroradiol 2010;31:1273–7.

29. Shrivastava A. The hot cross bun sign. Radiology 2007;245:606–7.

30. Loh KB, Rahmat K, Lim SY, et al. A hot cross bun sign from diffusion tensor imaging and tractography perspective. Neurol India 2011;59:266–9.

31. Ito M, Watanabe H, Kawai Y, et al. Usefulness of combined fractional anisotropy and apparent diffusion coefficient values for detection of involvement in multiple system atrophy. J Neurol Neurosurg Psychiatry 2006;78:722–8.

32. De Simone T, Regna-Gladin C, Carriero M, et al. Wallerian Degeneration of the Pontocerebellar Fibers. AJNR Am J Neuroradiol 2005;26:1062–5.

Imaging Approach to the Cord T2 Hyperintensity (Myelopathy)

Allison M. Grayev, MD[a], Jennifer Kissane, MD[b], Sangam Kanekar, MD[c,d,e,*]

KEYWORDS

- Myelopathy • Acute transverse myelitis • MS • ADEM • Vascular malformation • MRI

KEY POINTS

- In clinically suspected case of myelopathy, MR imaging without and with gadolinium remains the modality of choice.
- The first and best imaging approach in the evaluation of myelopathy is to identify whether the cause of myelopathy is compressive or noncompressive.
- The commonest imaging finding in myelopathy is either focal or diffuse cord hyperintensity on the T2-weighted MR imaging images.
- Detailed clinical history, acuity of symptoms (acute vs insidious onset), distribution of the signal abnormalities, including length of cord involvement, specific tract involvement, and the region of the spinal cord that is affected, are very useful in making the diagnosis.

INTRODUCTION

Myelopathy is defined as a neurologic deficit related to a spinal cord pathologic abnormality. The commonest imaging finding in myelopathy is either focal or diffuse cord hyperintensity on the T2-weighted magnetic resonance (MR) images (T2 WI). Intramedullary T2 hyperintensity can pose a serious dilemma in spinal imaging because it has a myriad of causes, which can be difficult to differentiate. The clinical symptoms of myelopathy can be insidious in onset and vague in presentation. In addition, the numerous patterns of tract decussation can lead to confusing physical examination symptoms and difficulty in pinpointing a level of pathologic abnormality. The radiologic appearance of myelopathy is no less confusing, as many pathologies present with T2 hyperintensity. A systematic approach that incorporates history, physical examination, and radiologic findings is imperative to narrow the differential diagnosis. Contrast-enhanced MR imaging remains the primary investigation in the evaluation of a myelopathic patient. The first and best imaging approach is to identify whether the cause of myelopathy is compressive or noncompressive, because evaluation of compressive causes is often straightforward with a specific

[a] Section of Neuroradiology, University of Wisconsin School of Medicine and Public Health, 1308 W Dayton Street, Madison, WI 53715, USA; [b] Department of Radiology, Penn State Milton S. Hershey Medical Center and College of Medicine, Pennsylvania State University, 500 University Drive, Hershey, PA 17033, USA; [c] Section of Neuroradiology, Department of Radiology, Penn State Milton S. Hershey Medical Center and College of Medicine, Pennsylvania State University, 500 University Drive, Hershey, PA 17033, USA; [d] Department of Neurology, Penn State Milton S. Hershey Medical Center and College of Medicine, Pennsylvania State University, 500 University Drive, Hershey, PA 17033, USA; [e] Department of Otolaryngology, Penn State Milton S. Hershey Medical Center and College of Medicine, Pennsylvania State University, 500 University Drive, Hershey, PA 17033, USA
* Corresponding author. Department of Radiology, College of Medicine, Penn State Milton S. Hershey Medical Center and College of Medicine, Pennsylvania State University, 500 University Drive, Hershey, PA 17033.
E-mail address: skanekar@hmc.psu.edu

Radiol Clin N Am 52 (2014) 427–446
http://dx.doi.org/10.1016/j.rcl.2013.11.002

cause identified on MR. In contrast, negotiating the exact cause of noncompressive myelopathy may be very challenging. Detailed clinical history, acuity of symptoms (acute vs insidious onset), distribution of the signal abnormalities, including length of cord involvement, specific tract involvement, and the region of the spinal cord that is affected, are very useful in making the diagnosis.

Common causes of the myelopathy can be classified into compressive, infection, inflammatory, vascular, metabolic/toxic, and hereditary (Table 1).

COMPRESSIVE
Trauma

Trauma is one of the most common causes of compressive myelopathy, which may be secondary to osseous spinal canal compromise or epidural hematoma. This effect may be compounded in the setting of degenerative changes, especially in the cervical spine. Cord compression following trauma may be due to the presence of associated spinal fractures, subluxation, ligamentous injury, prevertebral swelling, and epidural hematoma. Following trauma, any neurologic symptom related to the cord is an indication for an MR imaging, especially when computed tomography (CT) is negative.[1] One of the common clinical presentations is that of the central cord syndrome, which consists of motor and sensory impairment. Central cord syndrome is most commonly seen in the cervical spine and, therefore, the symptoms are most pronounced in the upper extremities.[2]

In the setting of trauma, CT remains the primary modality because of its speed and sensitivity in the diagnosis of bony injury. Fracture fragment, subluxation, and extradural or subdural hematoma may cause severe canal compromise and cord compression (Fig. 1). MR imaging is more sensitive in identifying soft tissue, ligamentous, and cord injury. MR imaging may show mild to diffuse cord swelling, focal or diffuse edema, and in some cases, intra- or extramedullary hemorrhage. Cord edema is seen as focal or diffuse hyperintensity on T2 WI. Hemorrhagic contusion, defned as a discrete focus of hemorrhage within the spinal cord, is seen as foci of low signal intensities within cord edema, on T2, and on gradient echo sequence (GRE) images (Fig. 2). In the setting of trauma, the extent of cord edema and the presence of hemorrhagic contusion should be evaluated because edema spanning over 2 levels of vertebral segments is associated with a greater severity of neurologic deficits and cord edema alone has a more favorable prognosis than cord hemorrhage.[3]

It is not uncommon to see trauma to the cord following spine surgery or instrumentation; this may be a direct injury to the cord with the surgical instruments or due to vascular compromise during surgical manipulation. Clinical presentation is fairly acute with sensory or motor deficit immediately following the procedure. On imaging, most of these lesions are focal and at the site of surgery (Fig. 3).

Spondylosis

Degenerative changes may cause myelopathy in the absence of trauma, secondary to direct cord compression or vascular compromise (mainly venous). Both disc herniation and osteophyte formation may cause compressive myelopathy and the problem may be compounded by superimposed spinal canal stenosis. In fact, cervical spondylotic myelopathy is the most common cause of myelopathy in patients older than 55 years[4] with C5-C6 followed by C6-C7 being the most common levels. There is no uniform prognosis or anticipated progression of disease with some patients presenting with progressive symptoms, whereas others have long periods of relatively little symptoms.[5]

Imaging, especially MR imaging, plays a very important role in the diagnosis of myelopathy due to spondylosis. The role of plain radiographs is debatable; however, in clinical practice radiographs remain the first investigation performed. Spinal canal narrowing can be assessed on lateral plain radiographs of the cervical spine by measuring the distance from the most posterior aspect of one vertebral body to the closest spinolaminar line. Measurements less than 13 mm are associated with an increased risk for myelopathy[6] and absolute/severe stenosis is defined as measurement less than 10 mm. Cross-sectional imaging CT and MR imaging are complementary to each other in diagnosis of compressive myelopathy. Bony changes such as early osteophytes and un-covertebral hypertrophy are better seen on CT, whereas MR imaging, due to its superior ability to image soft tissue, provides additional information regarding cord, disc ligaments, and cysts. GRE on MR imaging is very sensitive in distinguishing osteophytes from disc herniation because osteophytes show low signal intensity relative to higher signal intensity disc material. Canal measurements and cord signal intensity are best assessed on T2 WI images. Cord changes on MR imaging will depend on the duration of the compression.[6] In acute to subacute stages where the changes are predominately due to cord edema, T2 WI will show bright signal intensity focal at either the level of disc herniation or the long segment depending on the extent of stenosis

Table 1
Common causes of myelopathy

Compressive	Infection	Inflammatory	Vascular	Metabolic/Toxic	Hereditary
Trauma	Chronic	Transverse myelitis	Stroke	Nutritional deficiency	Spinocerebellar degeneration
Nonneoplastic	Fungal	MS	Spinal hemorrhage	B12 def	Motor neuron disease
Degenerative	HIV myelopathy	ADEM	(SAH, SD, ED)	Vit E def	Leukodystrophy
OPLL	Syphilis	NMO	Spinal malformation	Cu def	Krabbe disease
Neoplastic	TB	Postvaccinial	Cavernoma	Folate def	MLD
Metastasis	Acute	Sarcoidosis		Toxins	Adrenomyeloleukodystrophy
Meningioma	Viral	Paraneoplastic		Fluorosis	Distal motor axonopathies
Neurofibroma	Bacterial	syndrome		Lathyrism	Hereditary spastic paraplegia
Congenital spinal				Hepatic failure	Mitochondrial myelopathy
and cranio-vertebral				Heroin	
junction malformation				Superficial siderosis	
				Radiotherapy	

Abbreviations: def, deficiency; MLD, metachromatic leukodystrophy; TB, tuberculosis.

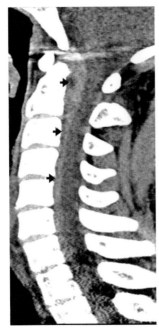

Fig. 1. Extradural hematoma. A 31-year-old male patient with a history of trauma and weakness in both upper extremities. Sagittal reformatted CT scan image shows hyperdense extradural hematoma (*arrows*) compressing the cervicomedullary junction and cervical cord.

increased signal intensity in the cord on T2 WI with corresponding hypointensity on T1 WI. Other findings that may be seen contributing to the myelopathy are bulging or herniated disc, osteophytes, facet and uncovertebral hypertrophy, and redundancy of the posterior longitudinal ligament and ligamentum flavum.

Ossification of the posterior longitudinal ligament (OPLL) is a degenerative disease of the spine that can cause severe compression of the spinal cord. It is one of the most common diseases that compress the posterior thoracic spinal cord and may cause either radiculopathy or myelopathy. Histologic study of OPLL has demonstrated the active stages of ossification, showing initial proliferation of small vessels in the ligament and subsequent bone formation.[7] On imaging this ossification can be classified into continuous, discontinuous, or segmental. Ossification of the ligaments is well demonstrated by plain radiography or CT scan as ossification just posterior to the vertebral bodies leading to narrowing of the canal. T1 WI noninvasively provides useful information about the degree and extent of spinal cord compression as well as the character of the ossification (**Fig. 5**). T2 WI sequences are most effective to evaluate both spinal cord compression due to the ossification and abnormal signal intensity of the spinal cord.[7] Chronic compression or minor trauma produces cord compression with various degrees of pathologic changes, including edema, demyelination, myelomalacia, cavitation, and necrosis.

(**Fig. 4**). If the cord compression is present over a long period of time, irreversible changes such as gliosis and myelomalacia develop within the cord. These changes present as focal areas of

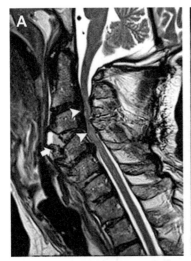
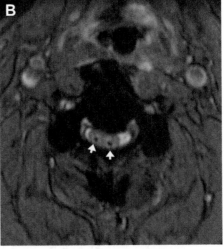

Fig. 2. Hemorrhagic contusion. A 66-year-old female patient in a motor vehicular accident presented with quadriparesis. (*A*) Sagittal T2 WI shows fracture dislocation of C4 vertebral body with tear of anterior longitudinal ligament (*arrow*). The spinal cord shows increased signal intensity from C3 to C4 level (*arrowheads*) with superimposed severe canal stenosis due to advanced degenerative changes. (*B*) Axial GRE image at C4 level shows diffuse cord edema with tiny hemorrhagic foci (*arrows*) consistent with hemorrhagic contusion.

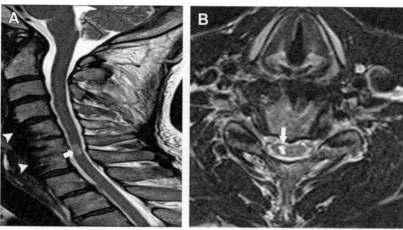

Fig. 3. A 55-year-old female patient presented with myelopathic symptoms immediately following the anterior cervical discectomy and fusion (ACDF) surgery. (*A*) Sagittal and (*B*) axial T2 WI show focal hyperintensity (*arrow*) within the right side of the cervical cord at C6-C7 level, suggestive of myelomalacia. ACDF changes (*arrowheads*) are seen from C5-C7 level.

Neoplasm

Tumors arising from any of the spinal compartments, extradural, intradural extramedullary, or intramedullary, can cause cord hyperintensity and myelopathic changes due to compression.[8]

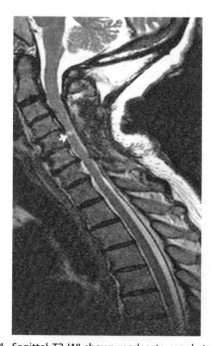

Fig. 4. Sagittal T2 WI shows moderate canal stenosis secondary to degenerative changes in the anterior and posterior elements of the cervical spine. Focal area of hyperintensity (*arrow*) is seen within the cord at the C5 level suggestive of myelomalacia, most likely from venous congestion.

Most of the extradural neoplasms are osseous in origin. Osseous tumors, such as osteoblastoma, aneurysmal bone cyst, multiple myeloma, lymphoma, and Ewing sarcoma, are all identified on MR imaging, but may be better evaluated with CT. In addition, extradural metastatic disease and lymphoma may also cause compression.

Intradural extramedullary tumors, such as nerve sheath tumors, meningiomas, or metastases, initially displace the cord before causing compression. Schwannomas are the most common intradural extramedullary mass, but may also occur in the extradural compartment or span the intradural and extradural spaces. The classic imaging appearance is a "dumbbell"-shaped enhancing mass. It is unusual for a nerve sheath tumor to calcify; however, cystic degeneration and hemorrhage may occur. These lesions are most commonly located in the thoracic region. They arise from the epineurium and have a true capsule. Schwannomas are usually eccentric with respect to the nerve root and displace the nerve root laterally. Differentiating schwannoma from neurofibroma may be difficult; however, schwannomas are more likely to demonstrate hemorrhage and cystic degeneration. In addition, schwannomas are usually more circumscribed and lobulated, whereas neurofibromas are more likely to demonstrate fusiform enlargement. Neurofibromas arise from the nerve fascicle and are rarely encapsulated. They are centrally located and cannot be easily separated from the involved nerve root. The classic imaging appearance of a neurofibroma is a T2 peripherally hyperintense, centrally hypointense lesion. Multiple lesions can be seen in the

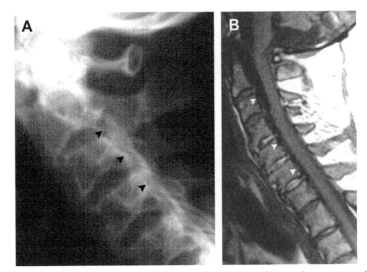

Fig. 5. A 63-year-old male patient presented with sensory and motor deficit in the upper and lower extremities. (*A*) Lateral radiograph of the cervical spine shows diffuse thickening of the posterior longitudinal ligament (*black arrowheads*) causing severe canal stenosis. (*B*) Sagittal T1 WI confirms the plain radiograph findings. There is severe compression of the cord at C2 level by a thickened hypointense posterior longitudinal ligament (*arrowheads*).

setting of type 1 neurofibromatosis, causing severe compression of the cord especially in the cervical region (Fig. 6).

The classic imaging appearance of a meningioma is an enhancing mass with a dural tail, which is isointense to the cord on T1 and T2 sequences. It often demonstrates calcification and is located within the intradural compartment 90% of the time (Fig. 7). Spinal meningiomas are most commonly found in the thoracic region[8]; however, in general, they are much less common than their intracranial counterparts (1:8).

INFECTION
Acute

Spinal osteomyelitis and epidural abscess (EA) with associated compressive myelopathy is an emergent condition that requires urgent diagnosis and treatment. The morbidity of EA is high and may range between 18% and 31%.[9] Risk factors for EA include diabetes mellitus, intravenous drug use, immunodeficiency, alcohol abuse, and chronic renal failure. Along with pain, fever, elevated peripheral leukocytosis, and erythrocyte

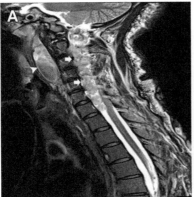
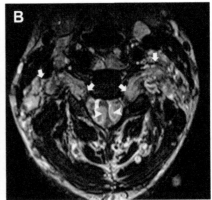

Fig. 6. Plexiform neurofibromatosis. A 21-year-old patient with NF1 presents with weakness and radicular pain in both upper extremities. (*A*) Sagittal T2 WI shows a large extramedullary intradural plexiform mass (*arrows*) causing severe compression of the cord. Plexiform mass is also seen in the prevertebral space (*arrowhead*). (*B*) Axial T2 WI shows bilateral widening of the neural foraminae (*arrows*) and compression of cord (*arrowheads*) from neurofibromas.

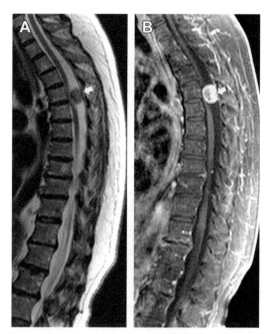

Fig. 7. Thoracic meningioma. (A) Sagittal T2 and (B) contrast-enhanced T1 WI images show an extramedullary-intradural intensely enhancing mass (*arrow*) compressing and displacing the thoracic cord anteriorly.

sedimentation rate, myelopathy is one of the frequent presenting symptoms of EA due to mechanical compression. *Staphylococcus aureus* is the most common causative organism found in 62% to 67% of the cases.[9,10] EA may be seen all the segments of the spine with thoracic (50%) more common than cervical (25%) and lumbar (25%).

MR imaging is the imaging modality of choice to identify the extent of infection and abscess, which is vital for surgical planning. Abscess is hypointense to slightly hyperintense compared with the cord on T1 WI and shows bright signal on T2 WI. In associated spondylodiscitis, disc and vertebral bodies show hypointensity on T1 WI and hyperintensity on T2 WI.[9,10] There may be associated destruction of the vertebral body as well as the prespinal and paraspinal soft tissues. On the contrast-enhanced scan, 2 patterns of enhancement may be seen with EA.[11] The most commonly seen is diffuse homogeneous or heterogeneous enhancement of the solid component of the abscess (Fig. 8). The second is a thin or thick rim of enhancement surrounding a collection of low signal intensity representing granulation tissue and pus. Gadolinium-enhanced sagittal and axial images are very important to define the extent as well as the location of the abscess, especially if they are multifocal and multiloculated. The cord may be severely compressed and displaced and demonstrate T2 hyperintensity, secondary to edema and inflammation.

Bacterial myelitis and intramedullary abscess are relatively rare and usually seen in the setting of bacteremia.[10,12] Early findings include edema and T2 hyperintensity within the cord, with the eventual development of a peripherally enhancing fluid collection. For patients with a high clinical concern, correlation with lumbar puncture is recommended. If infection is suspected, consideration of early empiric broad spectrum antimicrobial treatment is strongly recommended.[12]

Chronic

In *chronic fungal and tubercular infection*, myelopathy may result from spinal cord compression due to abscess formation, granulomatous tissue, or

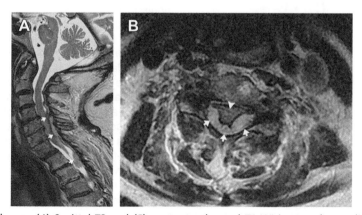

Fig. 8. Subdural abscess. (A) Sagittal T2 and (B) contrast-enhanced T1 WI images show a linear, hyperintense collection in the posterior subdural space (*arrows*) causing compression of the cord and mild edema. Axial image shows diffuse homogeneous enhancement of the abscess (*arrows*) causing severe compression of the cord (*arrowhead*).

osseous destruction. Chronic granulomatous infection may also lead to primary spinal cord involvement by other mechanisms.[9,13] They can lead to venous compression and stasis, producing edema within the border zones of the spinal cord. Arterial involvement from vasculitis can lead to ischemic myelomalacia and can progress to cord infarction from vascular inclusion. Finally, in endemic areas, direct involvement of the cord with intramedullary granuloma may be seen.

In most patients, myelopathy due to granulomatous infection is a compressive type. MR imaging shows decreased signal intensity in the involved vertebrae with or without involvement of the disc on T1 WI. T2 WI may show increased signal in the vertebrae, disc, and the paraspinal and epidural soft tissues. Thick granulation tissue may be seen surrounding the cord, causing loss of cord-cerebrospinal fluid (CSF) interface due to high signal intensity within the CSF on T1 WI.[9,12,14] Signal intensity of this granulation tissue is variable on T2 WI, ranging from isointense to hypointense. Granulation tissue shows thick, irregular, nodular, or contiguous enhancement on contrast-enhanced T1 WI (**Fig. 9**). The cord often shows hyperintensity on T2 WI due to either direct compression or myelopathy from vascular compromise. Spinal arachnoiditis is a frequent presentation in these infections, with thick exudates surrounding the cord, causing a variable degree of congestion and cord edema. In the chronic stage, collapse of the vertebrae may lead to kyphotic (gibbous) and angulation deformity with canal compromise.

Very rarely, fusiform swelling of the cord may be seen due to intramedullary granuloma, which is isointense or hyperintense on T1-WI images and shows a central hypointensity with surrounding hyperintense edema on T2 WI. Granuloma shows either solid or ring enhancement on postcontrast images. Candida and Aspergillus are the most common causes of spinal mycotic infections.[9,14] Although the final diagnosis is by pathology, a high index of suspicious is very important, especially in endemic areas and immunocompromised patients.

Chronic human immunodeficiency virus (HIV)-associated myelopathy (also known as vacuolar myelopathy) is pathologically characterized by vacuolization in the spinal cord from which it derives its name. There is predominant lateral and posterior column involvement with pathologic findings of edema and swelling of the myelin sheaths with an absence of demyelination.[15] Vacuolar myelopathy occurs in approximately 1% to 55% of patients with chronic HIV infection. The middle and lower thoracic regions are the most commonly involved areas of the spinal cord. The classic imaging findings include bilateral symmetric T2 hyperintensity within the dorsal and lateral columns, extending over multiple segments (**Fig. 10**).[16] A less common imaging appearance seen with HIV is high-signal-intensity abnormalities in the center of the cord on T2 WI, extending over multiple segments (**Fig. 11**).

INFLAMMATORY
Transverse Myelitis

Transverse myelitis presents with acute or subacute myelopathic symptoms with superimposed autonomic dysfunction. There are a myriad of causes of transverse myelitis, including demyelinating disorders, autoimmune disorders, infection, paraneoplastic syndromes, and isolated idiopathic transverse myelitis.[17] The overall incidence is approximately 4 cases per million people per year with a bimodal age distribution (second and fourth decades).[18] Although less than 10% of patients with transverse myelitis progress to multiple sclerosis (MS), transverse myelitis can be the sentinel event in a patient with MS. Patients who demonstrate smaller enhancing transverse myelitis lesions with less edema are more likely to develop MS.[19]

Idiopathic transverse myelitis is a monophasic inflammatory process that can be seen following viral infection or vaccination. Pathologic findings

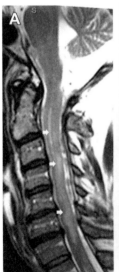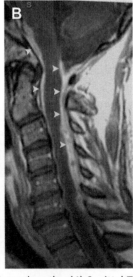

Fig. 9. Mucomycosis with myelopathy. (*A*) Sagittal T2 WI shows increased signal intensity within the cervical cord (*arrows*). There is mild effacement of the CSF space. (*B*) Contrast-enhanced sagittal T1 WI image shows thick enhancement (*arrowheads*) surrounding the cord.

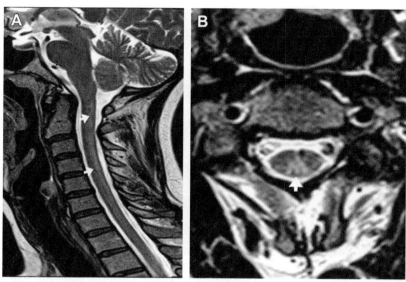

Fig. 10. Vacuolar myelopathy in HIV patient. (*A*) Sagittal and (*B*) axial T2 WIs show bilateral symmetric T2 hyperintensity within the dorsal and lateral columns (*arrows*), extending over multiple segments.

include perivascular monocytic and lymphocytic infiltration, demyelination, and axonal injury. Proposed diagnostic criteria for idiopathic acute transverse myelitis include sensory, motor, or autonomic dysfunction with bilateral (although not symmetric) signs and symptoms; clearly defined sensory level; exclusion of a compressive cause; inflammation (as documented by lumbar puncture or gadolinium enhancement); and progression of symptoms between 4 hours and 21 days following onset of symptoms.[20]

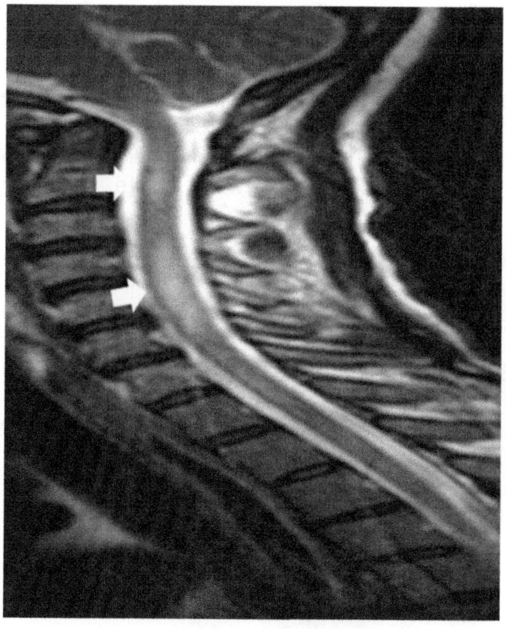

On MR, classic imaging findings include long segment, centrally located, increased signal on T2-weighted images. Increased signal intensity is seen usually occupying more than two-thirds of the cross-sectional area of the cord and extending more than 3 to 4 vertebral segments in length (**Fig. 12**).[21] Cord expansion may or may not be present. The thoracic and cervicothoracic cord is most commonly involved. Enhancement is variable and is most commonly seen in the subacute stages. Enhancement pattern may be diffuse, poorly defined, heterogeneous, nodular, or peripheral. Diffusion tensor imaging (DTI) studies of inflammatory myelitis show decreased fractional anisotropy (FA) values in the region of the T2 WI lesion and increased FA values in the periphery of the lesion.

MS

MS is a chronic demyelinating disease mediated by T cells, which activate macrophages, resulting in axonal loss and demyelination. Although the brain is classically involved, over three-quarters of patients are found to have spinal cord involvement at autopsy.[22] Up to 20% of patients may have isolated spinal involvement. MS patients with spinal lesions often present with ataxia with complaints of numbness in the lower extremities.[23] The incidence of MS varies geographically with a higher prevalence in northern countries, ranging from 1 to 80 cases per 100,000 people.

Fig. 11. HIV myelopathy. HIV-positive patient presented with gradual onset myelopathy. Sagittal T2 WI shows patchy hyperintensity (*arrows*) involving the central portion of the cord.

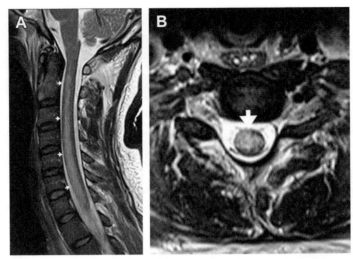

Fig. 12. Acute transverse myelitis. (A) Sagittal and (B) axial T2 WIs show diffuse enlargement of the cervical and visualized upper thoracic cord with abnormal hyperintensity (*arrows*) extending over more than 3 vertebral segments. Hyperintensity is seen occupying more than two-thirds of the cross-sectional area of the cord on axial section.

Patients usually present before the fifth decade and gender distribution depends on subtype. There are 5 recognized subtypes: benign, relapsing-remitting, secondary progressive, primary progressive, and progressive relapsing with secondary progressive being the most common. On pathology, acute lesions are characterized by fragmentation of myelin, relative axonal preservation, and microglial proliferation. In the subacute stage there is total loss of myelin and oligodendrocytes with marked proliferation of macrophages.

Spinal cord imaging with MR is very important in suspected cases of MS, particularly with the introduction of the MacDonald criteria for the early diagnosis of MS. There are 3 main imaging findings on MR: focal T2 hyperintense lesions, diffuse T2 hyperintensity with poorly demarcated borders, and atrophy (secondary to axonal loss in the chronic phases).[21] *Focal lesions* (demyelinating plaques) most commonly involve the cervical cord (~60%) followed by thoracic and lumbar cord. These plaques are hyperintense on T2-WI and iso-hypointense on T1-WI MR images. Focal plaques tend to be elongated in the direction of the long axis of the cord, characteristically peripherally located, and vary in length from a few millimeters to centimeters. Classic MS plaques do not extend over 2 vertebral segments in length and occupy less than half the cross-sectional area of the cord (**Fig. 13**). On axial MR images, plaques are peripherally located and generally do not respect boundaries between white and gray

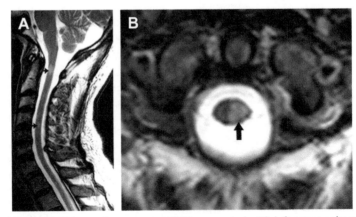

Fig. 13. A 31-year-old female patient, a known case of MS, presented with left arm weakness. (A) Sagittal T2 WI image shows focal hyperintense lesions (*arrows*) in the cervical cord at C2 and C4 levels. On the (B) axial T2 WI, the lesion is seen involving the left hemicord (*fat arrow* on axial).

matter. They may be wedge-shaped with the base over the cord surface or round if there is no contact with the cord surface. The cord is usually of normal size but may show swelling especially in the relapsing-remitting form of MS. Over half (56%) of acute plaques show enhancement on the post-contrast scans due to transient breakdown of the blood-brain barrier.[21] The enhancement may be homogeneous, nodular, or peripheral.

Diffuse abnormalities are more common in primary progressive and secondary progressive MS. It is characterized by mild, patchy, diffuse intramedullary hyperintensity on T2-WI MR images. *Focal or diffuse cord atrophy* with or without the presence of plaques has been recognized for many years.[24] Axonal degeneration, or an alternative atrophic process, is thought to be responsible for the cord atrophy. Plaques associated with cord atrophy have been reported in relapsing-remitting MS (possibly in greater number) than in secondary progressive forms of the disease. Imaging of the entire spinal cord is recommended when spinal symptoms are present in a patient with a known or presumptive diagnosis of MS.

Conventional MR has been able to diagnose cord abnormalities in only 35% of MS patients as compared with autopsy reports of greater than 90% of MS patients showing cord abnormalities. Newer imaging techniques such as DWI and DTI are used to increase the accuracy and understand the pathogenesis. MS lesions have been shown to have increased rates of diffusivity, with a significantly higher isotropic diffusion coefficient, compared with healthy control cords.[25,26] A significant decrease in FA is also seen on the DTI. These FA changes are thought to be due to loss of myelin from white matter fiber tracts, expansion of the extracellular space fraction, and perilesional inflammatory edema.[25,26] Although the exact role of DW imaging and DTI in MS of the spinal cord has not been completely evaluated, they appear to be promising in evaluating the symptomatic patients with a normal appearing cord on structural imaging.

Acute Disseminated Encephalomyelitis

Acute disseminated encephalomyelitis (ADEM) is an acute demyelinating disease that commonly affects children and adolescents following viral infection or vaccination. Patients often present with a rapid onset of encephalopathy and motor and/or sensory deficits with brainstem signs and symptoms and ataxia. The most probable pathophysiology is an autoimmune response to myelin basic protein, triggered by infection or immunization. Histopathology shows perivenular infiltrate of T-cell macrophages and occasionally plasma cells within the brain and spinal cord white matter associated with a corresponding zone of demyelination. Although this is classically considered a monophasic disease, recurrent or multiphasic forms of the disease have been reported.[27]

The MR imaging appearance of ADEM is nonspecific and indistinguishable from other inflammatory lesions like MS. Lesions are usually large, ill-defined, and hyperintense on T2 WI and extend over a long segment of the spinal cord (Fig. 14).[21,28] The cord shows mild expansion in the acute phase with variable enhancement.

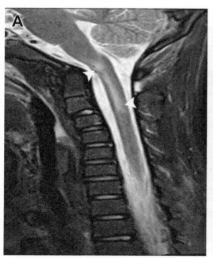 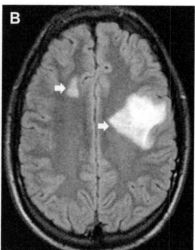

Fig. 14. ADEM. (*A*) Sagittal T2 WI shows a long segmented hyperintensity in the cervicomedullary junction and cervical cord (*arrowheads*). (*B*) Axial fluid attenuated inversion recovery image shows large areas of demyelinating plaques (*arrows*) in the bilateral frontal lobes.

ADEM predominately affects the thoracic cord. Imaging of the brain is indicated and, when positive, helps in the diagnosis of ADEM. In the brain, ADEM often demonstrates irregular T2 hyperintense lesions in the cerebral white matter, basal ganglia, thalamus, brainstem, and cortical regions.

Neuromyelitis Optica

Neuromyelitis optica (NMO; Devic disease) is a demyelinating disease characterized by bilateral visual disturbances and myelopathy with lesions restricted to the optic nerves and spinal cord. Patients are slightly older than those presenting with MS (mean age of onset 40 years) with a striking female predominance (9:1).[29] Approximately 80% of patients have a relapsing course with a worse overall prognosis than patients with MS. Pathologic findings include gray and white matter necrosis and cavitation with vascular hyalinization and fibrosis and a lack of inflammatory infiltrate. Diagnosis is usually confirmed by a combination of imaging findings and the presence of NMO-IgG in the serum or cerebrospinal fluid.[29,30] Imaging findings include a long segment expansion of the cord spanning over multiple segments with diffuse hyperintensity on T2 WI (**Fig. 15**). There may be areas of cavitation. Enhancement is variable and when present it is patchy. The manifestation of a longitudinally extensive lesion on spinal cord MR imaging is one of the most characteristic neuroimaging findings for NMO. Another classic sign seen on MR imaging is T2 hyperintensity and/or enhancement within the optic nerves and optic chiasm. A negative brain MR imaging has been long considered a major supportive criterion for the diagnosis of NMO. Over the last decade however it has been shown that brain abnormalities are not rare in NMO. Although brain lesions are less common at the time of presentation, most NMO patients develop nonspecific, clinically silent brain lesions on follow-up imaging. Brain lesions may be symptomatic or asymptomatic clinically. On T2 or fluid attenuated inversion recovery images they are seen as dotlike or patchy hyperintense lesions, commonly located in the cerebral deep white matter, brainstem, periaqueductal region, or cerebellum.[31] Although steroids may be beneficial in the treatment of MS, there is no known role in NMO.

Sarcoidosis

Sarcoidosis is a systemic disease that presents with central nervous system involvement in up to 10% of patients.[32] Spinal involvement is even more unusual, occurring in approximately 5% of all patients with central nervous system involvement (0.5% of all patients). The incidence of sarcoidosis is approximately 10 to 40 per 100,000 people with an onset of symptoms usually in the third to fourth decade. Although systemic sarcoidosis is more common in women, there is a slight predominance of male patients in spinal sarcoidosis. Diagnosis may be challenging because only half of the patients with neurosarcoidosis have an elevated serum angiotensin-converting enzyme level. Pathologically, spinal sarcoidosis presents as perivascular granulomatous infiltrates leading to demyelination in the dorsal and lateral columns.

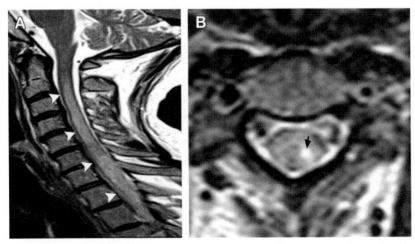

Fig. 15. NMO. (*A*) Sagittal and (*B*) axial T2 WIs show a long segment hyperintensity involving the cervical cord with mild expansion (*arrowheads*). On the axial section, the cord shows diffuse hyperintensity with a small area of cavity on the left side (*black arrow*).

Neurosarcoidosis has a predilection for the cervical and thoracic cord and lesions can involve any or all compartments of the spine (intramedullary, extramedullary-intradural, or extradural).[33,34] The imaging appearance of intramedullary sarcoidosis is nonspecific and may mimic neoplasms, MS, and fungal infections on MR imaging. MR imaging shows fusiform enlargements of the spinal cord with high signal intensity in T2 WI images, low signal intensity in T1 WI images, and patchy, multifocal nodular or rim enhancement on contrast-enhanced scan (Fig. 16). Associated diffuse or nodular dural or leptomeningeal enhancement is very common. Confirming the diagnosis of spinal sarcoidosis as a cause of myelopathy is very challenging. A high level of suspicion and other tests such as high-resolution CT of the chest, gallium scan, and CSF examination may be helpful.

Systemic Lupus Erythematosus

Systemic lupus erythematosus (SLE) rarely manifests as myelopathy (less than 5% of patients). In patients who present with clinical myelitis, up to one-third of patients will have normal spinal imaging. There are 2 subtypes of SLE myelitis: rapid onset (less than 6 hours) and subacute onset (24 hours to 30 days).[35] The patients with rapid onset tend to present with flaccid paralysis, hyporeflexia, and urinary retention and tend to have a poor outcome with persistent paraplegia. The subacute onset subtype presents with spasticity, hyperreflexia, and mild weakness, followed by a relapsing course. MR imaging of the spinal cord in SLE myelitis is variable and may be normal at presentation in 16% to 30% of patients.[35,36] The commonest imaging finding seen is a long-segment central T2 hyperintensity, expansion of

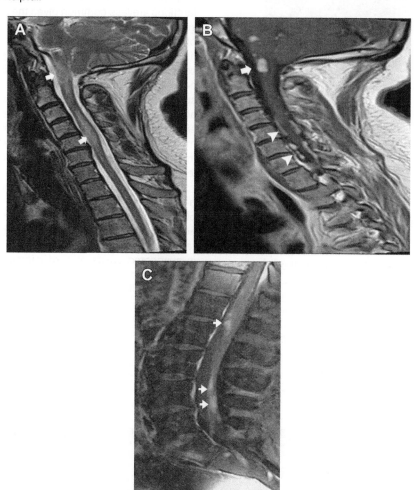

Fig. 16. Sarcoidosis. (A) Sagittal T2 WI shows patchy areas of increased signal intensity at the cervicomedullary junction and in the cervical cord (*arrows*). Contrast-enhanced sagittal T1 WI of the (B) cervical and (C) lumbar spine show nodular intramedullary (*thick arrow*), dural (*arrowheads*), and leptomeningeal (*arrows*) enhancement. The patient had diffuse sarcoidosis.

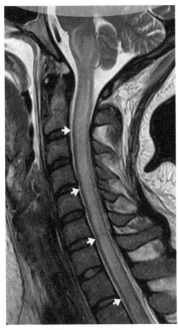

Fig. 17. Acute longitudinal myelitis in SLE. Sagittal T2 WI image shows a long segment central T2 hyperintensity and expansion of the cord (*arrows*).

the cord, and variable enhancement (acute longitudinal myelitis) (Fig. 17). On imaging these findings are indistinguishable from acute idiopathic transverse myelitis. Diagnosis largely depends on associated clinical and CSF findings.

Vascular

Vascular disease affecting the spinal cord cancause devastating neurologic morbidity; fortunately, these pathologic abnormalities are rare as compared with cerebrovascular events. Various pathologic abnormalities that may involve the cord or the spinal canal include infarction, dural arteriovenous fistula, arteriovenous malformation (AVM), cavernous malformation, compressive epidural hematoma, hematomyelia, vasculitides, and genetic abnormalities.

Spinal cord infarction

Spinal cord infarction has a variable clinical presentation depending on the vascular distribution involved (Fig. 18); however, the key is the hyperacute onset of symptoms. Spinal cord infarctions represent only 1% of all central nervous system infarctions (see Fig. 18).[37,38] The anterior spinal artery distribution is most often affected, leading to motor deficit and symptoms referable to the spinothalamic tracts (loss of pain and temperature sensation) with areflexia and bladder and bowel dysfunction. The anterior spinal artery is responsible for the arterial supply to the ventral gray matter horns, corticospinal tracts, and lateral spinothalamic tracts. The origin of the anterior spinal artery is divided into thirds from cranial to caudal with the upper one-third being supplied by the vertebral arteries (via ascending cervical radicular arteries), the middle one-third supplied by the artery of Adamkiewicz, and the lower one-third supplied by lumbar and sacral radicular branches from the aorta. Posterior spinal artery infarctions are less common given the paired arterial supply from the posterior spinal arteries that supply the dorsal columns and dorsal gray matter horns. Posterior spinal infarctions result in dorsal column or sensory symptoms (loss of proprioception and vibration sense) with paresis and sphincter dysfunction. Hypotensive events or aortic surgery can lead to central infarction (bilateral spinothalamic sensory deficit with preserved motor function) or complete transverse infarction (motor and sensory deficit referable to a focal level).

In the early acute phase, MR imaging may be negative on routine sequences. In less than 50% of the cases T2 hyperintensity similar to the acute myelitis may be seen. It is therefore important to incorporate sagittal and axial DWI images in suspected cases of cord infarction. Similar to cerebrovascular infarction, DWI shows areas of restricted diffusion in the involved territory of the infarcted cord (Fig. 19).[39] Variable contrast enhancement can be seen during the subacute phase and may persist for up to 3 weeks. There may be associated abnormal signal within adjacent vertebral bodies, representing osseous infarction in the setting of radicular artery occlusion.

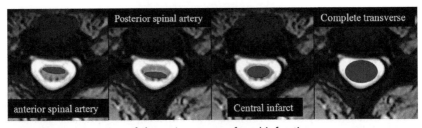

Fig. 18. Diagrammatic representation of the various types of cord infarction.

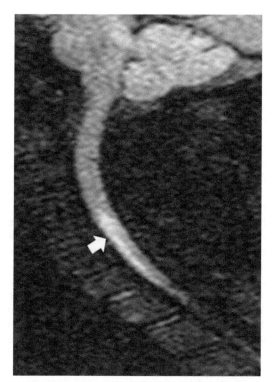

Fig. 19. Acute spinal cord infarction. Sagittal DWI image shows a linear area of restricted diffusion (*arrow*) suggestive of acute infarction. The patient presented with acute onset myelopathic symptoms following aortic repair.

Spinal hemorrhage

Epidural and subdural hemorrhages are rare but can lead to acute myelopathy secondary to compression. The most common causes are postoperative, especially after anticoagulation and trauma, but they can occur spontaneously.[37,38] The incidence of epidural hematoma is reported as high as 41% following trauma; however, patients are usually asymptomatic.[40] They result from tearing of the epidural venous plexus with focal extravasation of blood into the anterior epidural space. Large hematomas may cause compression of the cord leading to myelopathy. The imaging findings include an extradural heterogeneous mass that may encase or displace the cord. The T1 and T2 signal is variable and largely depends on the age of the hemorrhage. Acute epidural hematomas are the most difficult to diagnose because they remain isointense to the spinal cord on T1-WI and isointense with CSF on T2-WI sequences (**Fig. 20**). *Hematomyelia or spinal subarachnoid hemorrhage* is a frequent complication of intramedullary AVM. Anticoagulant therapy, trauma, cavernoma, hemorrhagic metastasis, and surgery may also lead to spinal subarachnoid hemorrhage or hematomyelia.[3] Evolution and degradation of the blood products, which are irritating/inflammatory to the neural tissue, may cause edema and hyperintensity of the cord with myelopathic symptoms. Imaging of the remainder of the spinal column is recommended to evaluate

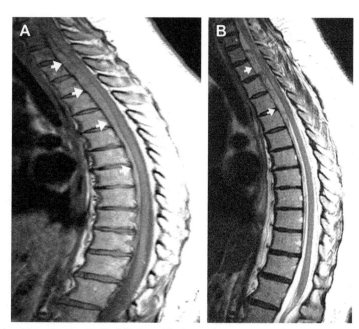

Fig. 20. (*A, B*) Subdural hematoma. Sagittal (T1) and (T2) WIs demonstrate a hyperintense signal (*arrows*) within the anterior spinal subdural compartment causing severe compression and displacement of the cord posteriorly.

for the extent of hematoma as well as the cause, particularly in the absence of antecedent trauma.

Spinal vascular malformations

Spinal vascular malformations are categorized according to the Spetzler classification.[41] The most common vascular malformation is type I (dural arteriovenous fistula), representing approximately 80% of all spinal vascular malformations.[38] These patients are generally men in their fifth to sixth decade who present with progressive myelopathic symptoms, usually referable to the T5 to L3 levels and are thought to represent acquired lesions with 60% occurring spontaneously and 40% occurring secondary to trauma.[38] On imaging, there is T2 hyperintensity and expansion of the cord with surrounding linear T2 hypointensities (consistent with dilated pial veins) (Fig. 21). The increased pial venous flow leads to increased venous pressure transmitted to the intramedullary veins, producing venous hypertension with a resultant decreased intramedullary arteriovenous gradient causing reduced tissue perfusion and ischemia.[42] Types II through IV vascular malformations are

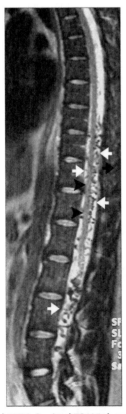

Fig. 21. Spinal AVM. Sagittal T2 WI shows dilated flow voids ventral and dorsal to the cord (*white arrows*). The lumbar cord and conus medullaris show hyperintensity suggestive of edema (*black arrowheads*).

thought to be congenital in origin and although they all present with T2 hyperintensity within the cord, they can be differentiated based on the presence and location of a nidus and associated findings. Type II vascular malformations are intramedullary glomus-type AVMs, similar to intracranial AVMs, and often occur in the cervical and upper thoracic cord, and can be seen in association with Klippel-Trenauny-Weber and Osler-Weber-Rendu syndromes. Type III vascular malformations are juvenile (metameric) -type AVMs that have extension intramedullary and extramedullary components, often extending to the paraspinal soft tissues. Type III vascular malformations may occur anywhere in the spine, but have a propensity for the cervical and upper thoracic cord. Type III vascular malformations are often the most severe lesions with a poor prognosis given the unresectability of the lesions. Fortunately, these are the rarest of the spinal vascular malformations, representing less than 10% of vascular malformations and can be seen in association with Cobb syndrome (metameric vascular malformation involving skin, bone, and spinal cord). Type IV vascular malformations are intradural extramedullary or peri-medullary arteriovenous fistulas, which can be divided based on location (type A and B occur at the conus; type C involves the thoracic cord).[43] Type IV-A represents a slow-flow small arteriovenous fistula; type IV-B is an intermediate arteriovenous fistula with higher flow rate, and type IV-C is a large arteriovenous fistula with both arterial and venous enlargement. These malformations can be seen in association with Osler-Weber-Rendu syndrome. Cord signal abnormality in spinal AVMs can be secondary to venous congestion as well as hemorrhage.[38]

Cavernomas

Cavernomas are discrete lesions composed of dilated, thin-walled capillaries lined by simple endothelium. Spinal cavernomas are rare and, because greater than 95% of cavernomas occur in the brain, it is imperative to image the brain when a spinal cavernoma is found.[37] Spinal cavernomas are most commonly located within the thoracic cord, followed by the cervical cord. There is a striking female predominance (7:1) with most patients presenting in the third to sixth decade. The clinical presentation is variable, ranging from slowly progressive myelopathic symptoms to acute quadriplegia, which is mostly due to new hemorrhage.[44] The classic imaging appearance is a well-defined, lobulated lesion with a T2 hypointense rim and heterogeneous center. The hypointense rim is due to hemosiderin deposition from prior hemorrhage (**Fig. 22**).[45] In the setting of acute hemorrhage, there may be variable surrounding T2 hyperintensity secondary to edema. Rarely, the MR imaging appearance of a cavernoma may be confused with intramedullary AVM and can be resolved with a spinal angiogram because cavernomas are angiographically silent.

METABOLIC/TOXIC

Metabolic, nutritional, and toxic agents can also affect the cord leading to myelopathic changes clinically and hyperintensities on T2 WI images. Long-term nutritional deficiencies of vitamin B12, folate, copper, and vitamin E can cause temporary or permanent neuronal damage leading to myelopathic symptoms. Various toxins (Lathyrism, cyanide, and fluoride), drugs, chemical agents, and hepatic and renal failure have also been described as causative agents for myelopathy and myeloneuropathy. Their imaging findings are rare and nonspecific and in most cases diagnosis is made by a high index of clinical suspicion and exclusion of other potential causes.

Subacute Combined Degeneration

Subacute combined degeneration presents with symmetric dysesthesia and loss of positional sense and vibration, which may progress to spastic paraparesis or tetraparesis. There may be additional findings of mood changes and psychosis.[46] Patients are usually in their fifth to eighth decade with a slight male predominance. Subacute combined degeneration is most commonly caused by B12 deficiency, usually secondary to malabsorption (pernicious anemia). It may be seen in strict vegans, patients with blind loop syndrome, fish tapeworm infestation, or nitrous oxide accumulation. Vitamin B12 is a coenzyme in the catabolic pathway of methylmalonic acid and in the absence of B12 methylmalonic acid accumulates and is directly toxic to myelin. The classic imaging appearance is T2 hyperintensities within the bilateral dorsal columns without significant enhancement. The lateral columns may also be affected. If the condition is not recognized and promptly treated, there may be permanent damage and axonal loss.[21]

Superficial Siderosis

Superficial siderosis results from hemosiderin deposition in the subpial layers of the brain and spinal cord and may be seen following trauma, surgery, tracking of an intracranial hematoma into the spinal cavity, and tumoral bleed. These changes are best visualized on gradient echo or susceptibility-weighted imaging where it shows a rim of hypointensity around the cord with or without edema on T2-WI images. Superficial siderosis may be complicated by arachnoiditis and demonstrate nerve root clumping on imaging. There may be diffuse or patchy pachymeningeal enhancement.

Both *radiation (RT)* and *chemotherapy* (particularly methotrexate) can cause a toxic myelopathy. The threshold radiation dose for the development of myelopathy is a total dose of 5000 cGy or daily fractions of greater than 200 cGy. There are 2

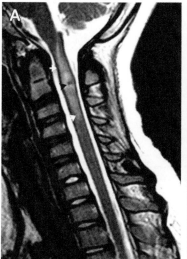
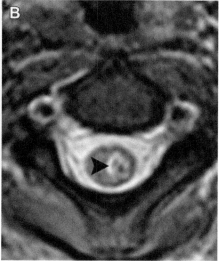

Fig. 22. Intramedullary cord cavernoma. (*A*) Sagittal T2 and (*B*) axial GRE show diffuse expansion of the upper cervical cord (*white arrows*) with hypointensity in the center (*black arrowhead*). Axial image shows dark signal within due to hemosiderin deposition (*black arrowhead*).

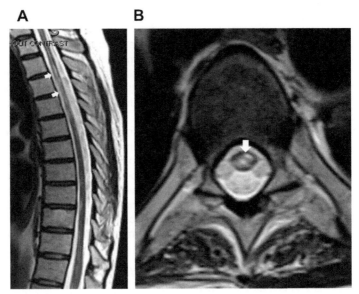

A **B**

Fig. 23. Radiation myelopathy. (*A*) Sagittal and (*B*) axial T2 WIs show mild atrophy and hyperintensity (*arrows*) in the upper thoracic cord. This patient had whole spine radiation 2 years back.

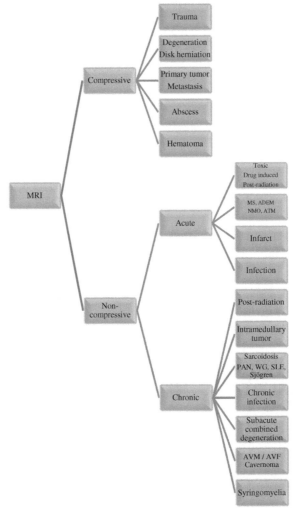

Fig. 24. Diagnostic algorithm for T2 hyperintensity within the cord. ATM, acute transverse myelitis; AVF, arteriovenous fistula; PAN, polyarteritis nodosa; WG, Wegener's granulomatosis.

phases of radiation injury—acute and chronic. Chronic, or delayed, radiation myelopathy results from direct injury to glial cells, myelin, and small blood vessels, leading to demyelination and axonal damage, which may present months to years following treatment.[47] T2 WI shows hyperintensity with or without atrophy of the cord within the radiation field (Fig. 23). Patchy, nodular enhancement may be seen in the subacute stages. Another finding that may help in diagnosing the RT-induced myelopathy is fatty marrow signal within adjacent vertebral bodies, with a sharp border correlating with the radiation portal. Intrathecal methotrexate can have a similar pattern of myelopathy, which is seen more commonly in patients with concurrent or prior spinal radiation therapy, multiple intrathecal chemotherapy injections, or a history of active central nervous system leukemia. Diagnosis of RT- and chemotherapy-induced myelopathy may be easy with prior history of therapy. However, if there is enhancement, as in the subacute stages, differentiating it from the recurrent or metastatic tumor may be difficult.

HEREDITARY

Hereditary causes of myelopathy are rare but should be considered in an appropriate clinical setting. Adrenomyeloneuropathy refers to spinal cord demyelination in patients with adrenoleukodystrophy, which is a peroxysmal disorder leading to progressive spastic paraparesis. Krabbe disease is due to a deficiency of galactosidase and results in galactocerebrosidase accumulation and resultant degeneration of corticospinal tracts.

SUMMARY

The radiologist is often faced with a common imaging presentation of T2 hyperintensity within the cord and may not be able to arrive at the correct diagnosis without a team approach, incorporating physical findings, patient history, and corroborative laboratory tests. The authors have found the following algorithmic approach (Fig. 24) extremely useful in their practice. In clinically suspected cases of myelopathy, MR imaging without and with gadolinium remains the modality of choice. Patients can then be divided into compressive and noncompressive groups based on imaging findings. Compressive myelopathy can often be adequately characterized on imaging; however, further refinement of the differential diagnosis of noncompressive myelopathy depends on patient history and clinical presentation. Noncompressive myelopathy can be broadly classified into acute and insidious onset and further categorized by distribution of

the signal abnormalities, including length of cord involvement, specific tract involvement, and the region of the spinal cord that is affected.

REFERENCES

1. Demaerel P. Magnetic resonance imaging of spinal cord trauma: a pictorial essay. Neuroradiology 2006;48:223–32.
2. Ishida Y, Tominaga T. Predictors of neurologic recovery in acute central cord injury with only upper extremity impairment. Spine 2002;27:1652–7.
3. Silberstein M, Tress BM, Hennessy O. Prediction of neurologic outcome in acute spinal cord injury: the role of CT and MR. AJNR Am J Neuroradiol 1992; 13:1597–608.
4. Toledano M, Bartleson JD. Cervical spondylotic myelopathy. Neurol Clin 2013;31:287–305.
5. Matz PG, Anderson PA, Holly LT, et al. The natural history of cervical spondylotic myelopathy. J Neurosurg Spine 2009;11:104–11.
6. Kaplan R, Czervionke L, Haughton V. Degenerative disease of spine. In: Atlas SW, editor. Magnetic resonance imaging of the brain and spine, vol. 1, 4th edition. Philadelphia: Williams & Wilkins; 2009. p. 1448–507.
7. Otake S, Matsuo M, Nishizawa S, et al. Ossification of the posterior longitudinal ligament: MR evaluation. AJNR Am J Neuroradiol 1992;13(4):1059–67.
8. Smith JK, Lury K, Castillo M. Imaging of spinal and spinal cord tumors. Semin Roentgenol 2006;41:274–93.
9. Mendonca R. Spinal infection and inflammatory disorders. In: Atlas SW, editor. Magnetic resonance imaging of the brain and spine, vol. 1, 4th edition. Philadelphia: Williams & Wilkins; 2009. p. 1448–507.
10. Murphy KJ, Brunberg JA, Quint DJ, et al. Spinal cord infection: myelitis and abscess formation. AJNR Am J Neuroradiol 1997;18:455–8.
11. Numaguchi Y, Rigamonti D, Rothman MI, et al. Spinal epidural abscess: evaluation with gadolinium enhanced MR imaging. Radiographics 1993;13:545.
12. Richie MB, Pruitt AA. Spinal cord infections. Neurol Clin 2013;31:19–53.
13. deRoos A, van Persijn van Meerten EL, Bloem JL, et al. MRI of tuberculous spondylitis. AJR Am J Roentgenol 1986;146:79–82.
14. Kwon JW, Hong SH, Choi SH, et al. MRI findings of Aspergillus spondylitis. AJR Am J Roentgenol 2011;197(5):W919–23.
15. Petito CK, Navia BA, Cho ES, et al. Vacuolar myelopathy pathologically resembling subacute combined degeneration in patients with the acquired immunodeficiency syndrome. N Engl J Med 1985;312:874–9.
16. DeSanto J, Ross JS. Spine infection/inflammation. Radiol Clin North Am 2011;49:105–27.
17. Beh SC, Greenberg BM, Frohman T, et al. Transverse myelitis. Neurol Clin 2013;31:79–138.

18. Goh C, Phal PM, Desmond PM. Neuroimaging in acute transverse myelitis. Neuroimaging Clin N Am 2011;21:951–73.

19. Campi A, Filippi M, Comi G, et al. Acute transverse myelopathy: Spinal and cranial MR study with clinical follow up. AJNR Am J Neuroradiol 1995;16: 115–23.

20. Barnes G, Benjamin S, Bowen JD, et al. Proposed diagnostic criteria and nosology of acute transverse myelitis. Neurology 2002;59:499–505.

21. Thurnher MM, Cartes-Zumelzu F, Mueller-Mang C. Demyelinating and infectious disease of the spinal cord. Neuroimaging Clin N Am 2007;17:37–55.

22. Ikuta F, Zimmerman HM. Distribution of plaques in seventy autopsy cases of multiple sclerosis in the United States. Neurology 1976;26:26–8.

23. Sheremata W, Tornes L. Multiple sclerosis and the spinal cord. Neurol Clin 2013;31:55–77.

24. Bergers E, Bot JC, de Groot CJ, et al. Axonal damage in spinal cord of MS patients occurs largely independently of T2 MRI lesions. Neurology 2002; 59:1766–71.

25. Valsasina P, Rocca MA, Agosta F, et al. Mean diffusivity and fractional anisotropy histogram analysis of the cervical cord in MS patients. Neuroimage 2005;26:822–8.

26. Hasseltine SM, Law M, Babb J, et al. Diffusion tensor imaging in multiple sclerosis: assessment of regional differences in the axial plane within normal-appearing cervical spinal cord. AJNR Am J Neuroradiol 2006;27(6):1189–93.

27. Schwarz S, Mohr A, Knauth M, et al. Acute disseminated encephalomyelitis: a follow-up study of 40 adult patients. Neurology 2001;56:1313–8.

28. Singh S, Prabhakar S, Korah IP, et al. Acute disseminated encephalomyelitis and multiple sclerosis: magnetic resonance imaging differentiation. Australas Radiol 2000;44:404–11.

29. Wingerchuk DM, Lennon VA, Lucchinetti CF, et al. The spectrum of neuromyelitis optica. Lancet Neurol 2007;6:805–15.

30. Ghezzi A, Bergamaschi R, Martinelli V, et al. Clinical characteristics, course and prognosis of relapsing Devic's neuromyelitis optica. J Neurol 2004;251: 47–52.

31. Sahraian MA, Radue EW, Minagar A. Neuromyelitis optica: clinical manifestations and neuroimaging features. Neurol Clin 2013;31:139–52.

32. Iannuzzi MC, Rybicki BA, Teirstein AS. Sarcoidosis. N Engl J Med 2007;357:2153–65.

33. Junger SS, Stern BJ, Levine SR, et al. Intramedullary spinal sarcoidosis: clinical and magnetic resonance imaging characteristics. Neurology 1993;43:333–7.

34. Smith JK, Matheus MG, Castillo M. Imaging manifestations of neurosarcoidosis [review]. AJR Am J Roentgenol 2004;182(2):289–95.

35. Birnbaum J, Petri M, Thompson R, et al. Distinct subtypes of myelitis in systemic lupus erythematosus. Arthritis Rheum 2009;60:3378–87.

36. Kovacs B, Lafferty TL, Brent LH, et al. Transverse myelopathy in systemic lupus erythematosus: an analysis of 14 cases and review of the literature. Ann Rheum Dis 2000;59:120–4.

37. Rubin MN, Rabinstein AA. Vascular disease of the spinal cord. Neurol Clin 2013;31:153–81.

38. Krings T, Lasjaunias PL, Hans FJ, et al. Imaging in spinal vascular disease [review]. Neuroimaging Clin N Am 2007;17(1):57–72.

39. Bammer R, Fazekas F, Augustin M, et al. Diffusion-weighted MR imaging of the spinal cord. AJNR Am J Neuroradiol 2000;21:587–91.

40. Kerslake RW, Jaspan T, Worthington BS. Magnetic resonance imaging of spinal trauma. Br J Radiol 1991;64(761):386–402.

41. Spetzler RF, Detwiler PW, Riina HA, et al. Modified classification of spinal cord vascular lesions. J Neurosurg 2002;96:145–56.

42. Bradac GB, Daniele D, Riva A, et al. Spinal dural arteriovenous fistulas: an underestimated cause of myelopathy. Eur Neurol 1994;34:87–94.

43. Mourier KL, Gobin YP, George B, et al. Intradural perimedullary arteriovenous fistulae: results of surgical and endovascular treatment in a series of 35 cases. Neurosurgery 1993;32:885–91.

44. Cohen-Gadol AA, Jacob JT, Edwards DA, et al. Coexistence of intracranial and spinal cavernous malformations: a study of prevalence and natural history. J Neurosurg 2006;104:376–81.

45. Weinzierl MR, Krings T, Korinth MC, et al. MRI and intraoperative findings in cavernous haemangiomas of the spinal cord. Neuroradiology 2004;46:65–71.

46. Schwendimann RN. Metabolic, nutritional, and toxic myelopathies. Neurol Clin 2013;31:207–18.

47. Schiff D, Wen P. Central nervous system toxicities from cancer therapies. Hematol Oncol Clin North Am 2006;20:1377–98.

Index

Radiol Clin N Am 52 (2014) 447–454
http://dx.doi.org/10.1016/S0033-8389(14)00010-4
0033-8389/14/$ – see front matter © 2014 Elsevier Inc. All rights reserved.

Printed and bound by CPI Group (UK) Ltd, Croydon, CR0 4YY

03/10/2024

01040378-0003